AF834741

From the Midwife's Bag to the Patient's File

CEU Press Studies in the History of Medicine

Volume IX

Series Editor: Marius Turda

Published in the series:

Svetla Baloutzova
Demography and Nation
Social Legislation and Population Policy in Bulgaria, 1918–1944

Christian Promitzer · Sevasti Trubeta · Marius Turda, eds.
Health, Hygiene and Eugenics in Southeastern Europe to 1945

Francesco Cassata
Building the New Man
Eugenics, Racial Science and Genetics in Twentieth-Century Italy

Rachel E. Boaz
In Search of "Aryan Blood"
Serology in Interwar and National Socialist Germany

Richard Cleminson
Catholicism, Race and Empire
Eugenics in Portugal, 1900–1950

Maria Zarimis
Darwin's Footprint
Cultural Perspectives on Evolution in Greece (1880–1930s)

Tudor Georgescu
The Eugenic Fortress
The Transylvanian Saxon Experiment in Interwar Romania

Katerina Gardikas
Landscapes of Disease
Malaria in Modern Greece

From the Midwife's Bag to the Patient's File

Public Health in Eastern Europe

Edited by

Heike Karge, Friederike Kind-Kovács and Sara Bernasconi

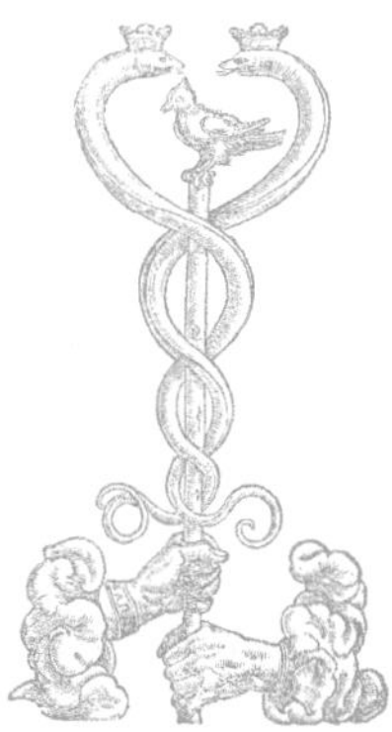

CEU PRESS

Central European University Press
Budapest—New York

© 2017 Heike Karge, Friederike Kind-Kovács, and Sara Bernasconi

Published in 2017 by
Central European University Press
An imprint of the
Central European University Limited Liability Company
Nádor utca 11, H-1051 Budapest, Hungary
Tel: +36-1-327-3138 or 327-3000 · *Fax*: +36-1-327-3183
E-mail: ceupress@press.ceu.edu
Website: www.ceupress.com

224 West 57th Street, New York NY 10019, USA
E-mail: meszarosa@press.ceu.edu

All rights reserved. No part of this publication may be reproduced, stored in a retrieval system, or transmitted, in any form or by any means, without the permission of the Publisher.

ISBN 978-963-386-208-7

ISSN 2079-1119

Library of Congress Cataloging-in-Publication Data

Names: Karge, Heike, editor.
Title: From the midwife's bag to the patient's file : public health in Eastern Europe / edited by Heike Karge, Friederike Kind-Kovacs, and Sara Bernasconi.
Description: Budapest ; New York : Central European University Press, 2017. | Series: CEU Press studies in the history of medicine, ISSN 2079-1119 ; Volume IX | Includes bibliographical references and index.
Identifiers: LCCN 2017043865 (print) | LCCN 2017047309 (ebook) | ISBN 9789633862094 | ISBN 9789633862087 (alk. paper)
Subjects: LCSH: Public health--Social aspects--History--Eastern Europe--19th century. | Public health--Social aspects--History--Eastern Europe--20th century.
Classification: LCC RA424 (ebook) | LCC RA424 .F76 2017 (print) | DDC 362.109437--dc23
LC record available at https://lccn.loc.gov/2017043865

Printed by Prime Rate Kft., Hungary

TABLE OF CONTENTS

LIST OF FIGURES

ACKNOWLEDGEMENTS

The present volume evolved from the international research network "Social Welfare and Public Health in Eastern and Southeastern Europe during the Long Twentieth Century" ("Sozialfürsorge und Gesundheit in Ost-und Südosteuropa im langen 20. Jahrhundert"). The network, led by Heike Karge (Regensburg University), Friederike Kind-Kovács (Regensburg University), and Sara Bernasconi (Zurich University), was funded by the German Research Foundation (DFG) between 2012 to 2015, whom we would like to thank for its generous support. We are thankful for the constructive feedback we received on earlier versions of the manuscript from Paul Weindling (Oxford Brookes University), Anelia Kassabova (Institute of Ethnology, Bulgarian Academy of Sciences), Hormoz Ebrahimnejad (University of Southhampton), Nancy M. Wingfield (Northern Illinois University), Maria Bucur (Indiana University Bloomington), Natali Stegmann (University of Regensburg), and Paul Lerner (University of Southern California).

We would also like to thank all the former network members who helped to initiate and delve into a fruitful debate on the state and transformation of public health in Southeastern and Eastern Europe. Only in the framework of this special research community could the ideas that are presented in this volume be developed and discussed. We are also thankful to all the institutions that hosted our various workshops in the last years, including the University of Regensburg and its Institute for East and Southeast European Studies, the Herder Institute in Marburg, the European University Institute in Florence, and the research network "Reluctant Internationalists" at Birkbeck College in London. Special thanks goes to Marius Turda from Oxford Brookes University, who, as the editor of the book series "CEU Press Studies in the History of Medicine," both encouraged the publication of this volume and gave substantial feedback. We are very grateful to Tudor Georgescu and Delphine Silberbauer for their help with the translation of a number of articles, as well as to Ed Hatton for his copy-editing of the volume. We would also like to thank our research assistants, Vera Spanner and Agnes Stelzer, for their help with managing the research network and preparing this volume. Lastly, we are greatly indebted to the editors of CEU Press for their help and support with this international book project.

We also wish to express our thanks to the libraries, museums, and archives that granted us permission to reprint the images in this volume. Despite thorough investigation, not all the copyright owners could be identified. In case the authors of this volume have by any chance and involuntarily infringed on any copyright, we hereby declare that the use of the images is entirely non-commercial and solely serves educational purposes. Therefore, we claim that the use of the images meets the requirements of the fair use statute.

Introduction

From the Midwife's Bag to the Patient's File: Public Health in Eastern Europe

Heike Karge, Friederike Kind-Kovács, and Sara Bernasconi

Health Turning Public

Andreas Vesalius's anatomical theater in the Church of San Salvatore in Bologna represents a historical site where a public discussion of health matters turned into an intimate encounter with a diseased and deceased body. Vesalius's first lecture with an audience of approximately 200 students, colleagues, and members of the elite took place in 1540 in the sacred protection of the church. Here, the pathological body was dissected, exhibited, and stared at. In this and many other medical settings, the body, as Hancock put it, came "to be recognized as a contested terrain on which struggles over control and resistance are fought out."[1] The "highly ritualized ceremony" of anatomical dissection allowed the anatomist not only to perform, but also to exhibit the knowledge of his profession and, thereby, his power to the audience.[2] At the same time, the anatomical theater represented an "early form of mass entertainment—of public spectacle."[3] In this setting, the single, dissected body served as a "body of [physiological] knowledge," thereby ac-

1 Hancock et al., *The Body, Culture and Society*, 1.

2 Dacome, "Women, Wax and Anatomy in the 'Century of Things,'" 54; Cunningham, *The Anatomical Renaissance*.

3 Van Dijck, *The Transparent Body*, 131.

quainting a "large audience with the advances of science."[4] Thus, it turned medical knowledge into public knowledge.

Though representing a premodern moment and site in the evolution of "public health," the anatomical theater ideally serves to visualize the aim of this collection of essays. In the contested terrain of the anatomical theater, all the actors and components at the core of this volume can be seen: a public component, although it is still far from what we mean by "public health"; the body on which medicine is performed, although not yet with the aim to prevent diseases on a large scale; and finally, the doctor, the medical specialist who demonstrates his professional skills to the public, although to a very limited audience.

The basic rupture that was to transform the contested terrain of the anatomical theater into the contested terrain of public health occurred at the moment of modern state and nation building. In the setting of the Renaissance, a single pathological body could stand for a multiplicity of diseased bodies, but public anatomy lectures did not lead to organized public health measures; that is, to a politics directed at preventing or curing collective diseases. Only in the nineteenth century, with the evolution of modern state projects, did the field of public health begin to emerge. No longer did the dead body dominate medical and scientific attention; it was now the living person with all of his or her diseases and impairments that became the focus.[5] The fear of epidemic diseases and of physical or mental degeneration paved the way for the emergence of discourses and practices aimed to prevent diseases and to maintain life. According to the World Health Organization,"[p]ublic health" came to be considered "a social and political concept" that was "aimed at the improving health, prolonging life and improving the *quality of life* among whole populations through *health promotion, disease prevention* and other forms of health intervention."[6]

Therefore, from the nineteenth century onward, the body in the theater must be imagined as the collective body of the population, a body that at-

4 Ibid., 123 and 134.

5 Foucault, *The Order of Things*. The turn to the "living" does not mean the development of new research techniques; for the whole of the nineteenth century, dissection remained the main source of new findings in medicine. See Buklijaš, "Public Anatomies in Fin-de-Siècle Vienna."

6 Definition of Public Health by the World Health Organization, in "Health Promotion Glossary," Geneva 1998. Online at: http://www.who.int/healthpromotion/about/HPR%20Glossary%201998.pdf?ua=1 [last accessed: April 11, 2017].

tracted the attention of the state. Besides medical agents, political agents started to care about the people living in the state's territory and to be concerned about their health, their productivity, and their reproduction. The new arena in which the treatment was to be performed was no longer the theater, but the state. This new arena was no longer a site of public medical self-display, but instead a biopolitical governmental site that involved many different actors.

By means of a great diversity and multiplicity of local case studies, the authors of this volume argue that public health issues represent a core element of modern state and nation building. Marius Turda recently suggested that social historians of medicine should integrate their research on medicine "within wider historiographic discussions if they want to overcome the reservations of their detractors."[7] With this volume, we seek to contribute to the slowly increasing body of corresponding and comparative studies in the humanities which use the lens of public health to bring into focus not only the cultural and social, but foremost the biopolitical dimensions of state and nation building in Eastern and Southeastern Europe from the nineteenth century onward.[8] In our research on the region, we observe close links between an evolving professionalizing elite and its understanding and use of scientific-professional knowledge and the modern state, which—in a very ambivalent manner—makes use of and instrumentalizes medical knowledge as a political tool for its own advancement.[9]

This was never an uncomplicated process. In Greece, for instance, wars, obsolete legislation, and constant shortages in the health budget hindered medical and hygienic modernization from the nineteenth century onward. The picture becomes even more complex when comparing the Greek example to the Prussian province of Posen, where medical modernization at the beginning of the twentieth century became a political tool of compet-

7 Turda, "Private and Public Traditions of Health Care in Central and South-Eastern Europe, from the Nineteenth to the (Mid-)Twentieth Centuries," 117.

8 Marks and Savelli (eds.), *Psychiatry in Communist Europe*; Pinnow, *Lost to the Collective*; Promitzer, Trubeta, and Turda (eds.), *Health, Hygiene and Eugenics in Southeastern Europe to 1945*; Turda, "Focus on Social History of Medicine in Central and Eastern Europe"; Michaels, *Curative Powers*; Turda (ed.), *The History of East-Central European Eugenics, 1900–1945*; Hering and Waaldijk (eds.), *Guardians of the Poor*; Zylberman, "Fewer Parallels Than Antitheses: René Sand and Andrija Stampar on Social Medicine, 1919–1955."

9 For a discussion of the interplay between science, society, and the state, see Ash, ed., *The Nationalization of Scientific Knowledge in the Habsburg Empire*; Duraković, *Serbien und das Modernisierungsproblem.*

ing local German and Polish elites, who strove to realize their own local ethno-national projects through health politics. By focusing on the implementing agents, using a genuinely innovative set of historical sources, asking new questions, and viewing the issues from new perspectives, the intentions, characters, and strategies of the different actors emerge. In court trials against midwives in Bosnia and Herzegovina around 1900, statistical files from early-twentieth-century Russia, or psychiatric patient files from the GDR of the 1960s, the ambivalences inherent in the modernizing projects, striving toward homogenization, become apparent.[10] Seeking to understand the place of public health in the processes of the modernization of state and societies, as well as the professionalization of its experts and institutions, can offer intriguing answers to the question of how public health was used and instrumentalized for the building and the legitimization of states and nations.

Secondly, we ask how challenges to the health of populations and societies triggered not only responses from the side of the state (empires or nation-states), but also international responses. New questions emerge about the interdependencies and entanglements of the national, transnational, and global dimensions of public health. The question of international humanitarianism after the First World War in Hungary, for example, must be discussed in its global as well in its local dimension and cannot be reduced to an aspect of Hungarian state or Jewish nation building only. Also, the "homecoming" of Polish (Jewish) medical experts from abroad to a newly founded Poland in 1918, and their active contribution to the project of Polish state building, leads us to reconsider the relationship between expert knowledge gained in Western Europe and the processes of adopting this knowledge to the allegedly national contexts of Eastern Europe. Last but not least, the psychiatric treatment of war neuroses in post-1945 Yugoslavia cannot be read as an isolated national case study, since psychiatric knowledge of soldiers' mental breakdowns in war had been crossing national borders since 1914. Just as medicine and the human body went "public" in the anatomical theater of the Renaissance, health issues transgressed borders—went global—in the twentieth century. Reflecting on the transnational and

10 For an inspiring analysis of statistics as part of the evolution of governmentality, see Hoffmann and Timm, "Utopian Biopolitics. Reproductive Policies, Gender Roles, and Sexuality in Nazi Germany and the Soviet Union."

global entanglements in the sphere of public health, we seek to facilitate comparison on a regional, European, and global level.[11]

Finally, by focusing exclusively on public health in Eastern and Southeastern Europe but identifying it simply as "European," we are rejecting the ongoing trend to marginalize Eastern Europe within European history. This is both a perspective and a claim, which has also been postulated by other historians dealing with this region.[12] With our focus on public health, we argue that the paths to twentieth-century modern and late modern statehood(s) were, in fact, not so different between the "East" and the "West" of Europe. The contributions to this volume challenge the idea of different paths to modernity and late modernity of Europe's Western (liberal) and Eastern (socialist) countries. The social and cultural history of public health in East and Southeastern Europe, as this volume suggests, shows how a common European framework emerged for solving health issues and organizing societies.

In what follows, we begin with a discussion of the basic concepts and perspectives that form the analytical ground for all the case studies in this volume. We explore the challenges that were particular to the history of state and nation building in Eastern and Southeastern Europe from the perspective of public health, and we summarize briefly the three sections to this volume.

Public Health between Biopolitics and Agency: Basic Approaches

Biopolitics in Modern Times

For Michel Foucault, the merging of the categories of life (the body) and politics was one of the key markers of modernity.[13] When we speak of "modern" actors, we depart first of all from the self-descriptions of the historical agents. It was the actors who regarded themselves modern and progres-

11 Regarding the promotion of a comparative social history of medicine, see Löwy, "The Social History of Medicine: Beyond the Local." For recent cultural scholarship on health in non-European contexts, see McCrea, *Diseased Relations*; Prince and Marsland (eds.), *Making and Unmaking Public Health in Africa*; Ebrahimnejad (ed.), *The Development of Modern Medicine in Non-Western Countries*.

12 See Rutar (ed.), *Beyond the Balkans: Towards an Inclusive History of Southeastern Europe*; Van Meurs and Müller (eds.), *Institutionen und Kultur in Südosteuropa*; Ther, "Vom Gegenstand zum Forschungsansatz. Zentraleuropa als kultureller Raum."

13 Foucault, *Society Must Be Defended*.

sive, mostly in contrast to the perceived "backwardness" of the societies they belonged to. Their ideas, justifications, and concepts must be taken seriously, because only then can we understand what was modern or backward for an actor, a group of agents, or a society at a certain time in a given space. In most of the contributions to this volume, health agents were interested in what they thought were modern forms of governmentality, and in the respective tools and techniques for improving, organizing, and controlling the population through public health. Thus, in this source material "modern" refers to a social, cultural, and political project in which different actors at various levels of administration were involved. These actors all had their ideas about what modern health experts and modern medical concepts should look like, and they also had their ideas as to how to get there. Thereby, medical concepts and hygienic discourses—in nation-states as well as in multiethnic empires—began to use the language of medical metaphors to express the healthy, i.e., the modern condition of a state.[14] In other words, medical concepts and hygienic discourses became increasingly entangled with political arguments.

In his lectures at the Collège de France (1975–1984), Foucault framed the evolving relationship between the collective body of the population and the modern state since the late eighteenth century as "biopolitics."[15] In his understanding, biopolitics is first of all a historically specific way of governing liberal societies. This "governmentality" consists of technologies of power, repressive elements to control the "social" and productive elements, as well as techniques of the self.[16] The making of the population and the controlling of this very population thereby went hand in hand. Health crises in the nineteenth century (such as the plague in Greece or cholera in Russia) were key moments of danger and perceived as serious threats to whole populations. Since these diseases could not be cured, taking preventive measures and treating the supposed causes of these epidemics—the "bad social conditions and circumstances"—remained the only way to protect people.

14 See, for example, Berger, *Bakterien in Krieg und Frieden*.

15 Foucault, *Society Must Be Defended*. From Foucault's time until today, the concept of biopolitics has experienced a remarkable career in the social and political sciences and inspired historical studies into various forms of social and political power in the twentieth and twenty-first centuries. For an introduction to the concept, see Lemke, *Biopolitics: An Advanced introduction*; Lemm and Vatter, *The Government of Life*.

16 Foucault, "Governmentality," in *The Foucault Effect: Studies in Governmentality*, 87–104; Foucault, *The Birth of Biopolitics*; Foucault, *The Government of Self and Others*; Foucault, *The Courage of Truth*.

Arguments of preventive medicine and social hygiene became stronger in political discourses about the modern conditions of states and the ways of governing them. Here, public health served as a means to create knowledge about the physical and the political figure called "population," with the aim not only to cure and protect it, but foremost to "govern" and to control societies and states.[17] From the nineteenth century onward, throughout Europe regulatory mechanisms were applied to health and reproduction to increase the birthrate and life expectancy, as well as to lower the mortality rate of certain populations. Health turned into a site where the "power of regularization" could target "the population as such" and take "control of life in general—with the body as one pole and the population as the other."[18]

As public health was "done" to the body, the issue of how the body was envisioned, treated, and talked about is central to this volume. Taking up the challenge of the "somatic turn,"[19] which aims at understanding how bodies served as "tools of social, economic and political differentiation,"[20] the case studies presented here look at a variety of bodies. They attest to the assumption that in every historical setting access to healthcare services was conditioned, be it through nationality, ethnicity, gender, social status, or class. On the one hand, the techniques to control, discipline, and alter both the individual and collective body were closely linked to the making of empires and nation-states. While empires extended their colonizing policies to the bodies of the colonized,[21] the advancement of industrialization made the focus on the (work-)productive and reproductive body necessary. Since then, on the other hand, the body has served as the forum and ground to debate and implement health, labor, gender, and welfare policies. The interwar period witnessed how collective bodies became increasingly ethnicized and later racialized, a development that went hand in hand with processes of social disintegration and exclusion and which escalated in the Holocaust. However, the ethnicization of bodies and their consequent exclusion from health and welfare benefits were not a peculiarity of the interwar period. Instead, the process continued after 1945 and throughout the era of state so-

17 Hacking, "How Should We Do the History of Statistics?"
18 Foucault, "17 March 1965," 247, 151, and 253.
19 Cooter and Stein, *Writing History in the Age of Biomedicine*, 96–97. See also Degele and Schmitz, "Somatic Turn?"
20 Porter, *Health, Civilization and the State*, 281.
21 Ballantyne and Burton, "Introduction: Bodies, Empires and World Histories."

cialism—discussed in this volume with the example of Hungary. As part of the transformation process from the socialist to the postsocialist era, another contribution discusses the exclusions from Serbian welfare legislation that were not based on ethnic criteria, but rather on social status. Whatever the criteria, exercising biopolitics in modern societies means first of all defining the inner and outer borders of the figure "population" and of those (not) entitled to healthcare and welfare.

With the beginning of the twentieth century, defining borders and optimizing their inner parts became the main goal of social engineers. According to Thomas Etzemüller, social engineering describes a process that encompasses much more than biopolitics, since the latter is only one among many techniques to control and organize modern societies.[22] Others include the structuring of space through city planning[23] or the rational communitarization of individuals into the household, the family, or the work place. Biopolitical techniques were to remain one of the most powerful and effective means to socially engineer societies in the first half of the twentieth century though. As Etzemüller states, wars—in particular the First World War—served as a laboratory for exploring different techniques of social engineering, and thus, for optimizing societies.[24] But biopolitics and, more generally, the project of social engineering were forceful components in the development of state-socialist societies, too.[25] The biopolitical means and practices—especially its forms of social control—but also the forms of subjectivation used in each specific historical and regional context differed. Foucault discussed power relations in the field of public health in liberal societies, where repressive measures combined with productive elements of governmentalities started to work as inner orientations of subjects and contributed to the very formation of subjects, agents, citizens, and patients.[26] In the contributions dealing with the post-1945 period, we shed light on the question of whether this subjectivization, as a Foucauldian key marker of liberal societies, worked in a similar way in socialist societies.

22 Etzemüller (ed.), *Die Ordnung der Moderne. Social Engineering im 20. Jahrhundert.*

23 Behrends and Kohlrausch (eds.), *Races to Modernity.*

24 Etzemüller, *Die Ordnung der Moderne,* 30.

25 See Gestwa, "Social und soul engineering unter Stalin und Chruschtschow, 1928–1964"; Pinnow, *Lost to the Collective,* and Browning and Siegelbaum, "Frameworks for Social Engineering: Stalinist Schema of Identification and the Nazi Volksgemeinschaft."

26 Lengwiler and Madarász (eds.), *Das präventive Selbst.*

It has long been accepted that the primary aim of state socialism was the state's goal to completely control its people and society. Following this line of thought, early medical sociology stated that the growth of medicalization in the region increased social control so that "the regulation of bodies would be complete."[27] The official discourse on physically disabled veterans of the Second World War in the Soviet Union seems to confirm this finding, but only at first sight. What is explored in this contribution, which looks at the example of two former "poster boys" of the Soviet military, is, in fact, the state's aspirations toward total control and a total instrumentalization of the injured body. However, the limits of this aspiration become visible through the official state neglect of ordinary Soviet war invalids. In a much more expressive way, the limits of biopolitically motivated state control become visible in the examples of psychiatric practices in the Charité psychiatry and neurology clinic in East Berlin and the treatment of women alcoholics in Czechoslovakia. In these two contributions, we observe the opposite to what early medical sociology thought about the complete regulation of bodies in socialism: namely, we observe spaces of freedom from state control—spaces that were generated and used not only by the patient, but also by the health expert, as one of the agents of the state. The result is that in the sphere of public health, postwar Eastern European societies under socialist ideology were subjectivized in different ways than Western liberal societies. At the very least, there were limits to the socialist adoption of the self. Therefore we assume that in the sphere of public health, a space opened up for other interpretative patterns, justifications, and arguments than socialist-ideological ones. As these examples suggest, we reject the extension of the totalitarian paradigm onto the field of public health, but instead we see the manifold ambivalent practices and *Eigensinn* among the actors involved.

Returning to the question of what is or was "modern," Katherine Pence and Paul Betts conclude with regard to the GDR, that "[a]fter all, it was precisely the regime's more comprehensive project of social engineering that qualified it as fundamentally modern."[28] Biopolitics and social engineering have been an intrinsic part of socialist societies and states; states that understood themselves as modern—although in a socialist sense. Pence and Betts

27 Turner, *Medical Power and Social Knowledge*, 210.

28 Pence and Betts, "Introduction," in *Socialist Modern: East German Everyday Culture and Politics*, 13.

call this different understanding of modernity an "alternative modernity," which cannot and should not be described and measured by Western standards, but which needs to be analyzed and understood from an internal position (of the contemporary actors). Accordingly, they describe the period after 1945 in the GDR as a "socialist modern" period. From the perspective of public health, however, we have settled on a different term. In order to describe the modern condition of state-socialist societies, we prefer the term "late modern."[29] This decision is grounded in two of our most important findings. The first, as outlined above, has to do with the evident fractures and gaps that characterized the adopting of the self in socialist public health systems. Socialist ideology was all encompassing in its claim, but when looked at through the practices of health experts and their "objects of expertise," it does not emerge as the main guideline for making decisions about inclusion and exclusion, or about defining what was normal and what was deviant. Instead, professional arguments and reasoning played a significant role. This, however, leads directly to our second finding, which is that public health perspectives are intrinsically linked to transborder communication and exchange. The reality that not even the Iron Curtain could entirely prevent the circulation of health knowledge indicates that health concerns were so essential to humankind that they transcended political barriers—at least much more easily than other societal concerns. The contributions dealing with the post-1945 period challenge the idea of an isolated socialist path toward modernity as it related to healthcare. Instead, they emphasize that at least from the end of the nineteenth century onward, there existed a European framework for solving public health issues that was not interrupted by the political division of Europe in 1945.

Tracing the Agents

Both during and before the twentieth century, the creation of a common European framework for public health concerns and standards can be attributed to a multiplicity of individual and collective health agents. As we

29 Employing the term "late modern" also ties in with a sociological debate, which interprets the last third of the twentieth century up to our present time as a radical stance and an intensification of modernity, instead of as a fundamentally altering postmodern condition. For this argument, see Giddens, *The Consequences of Modernity.*

approach diseases as cultural products, we consider public health not as something that people *have*, but as something that they *do*.[30] Doing requires agents—individual agents as well as collective ones. With our focus on the implementing agents on the ground, the agents "doing health," this volume pursues a praxeological approach. In the premodern "public" setting—characterized above by Vesalius's anatomy lecture—a diverse group of medical and social agents was "doing health." The dissection of a single dead body attracted medical practitioners, students, scientists, artists, and medical "tourists."[31] From the late nineteenth century onward, the professionalization of public health produced a different scale and diversity of involved agents. In order to represent this diversity, the volume focuses in a comparative manner on collective as well as individual agents of public health, including the providers as well as the recipients, or, in our language, the objects of public health.

Concerning the providers, the expert played a prominent role in the field of public health. As Lutz Raphael convincingly stated almost twenty years ago, it was the expert who was the main protagonist in the process of the "scientification of the social"[32] in modern societies since the late nineteenth century. These "social experts,"[33] as Isabel Heinemann would call them, possessed expertise from a variety of fields in the humanities and the applied sciences, and included psychiatrists, demographers, medical practitioners, and sociologists.[34] Public health experts were not just individual agents, such as medically trained professionals and practitioners, but also collective agents, i.e., healthcare institutions and related professional local, national,

30 This praxeological thought was first formulated in medical sociology. See Turner, *Medical Power and Social Knowledge*, 213.

31 "Leiden's Anatomical Theater: Pure Science or Vulgar Spectacle?" Leiden University website, July 15, 2014, http://www.news.leiden.edu/news-2014/anatomical-theatre.html [last accessed: April 21, 2017].

32 Raphael, "Die Verwissenschaftlichung des Sozialen als methodische und konzeptionelle Herausforderung für eine Sozialgeschichte des 20. Jahrhunderts." See also Trischler and Kohlrausch, *Building Europe on Expertise*.

33 Heinemann, "Social Experts and Modern Women's Reproduction: From 'Working Women's Neurosis' to the Abortion Debate, 1950–1980."

34 For a discussion of the individual agency of the psychiatric expert, see David Freis, "Curing the Soul of the Nation: Psychiatry, Society, and Psycho-Politics in the German-Speaking Countries, 1918–1939" (PhD thesis, European University Institute, 2015), https://www.academia.edu/19622366/Curing_the_Soul_of_the_Nation_Psychiatry_Society_and_Psycho-Politics_in_the_German-speaking_Countries_1918-1939 [last accessed: April 7, 2017]. For a biographical approach to female scientists in imperial Russia, see Creese and Creese, *Ladies in the Laboratory IV: Imperial Russia's Women in Science, 1800–1900: A Survey of Their Contributions to Research*.

or international authorities. Yet, what was common to all health experts was their involvement in and contribution to the professionalization of public health. This encompassed the improvement and standardization of public health practices and facilities.[35] Regarding the latter, studies in science, technology, and society as well as social anthropology show the importance of scientific and material "things"—technical artifacts, material objects, and techniques—to the actors' actions.[36] These "things" were not important just because they enabled health practitioners to treat the patient's body. Expert actors at an intermediary level of administration also used material things to communicate and report findings, needs, and problems to other public health experts in higher positions of the administration. In our volume, we observe this for instance in the example of the midwife's bag in the Habsburg Empire. Techniques and material objects, interwoven with the explanatory scientific figures and interpretative discourses, were thus important tools for modern communication and science.

When studying the development of the health professions, it becomes clear how heavily the state interfered with and controlled the field. In her studies on prerevolutionary Russian public health, Susan Gross Solomon has shown that the medical profession could only develop "within the rigid confines of the state's bureaucratic structures."[37] The state even commissioned professional experts in the humanities, medicine, and the social sciences for the project of state modernization. But governmental health practitioners were not exclusively and automatically representatives of the state. While "doing health," their role often became ambivalent. Christian Promitzer et al. convincingly state that on the one hand health practices—and, from our perspective, those practicing health—strive to provide care for the population, while on the other hand they strive to control and repress the individual rights of the members of this population.[38] Through our focus on the agent, we try to shed more light on this antinomy, emphasizing the agents' individual room for maneuver. We understand and approach health experts

35 From a critical sociological perspective, this has been explored since the 1970s through the concept of medicalization. For a recent assessment of this concept, see Conrad, *The Medicalization of Society.*

36 Latour, *We Have Never Been Modern.* For an analysis more focused on medicine, see Mol, *The Logic of Care: Health and the Problem of Patient Choice*; and Mol, *The Body Multiple: Ontology in Medical Practice.*

37 Gross Solomon, "The Expert and the State in Russian Public Health: Continuities and Changes across the Revolutionary Divide," 183.

38 Promitzer, Trubeta, Turda, "Introduction: Framing Issues of Health, Hygiene and Eugenics in Southeastern Europe," in *Health, Hygiene and Eugenics in Southeastern Europe to 1945*, 21.

as at least partly autonomous agents that had a voice of their own in the reciprocal process of professionalization and the making of public health.[39] Though acting as representatives of the state, certain health agents—such as, for instance, the hygiene institute in Poznan in the 1910s—first and foremost pursued local or territorial health policies. This room for maneuver also becomes visible in the case study of social workers in contemporary Serbia. Although expected to implement the exclusive welfare policy of the postsocialist Serbian state, these social workers appear to act with different motives, striving toward the inclusion of as many needy cases as possible in the local welfare system.

Several contributions to this volume move their focus beyond the expert and explore instead the experiences and perspectives of recipients and non-recipients, both, in fact, constituting the objects of public health. We use the term "object" first of all to convey the notion that from the point of view of the providers, designers, and experts of public health, the recipients of their healthcare measures were attributed a sole single function, namely to (not) receive these measures. The term "objects" describes this function of course solely from the perspective of the providers and the experts of public health. Yet, we deliberately decided to stick to this term, as we want to highlight the asymmetric power relation that was intrinsic to every aspect of public health politics. Those in positions of power normally did not constitute the objects, and, consequently, vice versa, the objects normally were not the ones in positions of power. But at the same time, our actor-centric perspective allows us to also shed light on the recipients' diverse reactions to patterns of power and control. Contributing to the writing of an "anti-heroic history of public health,"[40] we are interested in the ways the objects—the addressees of public health—struggled against their stigmatization and successfully (re)negotiated their position in society. Certainly, the relationship between the providers and objects of public health benefits cannot be understood as a one-way street. Although power was distributed asymmetrically, access to healthcare was negotiable. Here, the agency of the objects—the recipi-

39 Here we follow studies such as Vandendriessche, Peeters, and Wils (eds.), *Scientists' Expertise as Performance: Between State and Society, 1860–1960*; Trischler and Kohlrausch, *Building Europe on Expertise*; Kohlrausch, Steffen, and Wiederkehr (eds.), *Expert Cultures in Central Eastern Europe: The Internationalization of Knowledge and the Transformation of Nation States since World War I*; Engstrom (ed.), *Figurationen des Experten. Ambivalenzen der wissenschaftlichen Expertise im ausgehenden 18. und frühen 19. Jahrhundert.*

40 Porter, "Introduction," in *The History of Public Health and the Modern State*, 4.

ents—becomes visible, as they actively played their part in the processes of defining the borders and the very essence of the in- and out-groups.

Challenges in/to Eastern and Southeastern Europe

As outlined above, we argue for the existence of a shared European realm of thought, knowledge, and communication, as well as a joint European venue for interaction with regard to issues pertaining to public health from the mid-nineteenth century onward. We understand this shared realm or joint venue to be a nonphysical place, in which professional knowledge, administrative techniques, health objects, and the involved actors from (South-) Eastern and Western Europe—scientists, administrative authorities, physicians, and patients as well as political actors—merged. The image of merging does not imply here a fusing together; rather, all these elements and actors can be understood as permanently circulating, communicating, and acting with each other.

Of course, we do not propose that the joint European venue for interaction with issues pertaining to public health formed a homogenous and uniform platform. Though the development and the movement of medical knowledge and professional expertise had a strong pan-European dimension, the process of translating and adapting knowledge and expertise to each specific local and regional context bears its own peculiarities. Differences emerged because local and regional practices of implementing knowledge and expertise were accompanied by processes of translation and adaption. Differences emerged, too, because of the different strategies used by states, political elites, and professional groups to legitimize (non-)interventions in the sphere of public health. However, this finding should not lead to the assumption that these local and regional practices were more similar to each other because they were part of a common backward and lately—if at all—modernized European periphery, and that they therefore substantially differed from Western European practices. This has often been the underlying assumption of Western mainstream perception, which was rather quick to equate the history of Eastern and Southeastern Europe with markers that identified it as the uncivilized, troubled, and "dark" side of Europe. In fact, this assumption says much more about the idea and self-perception of Western Europe as the liberal, progressive, and therefore truly modern part of Europe.[41] However, the social and cultural history of Eastern and Southeastern Europe in the twentieth century was marked by three specific particularities, which in a decisive way affected the development of public health systems, social, medical, and welfare policies, and the accompanying discourses: the heterogeneity of the Ottoman, Habsburg, and Russian empires; the great impact of war; and the implementation of state socialism. Most of the regions we discuss in this volume belonged to the multi-ethnic empires (Ottoman, Habsburg, and Russian), which were governed in accordance with their heterogeneous realities: they covered large territories that contained large numbers of people belonging to different backgrounds, communicating in different languages, and moving within and outside the empires.[42] Their administrations were very complex because they had to deal with parallel and plural structures, governing competences at different levels of authority and responsibility, and a variety of cultures of communication and exchange.[43] From the middle of the nineteenth century onward, these imperial realities and operating modes were challenged by ideas of modern governance and a homogeneous (national) population, as well as by nationalizing concepts and movements.[44] Around 1900, we can observe the overlapping of imperial and nationalizing politics in most of the case studies here.[45] Imperial legacies and continuities—nationalizing policies and national homogenizing movements alike—can be followed in our regions throughout the entire twentieth century.[46]

---

41 Wolff, *Inventing Eastern Europe*; Todorova, *Imagining the Balkans*.

42 Steinmetz, "Empires, Imperial States, and Colonial Societies"; Berger et al. (eds.), *Nationalizing Empires*. On the Russian Empire, highlighting the role of transfers, see Aust, Vulpius, and Miller (eds.), *Imperium inter pares. Rol' transferov v istorii Rossijskoj imperii (1700–1917)*; Vulpius, "The Emergence of an Imperial Identity in the Russian Empire," in *Cultural Transfers: Encounters and Connections in the Global 18th Century*; Pravilova, *A Public Empire: Property and the Quest for the Common Good in Imperial Russia*. For the Ottoman Empire, see Wigen, "Ottoman Concepts of Empire"; for the Habsburg Empire, see Judson, *The Habsburg Empire: A New History*.

43 For the networks and traveling of medical knowledge, see the articles in the special issue of *East Central Europe* 40.3 (2013) on "Networks of Medical Knowledge in Eastern and Central Europe," as well as Sechel, *Medicine within and between the Habsburg and Ottoman Empires: 18th–19th Centuries*. For the concept of imperial biographies and the traveling of imperial experts and knowledge, see Buchen and Rolf (eds.), *Eliten im Vielvölkerreich: Imperiale Biographien in Russland und Österreich*.

44 For this argument, see Burklijaš and Lafferton, "Science, Medicine and Nationalism in the Habsburg Empire from the 1840s to 1918."

45 For this argument, explored through the relationship between territorialization and globalization, see Marung and Naumann (eds.), *Vergessene Vielfalt. Territorialität und Internationalisierung in Ostmitteleuropa seit der Mitte des 19. Jahrhunderts*. For the example of Warsaw, see Rolf, *Imperiale Herrschaft im Weichselland. Das Königreich Polen im Russischen Imperium (1864–1915)*.

46 Osterhammel, *The Transformation of the World: A Global History of the 19th Century*.

Both the homogenizing movements in empires and national territories and the multifold realities in these regions complicated the work of health workers. Large territories created a heterogeneity of people belonging not only to different social and economic strata, but also to varied ethnic and linguistic backgrounds. These differences complicated the design of a concept striving toward the making—that is, the homogenization—of the population through the rational language of statistics and science, as we can see in the example of the health administration of the railway population in imperial Russia. Therefore, the question of how medicine and public health—biopolitics—was used in the imperial setting belongs to one of the most intensely discussed and interesting questions in scholarship on postcolonialism today.[47]

Second, the two world wars and the many civil wars had important implications for the people and societies of Eastern and Southeastern Europe. No other region in Europe was in such a profound and durable way shaped by the disastrous effect of war and destruction. From our perspective, the impact of war on the development of public health is of twofold importance. On the one hand, wars not only produce destruction and death, but they also often result in new or fundamentally altered states. This was the case in Eastern and Southeastern Europe after the two world wars. The founding of new states, as well as the fundamental political, ideological, and social reshaping of already existing states was accompanied by manifold developments within the public health and sociopolitical spheres. The contributions to our volume, however, question the assumption that the world wars represented an absolute rupture between the prewar, wartime, and postwar societies. The idea to "optimize" populations through social engineering was not fundamentally altered by the world wars. Therefore, our focus has been on identifying the continuities that linked the prewar, wartime, and postwar periods. This perspective proves insightful, first of all, because the nature of the continuity between these periods was of major concern to the actors at the time. Indeed, the self-description and legitimization of postwar societies often relied on their claims of being radically distinct from their prewar predecessors. After 1918, the transition from an imperial to a national state context had to be legitimized, and after the Second World War

47 See Michaels, *Curative Powers.*

the same had to be done—with the exception of Greece—regarding the political-ideological transformation to state socialism.

On the other hand, the world wars triggered the sociopolitical development of public health and social welfare systems.[48] Besides causing destruction, wars can thus be read as an "enabling space" for the intensified transfer of knowledge and practices.[49] In Southeastern Europe, this intensified transfer implied for instance the advancement of eugenic ideas and practices.[50] Also, the wars of the twentieth century generated new social categories of the needy and the poor, such as the war disabled, veterans, widows, orphans, and other bereaved, as well as the sick. In the course of and after wars these were to become, on the one hand, the beneficiaries, i.e., the objects of public welfare (or were excluded from receiving it). On the other hand, these groups became visible as social actors, who in the postwar context negotiated their political, economic, and social position with regard to accessing public health, receiving social welfare, and being acknowledged by the public for their wartime-induced indigence and neediness.[51] Addressing the influence of war on the development of public health systems and discourses in postwar societies thus offers us a chance to compare issues of health and welfare in European postwar contexts and to contribute to the growing scholarship on the "cultural history of war"[52] as well as of postwar societies.

Third, times of war and crisis were followed by the implementation of state socialism, with striking consequences in all spheres of social, cultural, economic, and political life in Eastern and Southeastern European societies. With the exception of the Soviet Union—where the socialist project had

48 See Geyer, "Ein Vorbote des Wohlfahrtsstaates. Die Kriegsopferversorgung in Frankreich, Deutschland und Großbritannien nach dem Ersten Weltkrieg."

49 For this argument from the perspective of the advancement of anthropology, see Johler, Marchetti, and Scheer (eds.), *Doing Anthropology in Wartime and Warzones: World War One and the Cultural Sciences in Europe*.

50 Promitzer et al., *Health, Hygiene and Eugenics*.

51 Recent years have seen a rise in case studies with this perspective. See Newman, *Yugoslavia in the Shadow of War: Veterans and the Limits of State Building, 1903–1945*; Stegmann, *Kriegsdeutungen—Staatsgründungen—Sozialpolitik. Der Helden- und Opferdiskurs in der Tschechoslowakei, 1918–1948*; Karge, *Steinerne Erinnerung—versteinerte Erinnerung? Kriegsgedenken im sozialistischen Jugoslawien*. See also Boeckh and Stegmann, "Veterans and War Victims in Eastern Europe during the 20th Century: A Comparison"; Kienitz, *Beschädigte Helden: Kriegsinvalidität und Körperbilder 1914–1923*.

52 Following Ute Daniel, see the plea for a cultural history of war by Hirschfeld in his "Der Erste Weltkrieg in der deutschen und internationalen Geschichtsschreibung." For Russia and the Soviet Union, see Plamper, "Fear: Soldiers and Emotion in Early Twentieth-Century Russian Military Psychology;" and Merridale, "The Collective Mind: Trauma and Shell-Shock in Twentieth-Century Russia."

already resulted in a profound reshaping of society in 1917—and Greece, the countries of the Eastern Bloc experienced state socialism after the end of the Second World War. What followed was the division of Europe according to two opposing ideological systems, which within the totalitarian paradigm of historiography and political science have been approached as entirely separate realms. However, today's innovative studies on the Cold War period—while thoroughly historicizing Cold War cultures in Europe and beyond—deliver convincing arguments to reject this paradigm.[53] In line with these studies, our contributions dealing with the socialist period suggest that against all ideological logic, there existed a common space of communication and exchange of medical and public knowledge and expertise about health. Arguing that public health under socialism belonged to a common European realm of communication, practice, and negotiation, we understand the social engineering of socialist societies as a part of a common late modern approach to social and health issues, instead of a genuine socialist modern approach.

Structure of the Volume

Medical Agents and Modern State Building

Part I of this volume starts in the nineteenth century and addresses the close relationship between health and the modern state building processes that shaped most of Europe. At this time, various premodern concepts about the state were replaced by new forms of governing that required knowledge, techniques, and administrations associated with "modernity." Modern states were imagined as collective bodies, and states employed the new social method of statistics to control the shape of their populations. These changes were reflected in the medical metaphors that began to be widely used to describe the condition of a state.

Medical agents played an increasingly important role. They developed and prescribed public health procedures and led the process of professionalization of the healthcare sector by creating medical institutions and for-

53 See Mikkonen and Koivunen (eds.), *Beyond the Divide: Entangled Histories of Cold War Europe.* See also Vowinckel, Payk, and Lindenberger (eds.), *Cold War Cultures: Perspectives on Eastern and Western European Societies.*

malizing the health professions. They were also deeply involved in the making of states. Listening to medical agents, tuned in to the rhetoric and discourses they employed in designing and justifying their modern projects, reveals a great deal. For example, it allows us to observe that the question of whether an empire could be a "modern state" was not a real question to them. These medical agents imagined states and societies as modern, regardless of whether they were nation-states or empires. However, their efforts to homogenize the inhabitants of a territory in order to better govern and control them raised new legal and territorial questions. To build a health administration required medical agents to address a fundamental problem—who should belong to the healthy body?—and to take measures that resulted in the strengthening of governmental power. Obviously, this had broad consequences for both health workers and the objects of healthcare, as well as for their power relations within the state and society.

Maria Zarifi's chapter on nineteenth-century Greece examines the weak relationship between politics and science that hindered the implementation of the modernizing project with regard to medicine and public health. The powerful Greek Medical Council created an ideal setting for health workers by pushing through health legislation and institutionalizing the health professions in Greece. However, without consistent governmental support for these measures, many of the council's improvements could not succeed.

In this era, the use of statistics was an important tool to bring politics and health closer together. Statistics helped states to understand who the people living in their territory were and what they needed to become healthy members able to contribute to the state's wealth. In the context of the Russian Empire before 1914, Angelika Strobel observes that the state—the Ministry of Transportation—put great faith in statistics. Besides its descriptive strength, statistics were seen by state actors to have a prescriptive power. State authorities had great expectations that the use of statistics could, for example, help the empire's railway companies standardize their vast and important healthcare systems. These private and state railway companies were concerned to maintain and improve the strength and health of their workers, and they were interested in legal constructions to help them manage the imagined "railway population." But the application of statistics did not bring the expected homogenizing effects, because the generated facts turned out to be hard to interpret, multiplying the categories of representation year by year.

Sara Bernasconi discusses how, in Habsburg Bosnia and Herzegovina, a material object became the tool of administrative rule to create a modern institution of state midwifery and to establish closer connections between medical officers, political authorities, and the midwives. Midwifery prescriptions followed a routine in which the midwife had to present her bag for inspection every three months, produce a record of births, and refill the bag's medical supplies. If the bag was clean and the midwife had used disinfectants, she was approved and could continue her work as a midwife. These encounters took place regularly, from the time of the introduction of the midwifery bag in 1898 until the end of Habsburg rule. The bag became part of the midwife; a sort of professional extension—and the midwife also used the bag's condition to prove her morality. Extending the state's power over health workers by establishing formal relationships—in this case with the help of objects—did not only mean tightening their schedules, narrowing their working conditions, and establishing social control over them; it also had the potential to open up new arenas in which health actors could work, to empower them to use the new objects, and to provide conditions and arguments that they could use in their interest.

In her contribution, Justyna A. Turkowska shows how in the Prussian Empire, the central government relied on health institutions like the Institute of Hygiene or the Academy of Applied Medicine to strengthen both its medical influence as well as its political power in the province of Posen. While the majority of the people living in this Prussian borderland identified themselves as Polish, the central government pursued hegemonic and decidedly German aspirations, relying on medical expertise as the main tool. Tracing the debates on the Academy of Applied Medicine serves to uncover that the local elite also expressed its right to self-determination through medical claims. As such, they benefitted from the inconsistent and often ambivalent modernization politics of the center.

Public Health After Europe's World Wars

The articles in Part II focus on the biopolitical dimension of the processes of state building and state collapse in the periods following the two world wars in Europe. Each of the contributions sheds light on the ambivalent role of these world conflicts, both for the impairment and destruction as well as for the restructuring and professionalization of the region's health and welfare systems. The section starts by elaborating on how the First World War and the collapse of the multinational Habsburg Empire resulted in the transformation of the involved societies as well as the remaking of the local health and social welfare systems. The discontinuity of the region's empires and the making of the new nation-states went hand in hand with the employment of biopolitics for governing and improving the health of their populations. Yet biopolitical measures were seldom directed at a country's entire population, but rather at selective parts of it. This resulted in the marginalization and social exclusion of certain social and ethnic groups. The postwar period also represented a sociopolitical "enabling space" that allowed new social groups to participate and shape individual and collective conceptions of health and sickness.

The end of the Second World War and the implementation of state socialism were also accompanied by a reconfiguration of biopolitical perceptions, ideas, and practices. While the new socialist ideology saw the Partisan and resistance fighters as the incarnation of the (post)war hero, the war invalid and the physically or mentally damaged former fighter did not fit into this glorious image. Here, despite the socialist-idealist rhetoric of full social equality, new attitudes and practices of inclusion and exclusion emerged, which became visible in the marginalization of the ostensibly "unheroic" former fighter.

Tracing continuities in the field of biopolitics from the First to the Second World War, the four contributions in this section aim both to shed light on processes and practices of disciplining people through biopolitics, as well as to reveal the ability of societies to consciously appropriate so-called biopolitical "enabling spaces." They deal with the postwar period, and not with the actual war period. Hence, this section does not claim to discuss the violence and the physical destructiveness of the actual fighting[54] or the outbreak of certain (i.e., venereal) diseases or epidemics[55]; nor does

54 Newlands, *Civilians into Soldiers: War, the Body and British Army Recruits, 1939–45*; Böhler, Borodziej, and Puttkamer (eds.), *Legacies of Violence: Eastern Europe's First World War.*

55 A number of studies have examined the outbreak of epidemics or venereal diseases during wartime. See Röger, *Kriegsbeziehungen. Intimität, Gewalt und Prostitution im besetzten Polen 1939 bis 1945*; Fitzpatrick, "Prostitutes, Penicillin and Prophylaxis: Fighting Venereal Disease in the Commonwealth Division during the Korean War, 1950–1953."

it reflect on ideas and practices of eugenics or euthanasia in wartime.[56] Instead, each chapter looks at the short- and long-term effects of both world wars on the health condition as well as the public health systems of the involved societies.

Two of the chapters exemplify how the First World War not only impaired local health systems, but also made the (further) consolidation of transnational relief and international health networks indispensable. Katrin Steffen examines how the new "nationalizing" Polish state dealt with its internationally trained health experts, and considers what this tells us about the simultaneity of nationalization and internationalization processes of public health in the immediate postwar period. She furthermore deals with the place of ethnic minorities in the field of public health by studying the attitude of the Polish Army toward its ethnic minorities. She observes that the health sector revealed forms of a biopolitically motivated anti-Semitism. Through the lens of postwar child relief in Hungary, Friederike Kind-Kovács identifies patterns of ethnic marginalization that can be seen in the efforts to aid Jewish children. As her contribution shows, in response, international Jewish organizations, such as the American Jewish Joint Distribution Committee (JDC or the Joint), filled the gap and contributed to transatlantic interaction in the field of humanitarian relief.

The other two chapters in this section deal with the figure of the invalid soldier of the Second World War in postwar societies. Through the biographies of two celebrated war veterans in the Soviet Union, Alexander Friedman explores the discursive use of the physically injured and disabled body of the war veteran to legitimize the Soviet state. Heike Karge analyzes the psychiatric discourse on the mentally broken Yugoslav partisan fighter, pointing to the failure of the psychiatric attempt to provide the damaged veterans with a diagnosis that fitted Yugoslav socialist ideology. Her chapter demonstrates that in postwar Yugoslavia, the psychiatric practice of dealing with former soldiers who had been mentally affected during combat was not rooted in socialist ideology. Instead, it descended from the Central European interwar discourse on war neurosis. Juxtaposing these

56 On euthanasia, see Benedict and Shields (eds.), *Nurses and Midwives in Nazi Germany: The "Euthanasia Programs."* For eugenic movements and ideas in Eastern and Southeastern Europe, see Turda and Weindling (eds.), *Blood and Homeland: Eugenics and Racial Nationalism in Central and Southeast Europe, 1900–1940*; Turda (ed.), *The History of East-Central European Eugenics.*

four case studies, this section aims at exploring the problematic relationship between war and the professionalization of public health, while identifying historical continuities and discontinuities of local health discourses and practices from the aftermath of the First World War to the aftermath of the Second World War.

Regulating Societies After 1945: State-Socialist Policies and Legacies

Part III investigates the impact of state socialism on health and social welfare in Eastern and Southeastern Europe. Considering not only the different stages of state socialism, but also the presocialist legacies and the postsocialist period, this section covers an extended time frame, moving between legacies of the interwar period and developments at the very beginning of the twenty-first century. While each contribution presents a case study from a different region, they all ask the same questions: What were the socialist practices and legacies in the sphere of public health? Were there distinctly socialist practices at all? Recognizing that these questions are infinitely complex, the authors approach them from a number of perspectives.

First, two local case studies explore practices of inclusion and exclusion as an integral part of (post)socialist public health and welfare politics. From a Gender Studies perspective, Eszter Varsa explores these practices in Szabolcs-Szatmár County in Hungary from the 1950s onward. Focusing on pro- and antinatalist policies in socialist Hungary, Varsa addresses the regulation of health at the intersection of gender, race, and ethnicity, making visible how the stigmatization of certain groups of women (Roma) coincided with ethnic categories. She finds that the Hungarian socialist state carried a historical legacy stemming from the interwar period, when exclusion based on ethnic categories culminated in eugenic ideas and practices.

In the next case study, social anthropologist Andre Thiemann addresses practices of inclusion and exclusion in a medium-sized urban Center for Social Work in postsocialist Serbia. He is interested in how local social workers mediated social insecurity during postsocialism and analyzes the ways in which medical and welfare personnel sought to act in an inclusive way, often transgressing their prescribed discretionary responsibilities. By making use of the flexibility of the welfare system, they were able to influence the task and aim of more exclusionary state policies. Though addressing a post-socialist setting, Thiemann deals with the intriguing question of what kind of legacy the socialist ideology and welfare system actually produced. As he observes, a humanist approach toward the understanding of social welfare prevailed among social workers, which he argues is the legacy of the late socialist era of Yugoslavia.

Part III also focuses on the internationalization of professional standards. It shows how health and social workers were involved in developing and applying modern therapies and techniques, while meeting and even furthering pan-European and even global international standards. While Thiemann briefly sketches the role of international welfare actors in a globalizing world, the contribution by Esther Wahlen delivers convincing arguments for considering the depoliticized reading of social problems as a shared development of both Eastern and Western European states in the second half of the twentieth century. Analyzing the gradual "psychologization" of alcoholism in late Czechoslovakia, she argues that differences in professional practice were not linked to bloc affiliation. Instead, she uses the example of the professional treatment of alcoholism that in both parts of European health policy was the result of a common "late modern" form of governmentality, in which the individual was held responsible for social issues. Finally, Fanny Le Bonhomme offers an in-depth exploration of the professional practices and techniques of psychiatric experts at the Charité psychiatry and neurology clinic in the GDR. Her case study shows that public health practices often developed if not in contradiction to, then at least beyond official ideology. She identifies the enabling spaces that emerged in socialist psychiatric practice, which she examines through a close reading of psychiatric files.

PART I

Medical Agents and Modern State Building

CHAPTER I

Moving Backward Toward Modernity: The Role of the Medical Council in the Organization of Public Health in Greece, 1834–1924[1]

Maria Zarifi

> Today, no other discipline in medical science attracts and stimulates so much attention and the interest of both doctors and society as a whole than hygiene, [which was transformed by] the impact of microbiology.
>
> KONSTANTINOS SAVVAS (1900)[2]

With these words, Konstantinos Savvas, professor of hygiene and microbiology at the University of Athens, started his inaugural speech for the winter semester course in 1900, summarizing the importance of hygiene in modern societies. The Greek state was almost seventy year old, having survived a turbulent period marked by revolts, a radical change in demography and territorial gains of one-third of its initial size, insolvency, a humiliating war (the Greco-Turkish War of 1897), the establishment of a constitu-

1 This chapter is part of an ongoing project titled "The Quest for Modernity: Medical Networks and Knowledge Circulation between Germany and Greece, 1832–1952" and is largely based on the unpublished material of the *Proceedings of the Medical Council*, located at the private ELIA Archive in Athens. The archival material covers the period 1900–1949. Some years are missing, unfortunately: 1903, as well as the crucial years between 1906–1914 and 1917–1920. Information covering these gaps and the years before 1900 can be found in various primary and secondary sources of the time. I am grateful to Prof. George Antonakopoulos, who made available to me the 1884 and 1885 *Proceedings* volumes from his private collection.

2 Savvas Konstantinos, Λόγος Εναρκτήριος εις το μάθημα της Υγιεινής και Μικροβιολογίας, Εκφωνηθείς τη 15η Νοεμβρίου 1900 εν τη μεγάλη αιθούσι της Νομικής Σχολής (Athens, 1900), 3.

tion, and a new king (King George I). This extraordinary period, however, fanned Greek enthusiasm for modernity, which became a fundamental element of its national identity. The creation of a civilized modern state in accordance with Western standards was one of the ideals of the Modern Greek Enlightenment movement. It inspired the Greeks to rebel against the Ottomans and has ever since been a part of their imagination.[3]

One of the primary concerns of the newly born Modern Greek state after its liberation from the Ottomans was the improvement of the health of the nation, which had been decimated and exhausted by the struggle for independence. This imperative would also determine the identity of the state itself, as it was keen to become "civilized" and modern—in other words, European. In practical terms, this meant that ensuring the good health of the population should be the first step to be taken in order to put the country on a track of sustainability and development as quickly as possible. Therefore, in 1833, a Bavarian doctor, Karl-August Wibmer,[4] who was the personal physician to the first king of Greece, Otto von Wittelsbach, was given the job of establishing and organizing the national public health services. That effort went hand in hand with the establishment of medicine as a scientific discipline in Greece in accordance with Western standards, which only started after the first university in Greece was established in 1837.[5]

As in almost all of the new nation-states that had been created during the nineteenth century, knowledge—moreover, medical knowledge—was a domain controlled by a well-defined group of professionals.[6] Such an arrangement was regarded as a sign of modernity. In general, entry into the elite medical group in the making was always and everywhere dependent on acceptance by most of its existing members, who thereby exercised more or less strict control over recruitment and indeed over the new members' sub-

3 There is an extensive literature on the topic to be found in Apostolopoulos and Fragiskos (eds.), Νεοελληνικός Διαφωτισμός Βιβλιογραφία 1945–1995. Here I want to mention the classic works of Kitromilides, "Tradition, Enlightenment and Revolution: Ideological Change in Eighteenth and Nineteenth Century Greece"; Zakythinos, *The Making of Modern Greece*; Kitromilides, "'Imagined Communities' and the Origins of the National Question in the Balkans," in *Modern Greece: Nationalism and Nationality*; Kitromilides, *Enlightenment, Nationalism, Orthodoxy*; Zelepos, *Die Ethnisierung griechischer Identität 1870–1912*; Beaton and Ricks (eds.), *The Making of Modern Greece*.

4 In the Proceedings of the Medical Council, his name is written as 'Witmer.' *Proceedings of the Medical Council* (hereafter as Proceedings MC), April 11, 1915, in ELIA Archive, A.E. 19/01 Ιατροσυνέδριο 1.

5 Zarifi, "Modernizing through Medicine," 99–118.

6 Turczynski, *Sozial- und Kulturgeschichte Griechenlands im 19. Jahrhundert*, 229f.

sequent performance and behavior.[7] In the Greek case, the existing members were empirical doctors who had offered their services during the War for Independence and the Greco-Turkish War of 1897,[8] mostly educated or established doctors from the Greek diaspora working in central Europe, the metropolises of the Ottoman Empire, particularly Istanbul, and Smyrna (Izmir), as well as in Alexandria, the Danube principalities, Moldavia, and Wallachia. This group also included, of course, Philhellenes who either had fought on the site of the Greeks, like Heinrich Treiber, or had arrived with Otto's entourage.[9] The existing medical elite was dramatically increased after the Balkan Wars (1912–1913), when the Greek state almost doubled its territory. These medical scientists formed scientific and political networks within the state and also established contact with several European centers, particularly with those in which they had studied. They also contacted centers in nations regarded as being in the forefront of scientific advancement, such as Germany and France, which were held in high regard by the Greeks.

What is more interesting, though, are the domestic networks that were established to oversee the centralization of tasks and responsibilities, exert control over the discipline, and influence the decision-making processes. In other words, the Modern Greek state was gradually becoming a transactional reality of elites, a reality that relied on conceptual and normative maps, as Foucault would have said.[10] The content of these maps, though, could be detected not only in the West but also in the nation's past, i.e., antiquity and Orthodoxy, elements that shaped the Modern Greek identity. Both elements were present in the rhetoric of the Greek doctors in their public speeches, which stressed the Western and civilized orientation the new state had to follow, without forgetting the glorious elements of their ancient and Byzantine heritage, occasionally overstressing their direct link to their ancestors.[11] These "primordial codes" of collective identity[12] were employed by the modernizing elite of the state, including the physicians, in public

7 Lloyd, *Disciplines in the Making*, 81.

8 Lazaros Vladimiros, Το Υγειονομικό στον Ελληνοτουρκικό Πόλεμο του 1897 (Athens: Logothetis, 1997), 115–22.

9 On the Greek doctors in diaspora since the sixteenth century, see the brief review of Nikolaos Bouras, "Χρονικό της σύγχρονης ελληνικής ιατρικής διασποράς," *Archives of Hellenic Medicine* 26.2 (2009): 151–59.

10 Foucault, "Governmentality," in *The Foucault Effect*, 87–104.

11 Zarifi, "Modernizing through Medicine," 100–2.

12 Eisenstadt and Giesen, "The Construction of Collective Identity," 74, 77, 89ff.

speeches and writings, until they gave way to a rational rhetoric focusing on practical and scientific issues.[13]

In the field of medicine and public health, the modernizing elite took form in the Medical Council (Ιατροσυνέδριο) and its presidency, which in its regular meetings and contacts with government officials adopted a *realpolitik* rhetoric pointing to the Western nations Greece had to take as an example and follow if the state wanted to be part of the civilized world.[14] However, in such a turbulent period, did this rhetoric prove to be successful? Given that the young Greek state with its Bavarian king was aiming to become a modern, Western-oriented state, how did the institutional elite of the Medical Council contribute to this goal? How did this institution define modernity and what response did it find from the government? In the end, how much influence did the Medical Council have to implement its modernizing project? Focusing on its presidents, this chapter tries to follow the track of the modernizing process the Medical Council attempted to complete in a period that covers almost a century. It also discusses the obstacles they met, their successes and failures, challenging the accumulative and positivistic view of modernization, and highlighting aspects of this process that are not confined to state building per se but are also related to the development of the respective scientific discipline in Greece and the direct contacts with the international community, all of which are without doubt stages toward modernization.

The Medical Council: Authority with Limited Power

Created in 1834, the "Medical Council" was an institution that involved the existing major actors of the Greek public health system and created new ones over the next eighty years. Most of the names of the people involved appear in key policy and decision-making positions, almost until the end of the century, and after this period a new group of names appeared in most of the power positions, either in the government or in academia. This new elite should be in a position to influence the nature of its relationship with the

13 Until 1850, the emphasis on ancient Greece was particularly evident at the University of Athens. See Gazi, "'Europe': Writing an Ambivalent Concept in 19th Century Greek Historical Culture," in *Die Griechen und Europa*, 109.

14 This perception was also stimulated by the Western powers, which had, however, different content for them. See Herzfeld, "The Absent Presence: Discourses of Crypto-Colonialism," 902f.

state, as well as to determine the prevailing relationship between itself and the people and between the state and the people on health-related matters, albeit underneath the overall authority of the Ministry of the Interior. The Council's position was ensured by Article 8 of a Royal Decree, which mentioned the subjection of the Council to the secretary of the interior,[15] while giving it authority to control the implementation of health law and to instruct the health personal who had direct contact with the people (for example, in inoculation programs).[16] This was a new experience for the Greeks, not only because of the centralized nature of the authority—which they had only first experienced a few years earlier, when Ioannis Kapodistrias, a Greek foreign minister of the Russian Empire, was elected as the first head of state of independent Greece (1827–1831)—but also because this center of power was explicitly scientific in character.

The first body of the Medical Council included four doctors and two pharmacists, who were experts in both the theory and practice of medicine, surgery, obstetrics, and pharmacology.[17] Later on, according to the needs of the state, two veterinarians would be added. Employees of the Ministry of the Interior could also be members of the Council's body, while its president was regarded as an employee of the secretary of the interior and acted as the link between the government and the scientists. The Council had three major duties at first: to set oral, written, and practice exams for anyone qualifying as a doctor, surgeon, dentist, veterinarian, pharmacist, or midwife; to provide an official scientific opinion on forensic matters; and to confer over important health and medical issues and advise the minister of the interior in cases where health measures needed to be taken and laws needed to be drawn up or implemented.[18] It is interesting to note that the order of the above duties indicated the priorities of the Council's tasks, as well as marked the limits of its power. It is not strange, therefore, that the largest part of the Medical Council's *Proceedings* includes reports on the examination or licensing of professionals, particularly pharmacists. The Medical Council was also responsible for implementing legislation affecting public health

15 Royal Decree, "On the Creation of the Medical Committee," *Official Gazette of the Greek Government* (hereafter FEK) Nr. 24, July 12/24, 1834, Art. 8. The decree was published in Greek and German and the date of publication was indicated both in the Gregorian and Julian calendars.

16 See Foucault, *Security, Territory, Population: Lectures at the Collège de France 1977–1978*, 55ff., 343f.

17 Royal Decree, "On the Creation of the Medical Committee," FEK Nr. 24, July 12/24, 1834, Art. 2.

18 Royal Decree, "On the Creation of the Medical Committee," Art. 4.

safety; analyzing the quality of drinking and mineral water; carrying out experiments at its own microbiology laboratory to create drugs or vaccine serums and controlling all medical products of similar experiments being dispensed in private labs before going to the market; authorizing its members to attend international conferences and, most importantly, to further educate and train them in foreign institutions (e.g., at French, Swiss, German, and Italian sanatoriums); approving payments to doctors and chemists for conducting autopsies or chemical and toxicological analyses; and setting the fees the doctors could charge for their services.

These apparently bureaucratic responsibilities of the Council, which also included the gathering of data on the state of the health of the nation's population and the conditions in foreign ports during infectious disease outbreaks, delineate, on the one hand, the boundaries of its activities, and, on the other hand, its power to establish the medical and medical-related professions in Greece. This restriction of tasks was to prove to be quite painful every time a crisis broke out, particularly after the Balkan Wars (1912–1913) and the Asia Minor War (1919–1922) and their health consequences. Despite the limitations of its power in relation to the government, the Medical Council exerted a strong influence upon the Greek scientific community, as it was involved in the creation of the first two scientific societies in Greece (the Natural History Society of Athens and the Medical Society of Athens, both founded in 1835), the Theoretical and Practical School for Surgery, Pharmacy and Obstetrics, founded in 1835, and, ultimately, the creation of the University of Athens in 1837.[19]

The Medical Council's relationship with the state, however, was the main factor that determined whether its operation as an influential scientific body would be successful or not. The other factor was the president, who was elected by the members of the Council, usually with life tenure. This, however, was not the case from the beginning. This presidency factor was indicative of three major eras in the Council's efforts to modernize public health in Greece, advance medical science, and internationalize its profile. Its founder, Karl-August Wibmer, who also served as its president, marked the first era. He and the first members of the Council were appointed by the king; they included B. Roeser, A. Leukias, I. Nicolaidis-

19 For details, see Zarifi, "Modernizing through Medicine," 103ff.

Levadieus, P. Ipitis, Mann, H. Treiber, D. Maurokordatos, and X. Landerer.[20] Half of them were Bavarians and the other half were Greeks belonging to the diaspora who had been educated in Bucharest, Jena, Paris, and Vienna. Wibmer drew up a number of royal decrees based on Bavarian legislation during King Otto's Regency (1832–1835)[21] that initiated the organization of public health in Greece. Among them were the law that established the Medical Council, the law that created the School for Midwives,[22] a law covering the appointment of regional doctors,[23] and a law on infectious diseases and vaccination.[24] However, Wibmer caused dissention among the Greek scientific community when he published a report on the outbreak of the plague on the island of Poros in 1837,[25] refuting the view of a member of the Council, Petros Ipitis, who had witnessed the situation on the island and helped to tackle the disease, and criticized the two doctors sent by Otto to the island, Tompakakis and the French doctor Doumon, whose actions (following the irregular and incomplete measures ordered by the government) proved catastrophic.[26] Despite lacking firsthand knowledge of the events on the island, Wibmer attacked Ipitis for being vain and a liar and slandering the government. Ipitis was supported by his colleagues, who expressed their dismay that Otto put non-Greeks in charge of the nation's health, calling into question the merit of Wibmer's appointment, scorning and pushing aside the Greeks.[27] Ipitis, who was dedicated to the study and eradication of the plague, was later offered a chair at the University of Athens, but he declined it. These rivalries within the Medical Council, and further within the Greek medical community in the making, were strong indications of the troubled relations between government and scientists that

20 Antonakopoulos, "The Royal Medical Council of Greece, 1834–1922," 33.

21 The Otto era is divided into three periods: the years of regency from 1832 until Otto came of age in 1835; the years of absolute monarchy, from 1835 to 1843; and the years of constitutional monarchy from 1843 until his overthrow in 1862.

22 FEK Nr. 9, March 16, 1838.

23 FEK Nr. 7, February 8/20, 1834.

24 Cowpox vaccine (*Kuhpockenimpfung* in German). FEK Nr. 15, May 11/23, 1835; FEK Nr. 83, December 31, 1836; FEK Nr. 14, April 14, 1836; FEK Nr. 31, December 7, 1845; FEK Nr. 37, December 31, 1845.

25 Karl Wibmer, Ιστορική έκθεσις της εν Πόρω πανώλους κατά τους μήνας Απρίλιον, Μάιον και Ιούνιον του 1837 και των παρά της Κυβερνήσεως ληφθέντων μέτρων, εκδοθείσα κατά τα επίσημα της επί των Εσωτερικών Γραμματείας έγγραφα, και κατ' έγκρισιν της Α.Μ. υπό του Καρόλου Βίπμερ, Αρχιατρού της Α.Μ. ανωτέρου Ιατροσυμβούλου και Προέδρου του Βασιλικού Ιατροσυνεδρίου (Athens, 1837).

26 See Petros Ipitis, *Η πανώλη εις Πόρον ή ημερολόγιον των εις ταύτην την νήσον κατά τον Απρίλιον, Μάιον και Ιούνιον του έτους 1837 διατρεξάντων* (Athens, 1837).

27 See Kiatipis Vasilios, Η Πανώλιν εις Πόρον και ο Κάρολος Βίπμερ εις την Ελλάδα (Athens, 1837).

continued even after the appointment of Greek presidents and Otto's overthrow and exile in 1862.

The next president also came from Otto's court. It was the military doctor Heinrich Treiber, whose appointment seems to have been a compromise. In contrast to Wibmer, Treiber was an extraordinary figure, a genuine philhellene who arrived in Greece with the first volunteers in 1822. He offered his medical services at the front during the War for Independence and directed the small military hospitals in Nafplion and Salamina. After independence he became Otto's personal doctor and was later appointed professor of surgery at the University of Athens in 1837. In 1854, he organized the military pharmacy.[28] This was also the year that a cholera epidemic decimated Athens and Treiber again stood out for his services, which he offered free of charge. His name is mainly connected to the Greek army health service and its organization, but he was also one of the first modernizers of public health in Greece, and he enjoyed recognition and was appreciated by his contemporaries. However, what the exact reforms were that he promoted from his presidential post for the improvement of the new state's public health system are not recorded on the available archival material.

In 1840, Treiber was succeeded by Ioannis Vouros, a professor of pathology who was the first Greek to become president. He served in the post for the next three years. Having studied at the universities of Vienna and Halle, where he received his doctorate, Vouros continued to work along the Bavarian line. Three years later he resigned and was appointed royal doctor at Otto's court, only to become president again ten years later, in 1853,[29] a position he held until 1862. Vouros is regarded as one of the founders and reformers of modern medicine and public health in Greece, contributing to health legislation and publishing, among other topics, on the creation of a hospital institution in Paris in 1831 and the treatment of cholera, together with Treiber and other members of the Council, in 1854. Vouros dedicated most of his academic research to the history of the hospital and, quoting the philosopher Jean-Jacques Rousseau, he stressed from the very beginning its association to political society, i.e., the state, and to civilization.[30] The emer-

28 Vladimiros, Το Υγειονομικό, 44f.

29 Aristotelis P. Kouzis, Εκατονταετηρίς 1837–1937. Γ' Ιστορία της Ιατρικής Σχολής [Centenary, 1837–1937: The History of the Medical School] (Athens: Pyrsos, 1939), 23. Nikolaos Kostis must have been president between 1843 and 1853 (see page 52).

30 Ioannis Vouros, Περί Νοσοκομείων. Σχεδίασμα (Paris, 1831), 1.

gence of hospitals, argued Vouros, was the outcome of civilization, and its enormous advancement had been part of ancient Greek civilization, "from which derives everything that is good and useful for humanity."[31] The relief and cure of the poor, continued Vouros, and the learning of practical medicine (clinical medicine) were the primary achievements of the healing institutions.[32] This dual scope of hospitals was stressed also by the rectors-doctors in their inaugural speeches at Athens University, relating it to progress and in accord with Western civilization.[33]

The first town hospital (Αστυκλινική) was established for the poor in the Greek capital in 1857 and its first director was Dimitrios Orphanidis, who succeeded Vouros as the Council's president. To the Ministry of Education, Orphanidis reported the significance of the institution for public health and medical science. The hospital served as location for the study of critical and contemporary medical issues, contributing to the advancement of domestic medicine. Moreover, the hospital supplemented the education of young doctors who had to practice in order to gain experience. It was necessary for young doctors to have a certain amount of practical experience before taking their exams in front of the Medical Council. In other words, the town hospital was the link between the university and the Council, which granted the license to those practicing the medical profession.[34]

The most significant benefit of the hospital, though, was the treatment and, particularly, the relief of the poor, which could be improved with more funds from the state. The very existence of the hospital would also change the habits of the people and their attitude toward healing, and move them away from relying on charlatans and impostors. Perhaps the most remarkable contribution of the hospital to social welfare was its philanthropy, which was demonstrated not only with free medication and home visits to the poor,[35] who were unable to go to the hospital, but also with the nutritional care of foundlings.[36] If nutrition is a factor of civilization, to para-

31 Vouros, Περί Νοσοκομείων, 5.

32 See also, Dimitrios Orphanidis, Έκθεσις της εν Αθήναις Αστυκλινικής από της συστάσεως αυτής μέχρι του τέλους του έτους 1858 (Athens, 1859).

33 See: Miltiadis Venizelos, Λόγος εκφωνηθείς τη ΚΣΤ' Νοεμβρίου 1867, Παραδιδόντος την Πρυτανείαν (Athens, 1868), 20–24; Panagiotis Kyriakos, Λόγος αναγγελθείς εν τω Εθνικώ Πανεπιστημίω τη 17η Δεκεμβρίου 1882 (Athens, 1883), 18ff.

34 Orphanidis, Έκθεσις, 5ff.

35 Ibid., 18.

36 Ibid., 9ff.

phrase Henry E. Sigerist,[37] the town hospital not only fulfilled this condition but went beyond it, at least in design and intention, to function as a model welfare institution. The reality, however, was a different story, since the annual budget made no provision for the purchase of specialized medical tools (such as, for example, those needed to carry out surgery).[38] This shortage reflected the weak economy of the Greek state at the time, which was due in particular to the occupation of the port of Piraeus by the Anglo-French in 1854 to ensure Greek neutrality during the Crimean War.[39] In addition, the failed Greek revolt in Epirus and the uprisings in Crete during that period—carried out in the hope that a Russian victory in Crimea would help the Greeks to make territorial gains against the Ottomans—resulted in a terrible pandemic of cholera that affected many countries and broke out simultaneously in Piraeus and Athens due to the presence of foreign troops and left the population in tatters with many orphans needing care.

Vouros, who was president during that period for a second time, published with other members of the Council a guide designed to protect the population and seamen against cholera. The advice in the guide was drafted based on former international experience,[40] except the measures covering ship crews, which the authors took from the protective measures recommended by the English Health Council, which had been officially sent to the Greek government through the English embassy in Athens.[41] The measures concerned food, drink, clothing, protection against cold, housing, and labor. A number of vegetables were classified as very dangerous, including cucumbers, melons, figs, corn, turnips, radishes, cabbages, and cauliflowers. Less dangerous were okra, celery, greens, and fresh beans. Legumes of all kind should be avoided altogether. Vegetables should never be eaten alone or raw but always cooked, particularly with meat. Pies and other heavy, fatty, or spicy foods, as well as pickles and salted fish, should be avoided because they made people drink too much water. Milk should be consumed only in small quantities. In general, people should eat small but frequent meals. Ap-

37 Henry E. Sigerist, *Krankheit und Zivilisation* (Frankfurt, 1952), 19.

38 Orphanidis, Έκθεσις, 15f.

39 The occupation lasted until 1857, the year the town hospital was founded.

40 I. Vouros, H. Treiber, and B. Roeser, Διαιτητικά Παραγγέλματα εις προφύλαξιν από της χολέρας (Athens, July 8, 1854), 1, 5.

41 I. Vouros, H. Treiber, and B. Roeser, Παραγγέλματα εις τους έλληνας πλοιάρχους περί προφυλάξεως από της χολέρας και πρί προχείρου βοηθείας κατ'αυτής (Athens, July 9, 1854), 1.

parently, almost everything that made up the diet of the poor was regarded as dangerous, let alone commonly consumed types of alcohol, like raki or sour wine. Water and nonalcoholic beverages were all that one was allowed to drink.[42] It was also important to keep the body warm with suitable underwear and to avoid sitting outside in cafés, because sudden changes in body temperature could make a person vulnerable to cholera. It is noteworthy that people were advised not to go to the toilet, usually located outside the house, during the night, but instead to use "mobile" containers. Clean air was held to be one of the most important protective measures[43]; therefore, houses should be aired very well and meticulously cleaned. Villagers should keep their animals in a separate building away from their house. Last, heavy physical and intellectual work should be avoided because it irritated the nervous system and made the body weak and prone to cholera. It was also important to educate people to be cautious about quack medicines available on the market (such as the so-called German pills and aloe), some of which were even poisonous.[44] All these measures describe a state effort to protect and eventually control the poor population, the members of which, in particular, were more prone to illness. Even though prominent people also fell victim to the disease, their numbers were small and many of them were able to recover due to their better living conditions.[45] This particular outbreak of cholera, which severely affected the population of Athens, underscored the fact that drastic measures to improve public health had to be taken that were aligned with European modernity, i.e., social control and state intervention.[46]

It is striking that even as knowledge of microbiology was growing (the British physician John Snow unveiled the link between cholera and contaminated water in 1854, for example[47]), the Medical Council was still implementing outdated preventive measures to the population based on their members' own medical experience and not on recent scientific discoveries.

42 Vouros, Treiber, and Roeser, Διαιτητικά Παραγγέλματα, 1–3.

43 Ibid., 4.

44 Ibid., 6.

45 Christos Loukos, "Επιδημία και Κοινωνία. Η Χολέρα στην Ερμούπολη της Σύρου (1854)," *Mnimon* 14 (1992): 58f.

46 See: Giorgos Nikolaidis and Spyros Sakellaropoulos, "Κοινωνική πολιτική στην Ελλάδα τον μεσοπόλεμο: γεγονότα, συγκρούσεις και εννοιολογικοί μετασχηματισμοί," in Δημόσια Υγεία και Κοινωνική Πολιτική: Ο Ελευθέριος Βενιζέλος και η Εποχή του. Πρακτικά Συνεδρίου, ed. John Kyriopoulos (Athens, 2008), 436ff.

47 Snow proposed a microbial origin for epidemic cholera in 1849, but he could only prove it in 1854, when two major epidemics broke out in London.

It is also striking that the use of clean water is not recommended to the public, even though that advice is given to ship captains. It seems that in spite of recent discoveries, no updated measures had been enacted. This side of modernity was still either unknown to, or not accepted by the Greek specialists, which not only indicates the wide variety of ways in which medical practitioners embraced modern developments,[48] but also the fact that debates within the international scientific community throughout the nineteenth century over the infectious or noninfectious nature of the disease left space for political and economic interests to influence public health policy. It was only after 1883, when the German physician Robert Koch identified the cholera bacillus with a microscope, that the international community, through the International Sanitary Conferences, made an effort to professionalize science and set universal standards to tackle infectious disease like cholera. Until then, the disease would continue to be associated with lifestyle, which held that those who lived immoderate and excessive lives were more likely to become infected or die in contrast to those who lived abstemiously.[49] The published orders, which were addressed to physicians and captains, also make it clear that the poor were the most vulnerable to the disease. For this reason, in order to protect the royal family, workers at the royal court were given special warm "cholera" clothing to wear that was supposed to protect them from infection.[50]

Between Modernity and Backwardness

The two remaining presidents of the Medical Council before 1908 were Dimitrios Orphanidis, a professor of pathology educated at the University of Athens and in Paris, and Michail Chatzimichalis,[51] a professor of pathologic anatomy who was educated in Germany. Orphanidis was distinguished for his efforts during the cholera outbreak, serving as the leading doctor in Attica. For his services he was decorated by King Otto himself.

48 On this problematique, see Eisenstadt, "Multiple Modernities;" Wittrock, "Modernity: One, None, or Many?"

49 Vouros, Treiber, and Roeser, Διαιτητικά Παραγγέλματα, 6; Vouros, Treiber, and Roeser, Παραγγέλματα εις τους έλληνας πλοιάρχους, 2.

50 B. Roeser to the Royal Court, July 21/9, 1854 and August 23/11, 1854, General State Archives (GAK), Ανακτορικά. Ιατρική Υπηρεσία Ανακτόρων (Royal Documents, Royal Medical Service), File 184.

51 Dimitrios Orphanidis was president from 1862 to 1897–1898 and Michail Chatzimichalis from 1897–1898 to 1908.

Both presidents concentrated on tackling infectious diseases, particularly cholera and the plague, which infested Europe throughout the nineteenth century and beyond. Greece was especially vulnerable, due to its geographic position and the constant social disturbances associated with numerous rebellions against Turkish authority, which not only forced large numbers of people (in armies and in the general population) to move across borders and to live in squalid conditions, but also served to damage and undermine the elements of the already primitive public health infrastructure, such as the obsolete water supply system.[52]

Purification, fumigation, and quarantine measures were the basic means used to prevent the spread of disease. These measures were followed in all the affected European countries as well as in Russia and Turkey, and they managed *grosso modo* to provide a measure of protection for the population, but with a cost to international trade. For this reason, Chatzimichalis suggested the minimization of the quarantine measures applied to ships approaching Greek ports.[53] The previous president, Orphanidis, had supported the strict implementation of quarantine measures, both on land and on sea, as agreed at the Vienna International Sanitary Conference in 1874.[54] It was at this conference that the idea of "Fortress Europe" was generated, providing a chance for the peripheral states, such as the Ottoman and Russian Empires, "to fashion themselves as crucial partners in the protection of Europe's richer nations."[55]

Greece embraced its role as a peripheral state and an important trade maritime gate to the rest of Europe, and tried to establish itself as an equal interlocutor and a modern state. This policy, however, proved unrealistic and was gradually relaxed, satisfying Britain, which had long opposed what it felt to be excessive quarantine periods (usually lasting 30 to 40 days), which slowed down its overseas communication with its colonies and commerce. The British in particular benefited from the debates over the diverging scientific theories regarding the causation of cholera, which gave diplomats an

52 On the history of the water supply in Athens and its social character, see Georgia Mavrogonatou and Konstantinos Chatzis, "Τεχνολογία και Δημόσια Σφαίρα: Το ζήτημα της Υδροδότησης της Αθήνας υπό το Πρίσμα της «Δημοποίησης» 1880–1914," part I in Τα Ιστορικά 55 (2011): 323–42, part II in Τα Ιστορικά 56 (2012): 145–70.

53 Proceedings MC, April 15, 1915. ELIA Archive, A.E. 19/01 Ιατροσυνέδριο 1.

54 Kouzis, Εκατονταετηρίς 1837–1937, 30.

55 Huber, "The Unification of the Globe by Disease?" 475.

excuse to continue promoting their economic agenda of open trade.[56] The decision on relaxed quarantines was eventually taken at the Sanitary Conference of Venice in 1892 and followed the scientific and technological advancements of the time. It adopted modern health measures, such as the implementation of on-the-spot bacteriological tests, and endorsed chemical disinfection with scientific devices like the Clayton machine.[57] Greece, too, supported these measures, abandoning its former strict quarantinist position and adopting modern scientific developments: "The science of our days," argued George Argyropoulos,[58] Greece's delegate at the Venice Conference, "is able to suffocate the germs of the scourge on the spot; and that is why we all agree upon protecting ourselves against the danger of propagation by measures based on disinfection in place of quarantine."[59] It seems that the Venice Conference was the beginning of the end of the long conflict between the quarantinists (Russia, Austria, Prussia) and the sanitationists (Britain, France).[60]

President Chatzimichalis followed this liberal scientific position but, like his predecessors, failed to show any reform zeal regarding public health legislation, which was not seriously updated until 1922, when the Greek government passed a milestone law that changed the name of the Medical Council to the Supreme Hygiene Council and updated its responsibilities.[61] However, the long pause in health legislation was also due to the turbulence that occurred in Greece during Chatzimichalis's presidency. In 1897 alone, some of the most significant episodes of modern Greek history occurred, such as the Cretan Rebellion (which culminated in the Greco-Turkish War),

56 Huber, "The Unification of the Globe by Disease?" 460; Harrison, "Disease, Diplomacy and International Commerce."

57 Huber, "The Unification of the Globe by Disease?" 467; Proceedings MC, 09.09.1914. ELIA Archive, A.E. 19/01 Ιατροσυνέδριο 1.

58 Argyropoulos was the diplomatic agent of Greece in Egypt. A second delegate that also represented Greece at the conference was Dr. George Zancarol, surgeon to the Greek Hospital in Alexandria and delegate of Greece at the Egyptian Council for Sanitary, Maritime and Quarantine. See *International Sanitary Conference. Protocoles et procès-verbaux de la Conférence sanitaire internationale de Venise, inaugurée le 5 janvier 1892* (Rome: Impr. nationale de J. Bertero, 1892), Délégués à la Conférence Sanitaire Internationale De Venise, x.

59 Ibid., Protocol No. 10, January 23, 1892, 175 (cited in Huber, "The Unification of the Globe by Disease?" 467).

60 A classical study that thoroughly discusses this issue is Baldwin's *Contagion and the State in Europe*, 10–60, 206–10. See also Sechel, "Contagion Theories in the Habsburg Monarchy (1770–1830)."

61 FEK Nr. 122, 1922. See also Theodoros Dardavesis, "Η οργάνωση της κεντρικής διοίκησης για την υγειονομική πολιτική στην περίοδο του μεσοπολέμου," in Δημόσια Υγεία και Κοινωνική Πολιτική Ό Ελευθέριος Βενιζέλος και η Εποχή του. Πρακτικά Συνερίου, ed. John Kyriopoulos (Athens, 2008), 101.

the beginning of the struggle for Macedonia, and the assassination of Prime Minister Theodoros Deligiannis. Despite the lack of modern health legislation, the updated 1845 laws on infectious diseases and vaccination that remained in force were vital protections of the state's existence for many years to come, not only because the health of the population was constantly under threat (Greece being in the maritime crossroad between East and West), but also because the country was constantly in conflict with its neighbors, Turkey and Bulgaria, which led to a number of wars in the next quarter century, i.e., the Balkan Wars, the First World War, and, ultimately, the Asia Minor War. This last conflict shaped not only the state's current borders and radically changed its demography, leaving deep scars on the people's psyche, but also determined its political and cultural landscape and the path of its economic development; and, in the end, it transformed the whole society of the Greek state. Within these prolonged dire and unstable circumstances, every modernizing effort was not only an enormous challenge for Greece but also a matter of existence as a state.

During the Balkan Wars, another cholera epidemic broke out in the country. The Medical Council was responsible for immunizing the soldiers, securing in this way the victory of the Greek army over the nation's enemies.[62] Greece decided to immunize its army after having seen the Serbian population be decimated by cholera during the first Balkan War in 1912. In addition to purchasing immune serum and hiring the personnel to carry out the immunization, Greece also invested in dispensing its own vaccine formula. This took place at the Medical Council–affiliated microbiological laboratory, where Greek scientists created a cholera vaccine based on the technique developed by the German bacteriologist Wilhelm Kolle.[63] Even though the new vaccine did not completely protect those who received it—failing to prevent many deaths, particularly in the general population—it offered enough protection to the soldiers. In 1915, the Medical Council was ready to dispense a new, safer vaccine and asked for financial support to purchase animals for the experiments.[64] A year later, Serbian soldiers brought cholera to Corfu. The epidemic was effectively confined on the island, even

62 Antonakopoulos, "The Royal Medical Council," 35.

63 In 1896, Kolles developed a heat-inactivated cholera vaccine that was widely used during the twentieth century. See Indira Duraković, "Experimentierfeld Balkan. Ärzte am Schauplatz der Balkankriege von 1912–1913," *Südost-Forschungen* 68 (2009): 313ff.

64 Proceedings MC, April 15, 1915. ELIA Archive, A.E. 19/01 Ιατροσυνέδριο 1.

though it is not reported whether a program of immunization was delivered to the population.[65]

Before 1917, Greece had no autonomous ministry of public health—just a Health Department that was subject to the Ministry of the Interior. The extensive damage to the country, particularly in the north, the population movement that followed the Balkan Wars, and the entry of Greece into the First World War that year forced the country to establish the Ministry of Public Care, which, after several changes to its name and status, was reestablished in 1929 by the government led by Eleftherios Venizelos.[66] Perhaps the most important reformist of the Greek public health system died that year—Professor of Hygiene and Microbiology Konstantinos Savvas, who had been president of the Medical Council since 1908. Reviewing the health situation in 1915, Savvas determined that the health services in Greece were initially well organized with no shortages of staff. In addition to the Royal Medical Council, the regional doctors and the vaccinators, there were two health inspectors, twenty-six health centers, sixty-four health stations, sixty-two health outposts, eleven lazarettos, and many more municipal quarantine spots. Five hundred employees worked at the health services and an additional 500 doctors worked at thermal springs and therapeutic baths. Healing centers for those who suffered from leprosy and syphilis had been established.[67] These facts are indeed very impressive, given the fact that the territory covered by the new Greek state over the first thirty years of its existence amounted to about 50,000 square kilometers.

Despite placing solid foundations for the transformation of Greece in a Western-oriented state during Otto's reign, bringing to fruition the ideals of the Modern Greek Enlightenment, the change lasted only a few decades. From 1863, after Otto was forced to leave the county and Prince William of Denmark became King George I of the Hellenes, health services deteriorated. In 1870, for example, provisions for prefectural and regional doctors, vaccinators, and health centers were erased from the public health budget, even though the relevant law was still in force. In addition, spending on health was gradually reduced until 1908, despite a ninefold increase in the budget of

65 See the Proceedings MC of a number of series from January 1916 until May 1916. ELIA Archive, A.E. 19/01 Ιατροσυνέδριο 1.

66 Dardavesis, "Η οργάνωση της κεντρικής διοίκησης για την υγειονομική πολιτική," 101ff.

67 Proceedings MC, April 11, 1915. ELIA Archive, A.E. 19/01 Ιατροσυνέδριο 1.

the Ministry of the Interior.[68] This setback put Greece's modernizing project on hold at a time when its neighbors, such as Bulgaria, were spending much more on public health.[69] Moreover, Greece's obsolete legislation placed it in a backward position, failing to protect its population against infectious diseases; as a result, the country experienced an increase in mortality. The state became even more vulnerable every time a war broke out.

Even though Greece almost doubled not only its territory but also its population after the Balkan Wars, the state did not increase its spending on health. Until 1915,[70] no new law on infectious diseases was passed by the Greek parliament, except the 1908 law on the purchase and use of quinine, which did prove to be highly beneficial for the people. The lack of appropriate and updated legislation meant that in terms of healthcare, Greece remained a "primitive" place, as Savvas pointed out, where responsibility for overseeing the health of the public fell to the police authorities, who lacked even the basic knowledge needed to carry out governmental health directives.[71]

Almost eighty years after its establishment and with new discoveries and advancements in medical science accelerating pace, the Medical Council was still struggling to achieve the basics of public health in Greece.[72] The negligence of public health by the Greek state dramatically affected the living standards of Greeks, despite the fact that their country had a temperate climate and was sparsely populated, and people lived in a frugal and moderate way. A number of infectious diseases (such as smallpox, abdominal typhus, diphtheria, dysentery, meningitis, and scarlet fever) continued to decimate the young population, while venereal diseases, trachoma, and tuberculosis had a negative effect on the Greek economy by attacking the members of the work force most likely to be productive. A population that was excluded from the labor market and unable to create or retain the bonds of healthy family relations was a serious social problem and consequently a feature of an uncivilized society.[73] In addition, cholera and the plague con-

68 Proceedings MC, April 11, 1915. ELIA Archive, A.E. 19/01 Ιατροσυνέδριο 1.

69 This statement by Savvas is not supported by any concrete data and it could only be an argument strategy.

70 FEK Nr. January 2, 1915. Law 346 "Περί επιβλέψεως της Δημόσιας Υγείας" [On public health surveillance].

71 Proceedings MC, April 11, 1915. ELIA Archive, A.E. 19/01 Ιατροσυνέδριο 1.

72 Ibid. K. Savvas, Λόγος Εναρκτήριος εις το Μάθημα της Υγιεινής και Μικροβιολογίας [Inaugural speech for the course on hygiene and microbiology] (Athens: Estia, 1900), 25f.

73 Sigerist, *Krankheit und Zivilisation*, 57ff. See also Savvas, Λόγος Εναρκτήριος, 13ff. On the diseased working class and vocational health in Greece, see the short but comprehensive overview by Lida Pa-

tinued to threaten the entire population as long as there was constant movement of soldiers and people across Greece's borders.

Savvas eventually proposed modern legislation. His zeal to change the poor health situation of his country was manifested from the very beginning, when he became full member of the Council in 1895. He traveled several times to the Levant and studied the health legislation of other countries. His experience was ultimately converted into a detailed and extensive draft bill that was discussed by the members of the Council and published in 1910.[74] The draft legislation suggested the creation of seven health departments, criteria for practicing in the medical and the allied professions, and measures to be taken to prevent human and animal infectious diseases. Its articles described the rules for repeat vaccinations, the creation of health institutions, a framework for treatment and preventive medicine, as well as addressed health matters relating to food, beverages, and deceased individuals.[75] Despite the necessity to modernize the law, the ratification of this draft law proved to be a difficult task. Despite repeatedly writing to the government and personally visiting the minister of the interior, Savvas and the Medical Council did not succeed in transforming the draft into law until 1915, and even then only a part of it was accepted. The articles that according to Savvas's opinion would immensely improve Greece's health system remained unratified: the appointment and the tasks of municipal doctors, the reform of the health department of the Ministry of the Interior, and the measures on human infectious diseases and compulsory inoculation.[76] The appointment of municipal doctors should become a priority for the government, argued Savvas, and it should be done according to the rules followed by other countries, namely by requiring the candidate doctor to hold a medical degree and to pass additional exams set by the Medical Council.

The second priority was the reorganization of the Health Department at the Ministry of the Interior. One of the reforms should be the appointment of a doctor who specialized in hygiene as head of the department. This ap-

pastefanaki, "Από την 'Υγιεινή των Επιτηδευμάτων' στην 'Ηυξημένην Νοσηρότητα της Εργατικής Τάξεως': Η επαγγελματική υγεία στην Ελλάδα, 1870–1940," in Δημόσια Υγεία και Κοινωνική Πολιτική¨Ο Ελευθέριος Βενιζέλος και η Εποχή του. Πρακτικά Συνερίου, ed. John Kyriopoulos (Athens, 2008), 263–288.

74 At the time of writing this chapter, I have yet to locate the draft in question.

75 Proceedings MC, April 11, 1915. ELIA Archive, A.E. 19/01 Ιατροσυνέδριο 1.

76 Ibid.

pointment was crucial, as it was the missing link between the scientists and the government that would enable the turning of scientific knowledge into real policy. The person in this key role, already an institution in almost all other European states, was primarily responsible to explain to the minister the hygienic measures to be implemented following new scientific advancements. This figure also had to monitor the activities of the health services and the implementation of the relevant law, and when necessary suggest improvements or modifications. However, the actual interaction between science and power in the modern Greek state continued to take place in an uncoordinated and indifferent manner. While it was sometimes confrontational and occasionally compatible, the relationship was always difficult and problematic. The lack of a doctor chief director in the health department of the Ministry of the Interior since 1865 brought the organization of health in Greece to a critical stage. The Medical Council, despite trying very hard, particularly during Savvas's presidency, to influence the ministry, did not have much success, mostly due to the fact that its role, according to its royal founding decree from 1834, was merely advisory and with very limited political influence. When Orphanidis decided to leave his position as chief director of health at the Ministry of the Interior (which he continued to hold until 1865) in order to assume the presidency at the Medical Council in 1862, public health started to deteriorate. The chief director position at the ministry was occupied afterward by administrative civil servants, who acted merely as bureaucrats.

A third priority for the improvement of the country's public health system was the ratification of an updated law on infectious diseases.[77] The law officially still in force dated from 1836 (with minor changes made in 1845), and included a number of outdated protective measures, such as the use of chlorine incense and purification, the washing of clothes and furniture of the diseased with oxide, and fumigation with nitric acid, many of which were dangerous. It was only due to a gap in the 1835 law on inoculation that the Medical Council was able to suggest measures following modern scientific advancements against cholera, plague, typhus, and smallpox, which protected the population effectively.[78] For other infectious diseases,

77 Proceedings MC, April 11, 1915. ELIA Archive, A.E. 19/01 Ιατροσυνέδριο 1.

78 The nature of this gap, which left the Council some margins of action, is not specified.

though, no measure based on modern microbiology could be ratified under the framework of the existing law, increasing mortality rates at a time when all the other European countries had dramatically reduced them. Savvas, using the example of progressive foreign legislation and in particular the law in Germany, drew up a draft law on contagious diseases. In addition, he insisted on the resumption of the vaccination of children at age eleven. France, argued Savvas, was particularly in favor of that measure, repeating inoculation when the young person had reached twenty-one. Savvas's dramatic tone reinforced his effort to charm the Minister of the Interior, who was present at the Council's meeting on November 4, 1915, into supporting his measure. He argued that if the minister succeeded in getting the new health law accepted by the parliament in its entirety, he would be regarded as a national benefactor, be written into history, and receive the gratitude of the nation. Despite the minister's promises of action, however, the law had to wait for another seven years.

The reason for the delay was partly because a great number of health personnel were enlisted in the military during the wars Greece fought until 1922. When the Asia Minor War came to its end with the humiliating defeat of Greece, it created one of the largest waves of refugees in Europe in the twentieth century. It is estimated that in only two years (1922 and 1923), about 1,200,000 refugees arrived in Greece,[79] putting even more pressure on the already diminished capacity of the state health system. Typhus and malaria were the common infectious diseases among the refugees, who were living in the kinds of dreadful conditions that favored the transmission of the diseases and threatened the health of the whole population. At the same time, a pool of new medical staff arrived in the country and applied to be licensed by the Council. Educated in Paris, Berlin, Florence, Naples, Padua, and at the Royal Medical School in Istanbul, they contributed to the relief of the diseased. The forced increase of population was in principle a positive thing, but it also created tensions between different ethnic groups, which, as Savvas implied, could be overcome with modern, comprehensive, and fair health legislation.[80]

79 Κοινωνία των Εθνών. Η εγκατάσταση των Προσφύγων στην Ελλάδα. Γενεύη 1926 [Report of the League of Nations: The settlement of refugees in Greece, Geneva, 1926] (Athens: Trochalia, n.d.), 21.

80 Proceedings MC, April 11, 1915. ELIA Archive, A.E. 19/01 Ιατροσυνέδριο 1. See also Kontogiorgi, *Population Exchange in Greek Macedonia*, chapter 6.

Despite his reform efforts being blocked as president of the Medical Council, Savvas did admirable work in other posts, and he is remembered as one of the most important doctors who fought for the eradication of malaria in Greece.[81] From the beginning of the twentieth century, even before he became president of the Medical Council, Savvas established the Greek Anti-Malaria League in 1905 (together with the pediatrician and later professor of tropical diseases, Ioannis Kardamatis). The League played a central role in Greece throughout the first half of the twentieth century, when the disease was endemic. In 1903, already a member of the Medical Council, Savvas was responsible for the instructions for protection against malaria that were approved by the Council, and later he published a number of studies on malaria in Greece.[82] He also went to Italy to study the organization and administration of the Italian system for dealing with malaria, which he wanted to bring to Greece. After the Asia Minor War, he promoted close cooperation with the Rockefeller Foundation, which arrived in Greece in 1925.[83]

Conclusion

Throughout the long nineteenth century, the Greek state was affected by what I call "moments" of crisis, mostly translated into wars, which resulted in demands for the destruction of the old and the creation of something new. This turbulent and transitional period was the setting for Greece's initial foray into "modernity."[84] The modernizing project of the Greek state, as the Medical Council understood it, starting in the early nineteenth century, was not a smooth or continuous process, and it was not completed until 1922. The modernizing efforts were primarily focused on health legislation, the institutionalization of the health professions, and the advancement of medicine, in all cases following Western standards. The representative

81 For latest study on malaria in Greece, see the work of Gardikas, "Relief Work and Malaria in Greece, 1943–1947"; ibid., "Health Policy and Private Care: Malaria Sanitisation in Early 20th Century Greece," in *Health, Hygiene and Eugenics in Southeastern Europe to 1945*; see also Gardikas's *Landscapes of Disease*.

82 Konstantinos Savvas, Οδηγίαι προς προφύλαξιν από των ελωδών πυρετών (Athens, 1903); ibid., Η ελονοσία εν Ελλάδι και τα Πεπραγμένα του Συλλόγου (Athens, 1907); ibid., Περί της εν Ελλάδι και Κρήτη συχνότητος της ελονοσίας (Athens, 1909); ibid., Περί των ελών της Ελλάδος και της Κρήτης (Athens, 1909); K. Savvas and I. Kardamatis, Η ελονοσία εν Ελλάδι και τα Πεπραγμένα του Συλλόγου (1914–1928) (Athens: Greek Anti-Malaria League, 1928).

83 K. Tsiamis, E. Th. Piperaki, and A. Tsakris, "Σταθμοί στην ιστορία του ανθελονοσιακού αγώνα στην Ελλάδα (1905–1940)," Ιστορία Μικροβιολογίας 58.1–2 (2013): 62f.

84 See Blix, "Charting the 'Transitional Period,'" 52.

discipline of the age was microbiology, which brought with it all the elements of modern scientific progress at the time. Using modern instruments (like the microscope) and techniques, microbiologists aimed to identify the causes of infectious diseases and to find preventative and curative solutions. It is not a coincidence that one of the most successful health reformers in Greece in this period was a professor of microbiology. Savvas was a world-class scientist, full of passion to materialize the ideology of modernization in Greece that was shaped during the Modern Greek Enlightenment. He stood among Max Joseph Pettenkofer, Robert Koch, Louis Pasteur, Edward Jenner, Waldemar Haffkine, and Emil von Behring—the scientists who connected hygiene with microbiology, empirical practice with science, and civilization and modernity.[85] The use and application of statistical methods to address health problems was the second advancement that connected hygiene with modernity.[86] For Savvas, hygiene was closely connected with civilization; they were two sides of the same coin, a criterion to classify a nation as civilized or uncivilized. A civilized state was a state with a well-established public health system that embraced advances in medical science. Therefore, hygiene was also closely related to national identity, carrying all the old elements of the glorious past and gathering the new ones of the Western world. Modern health legislation was part of that world, demonstrating the successful modern and civilized identity of the state. Despite all the efforts made by the Greek medical elite to improve the health of the state, the domestic health infrastructure remained poor. The changes in the legislation were small, slow, and often made after emergencies, and therefore fragmented and nearly outdated before they were enacted. This was the result of the difficult relationship between the representatives of science and political power in the state, who never found a way to interact positively. The rivalries over public health control between the state mechanism and the medical community, represented by the Medical Council, was also nourished by the scattered hygiene services and the lack of a Health Ministry, i.e., the lack of a mature and well-structured health policy and a comprehensive health legislation, but also by the deficient implementation of the existing laws, mainly due to the unstable political conditions, the continuous wars, and the con-

85 Savvas, "Λόγος Εναρκτήριος," 6–9.
86 Ibid., 13.

stant lack of funds. In addition, the fact that the liberal party of Eleftherios Venizelos, which dominated the political scene in Greece during most of Savvas's incumbency as president of the Medical Council, combined with the fact that he served as chief doctor of the king and therefore was regarded as a royalist, leads us to speculate that political sympathies may have played a part in the fact that his strenuous efforts were either ignored or only partly materialized.[87]

The quest for modernity proved to be a Sisyphean task during the long nineteenth century in Greece, a constant struggle between the state and the intellectuals, the bureaucrats and the men of action. Modernization in the Greek state remained incomplete, "hovering," something in-between, a blocked process,[88] perhaps because there was no political modernization, either. The well-known scandal over the embezzlement of a large quantity of quinine that involved a director of the Ministry of Hygiene in 1929, shortly before Savvas died, is perhaps the best illustration of this handicap. It crystallized his idea for creating a health body independent of political change and free from political intervention.[89]

The end of the Asia Minor War marked the end of a constant crisis era, giving way to a new period characterized not only by enormous demographic, political, and economic challenges, but also by creativity, novelty, and a desire for reform, all due to the arrival of the postwar refugees. A long era of health reform guided by the Medical Council ended and a new one began in which the organization of public health in Greece eventually realized many of the Council's dreams and ambitions.

87 A definite conclusion regarding this political aspect can only be drawn after the completion of the ongoing project.

88 On the ideological background that binds together politicians and intellectuals and the coining of the term "hovering modernization," see Vasilis Bogiatzis, "Μετέωρος μοντερνισμός. Τεχνολογία, ιδεολογία της επιστήμης και πολιτική στην Ελλάδα του Μεσοπολέμου (1922–1940)" (Athens, 2012). Also see Tampakis, "Onwards Facing Backwards."

89 Tsiamis, Piperaki, and Tsakris, "Σταθμοί στην ιστορία," 62.

CHAPTER II

Creating the "Railway Population": Public Health and Statistics in Late Imperial Russia[1]

Angelika Strobel

In 1914, the renowned Russian statistician Aleksandr Kaufman, facing "an unprecedented expansion in the remit of social policy," declared statistics to be the "only tool toward a quantitative knowledge of the phenomena of social life."[2] Seven years earlier, a railway physician had similarly promised that statistics alone could reveal the state of the health of the "railway population" and its relationship to the conditions in which the people lived and worked.[3] This chapter focuses on the specific significance of statistics as a technology of governance and as a form of the representation and production of social objects in the health domain through the emergence of "railway medicine" in the late Russian Empire. I argue that its social product was the "railway population" (železnodorožnoe naselenie) formed of employees and their families.

During the course of the nineteenth century, statistical knowledge, pushed by advocates from science and public administrations keen to describe and represent social realities through numbers, achieved a dominant status throughout Europe. Numerical data became the very incarnation of the "modern fact," as it was deemed to be pre-interpretive and hence the

1 This chapter was translated by Tudor Georgescu.

2 Aleksandr Kaufman, "Čem dolžna byt' vtoraja vserossijskaja perepis'," *Vestnik Evropy* 3 (1914): 272.

3 V. M. Michajlov, "O pravil'noj postanovke sanitarnoj statistiki na železnych dorogach," *Obščestvennyj vrač* 4 (1907): 302.

very foundation for any kind of systematic knowledge of the world.[4] Governments demanded such facts and statistic regularities in order to control, measure, and compare their political actions and management of social and economic resources.[5] The practical reality of statistics was always guided by specific (political) interests and theoretical assumptions about what should be counted and how its quantification could contribute to a systematic form of knowledge. Statistics, both descriptive and prescriptive, generated the objects it described.[6] Statisticians could create social groups and aggregates that had not previously existed. When their categories and classifications were codified through institutions, discourses, and practices, though, they could have implications on daily life.[7]

Matters surrounding public health were important engines for statistical generalizations and social policies. A new perception of disease as a collective phenomenon followed from the cholera epidemics of the early nineteenth century in Europe. Seeking to prevent them, hygienists and physicians surveyed social conditions and realities, in addition to the disease itself. Also, the emergence of medical infrastructures, such as clinics and institutions, required a calculation of demand, supply, and resources grounded in data.[8] Finally, techniques of measurement and statistics for the formulation of quantitative norms gained increasing importance as

---

4 See Poovey, *A History of Modern Fact*. Poovey studies the historic moment when the history of description appeared as something distinct to the history of interpretation or theoretic analysis; that is, how a means of representation (numeric data) began to be considered immune to theory or interpretative analysis. On the history of statistics in relation to state power, economics, and moral sciences, see Desroisères, *Die Politik der großen Zahlen*.

5 See Patriarca, *Numbers and Nationhood*, 1–18. Patriarca discusses "statistical surveillance" in relation to the entanglement of statistics with problems of governability. On the concept of political interests and their tense relationship with scientific self-perception, see Porter, "Statistical and Social Facts from Quetelet to Durkheim," 19. On the political power of data within technologies of governance, see Rose, *Powers of Freedom*, 197–232.

6 Since the 1990s, scholars in the social sciences and humanities working on the history of (scientific) knowledge have been pointing out that statistical knowledge can also be construed, that is, prescriptive. For example, the philosophy of science: Hacking, *The Taming of Chance*; the sociology of knowledge: Desroisères, *Politik*; historic-epistemological: Poovey, *Making a Social Body*.

7 Ian Hacking talks of interactive classification types in the social sciences. The interaction between classifiers and the classified generated looping effects that constantly keep the objects of the social sciences in motion. Hacking, *The Social Construction of What?* 160f. See also Hacking, "Making up People."

8 Desroisères, *Politik*, 93–8; Hacking, *Taming of Chance*, 47–54; Bulmer et al., "The Social Survey in Historical Perspective," 7–9, on the statistics movement within the sanitary movement in Great Britain; see also Poovey, *Making a Social Body*, 115–31, on the importance of Edwin Chadwick's sanitary report to state formation.

reference points to medical practice itself, with medicine seeking to become an exact natural science at the end of the nineteenth century.[9]

In Imperial Russia (as elsewhere in Europe), from the second half of the nineteenth century onward statistical research became ever more important, accompanied by the growing complexity of social and economic administrative tasks.[10] With modernity, the social became a key to governability, and in this process health policies had a relevant function.[11] In contrast to other European states, which used statistics and social institutions such as medical provision, public transportation, or education to create a homogenous nation-state and a nationalized social body, in the Russian Empire statistical rationalizations and representations strengthened and proliferated the variety of institutions and objects.[12] A heterogeneously grown, imperial administration of territory, things, and people, I argue, preconditioned the development of a particular "railway population."[13]

First, I outline the structures and processes within which railway medicine emerged as a social institution. Then, using annual medical reports, I demonstrate how statistical information made heterogeneity visible and how this became a problem for central planning. This problem of heterogeneity was amplified when railway medicine tried to fashion a homogenous administrative social object through the execution of population counts. Finally, I discuss how the process of defining a "railway population" meant that various legal practices conflicted with each other as well as the principle of territoriality, which became important to the expansion of medical infrastructure.

9 See, for example, the contributions in Hess (ed.), *Normierung der Gesundheit*, which engage with the mathematical aspects of blood, urine, and cardiac health, or with physiological base values.

10 Statistics as a tool of social politics was particularly important in the local, self-government in European Russia, the *zemstva*. Their statisticians, inspired by the social sciences, collected a mass of data on the economic, demographic, and health conditions of the peasantry in their administrative territories. See Kingston-Mann, "Statistics, Social Science, and Social Justice"; Mespoulet, *Statistique et révolution en Russie*; Mespoulet, "Pratique de l'enquête et construction du savoir statistique en Russie à la fin du XIXe siècle"; Mespoulet, "Professional'naja etika zemskich statistikov i formy ich otnošenija k vlasti (1880–1922)."

11 The great famine and cholera epidemic, as well as the subsequent social unrest of 1891–1893, are considered by historians to be a watershed in healthcare and social politics. See, for example, Henze, *Disease, Health Care and Government in Late Imperial Russia*. Others have focused on how, with modernity, the social became a key to governability—for example, school lunches as a modern social institution. See Vernon, "The Ethics of Hunger and the Assembly of Society."

12 On statistics and state building in France, Great Britain, Germany, and the USA, see Desroisières, *Politik*, 165–234; on Great Britain: Poovey, *Making a Social Body*; on Italy: Patriarca, *Numbers*.

13 On Russian administrative structures, see for example Rowney and Huskey (eds.), *Russian Bureaucracy and the State*.

The Invention of Railway Medicine

Around the turn of the century, state and private railways became the most important means of transportation and communication in the multi-ethnic Russian Empire, and increasingly important to the imperial policy of the autocracy.[14] They were also of economic importance to the empire, in that they constituted large financial and labor-intensive enterprises with over half a million employees and workers along 55,000 kilometers of track.[15] The local companies organized the labor in different services that, for the most part, corresponded to their individual trades, such as communications, train services, the production of engines and rolling stock, or the construction and maintenance of railway tracks.[16] The employees and workers of the respective services, all the way up to the directors of the local train lines, were tied into a complicated hierarchical system in which every representative could autocratically rule the rung below and bore sole responsibility to that above.[17]

The railways, along with all the other (private) enterprises after 1866, were by law responsible for the provision of free medical care to their em-

14 Marks, *Road to Power*; Cvetkovski, *Modernisierung durch Beschleunigung*, 184–274; Schenk, *Russlands Fahrt in die Moderne*.

15 The data are for the year 1901. Bespalov and Eliseeva, *Železnye dorogi Rossii v XX veke v zerkale statistiki*, 75 and 92. In 1913, the railways had about 815,000 workers and employees along 68,000 kilometers of track. See Laverychev, "Trends Towards State Monopoly in Pre-Revolutionary Russia's Railways"; Solovyova, "The Railway System in the Mining Area of Southern Russia in the Late Nineteenth and Early Twentieth Century."

16 The administrative organization of the work was not equally differentiated along all lines and across all services. See the extensive discussion in Reichman, *Railwaymen and Revolution*, 49–70. The medical services organized the employees and workers, from a healthcare perspective, into nine groups, whereas the decisive criteria were income and the material and physical working conditions. The archival material of this chapter is from the Rossijskij Gosudarstvennyj Istoričeskij Archiv (hereafter RGIA), Ministerstvo Putej Soobščenii (Ministry of Transportation, hereafter MPS), Upravlenie železnych dorog, Vračebno-sanitarnaja čast' (Department of Railways, Public Health Section), hereafter with the signature f. 273, op. 8. See RGIA, f. 273, op. 8, d. 354, l. 77, "Forma otčetnosti po vračebno-sanitarnoj službe na železnych dorog, 1910–1916: "Obščaja vedomost' o boleznosti i smertnosti lic, polzovannych vračami, fel'dšerami i akušerkami ambulatorno, na domu, v bol'nicach (v svoich i postoronnich), priemnych pokojach i proč. i ob iskljucennych po nesposobnosti k železnodorožnych službe."

17 With regards to the railways, the contemporary interpretation compared the system of government to serfdom. From a socialist perspective, see V. Dmitriev, "Byt' služaščich i rabočich na železnych dorogach," *Sovremennyj mir* 1 (1912): 281–302; from the perspective of a railway physician, A. G. Bočarnikov, "O roli vrača v bor'be za trezvost' na železnych dorogach," *Vestnik železnodorožnoj mediciny i sanitarii* (hereafter *VŽMiS*) 3 (1914): 36–42. The power relationships were complicated, especially in the upper echelons, by the growing leadership role of the state. Laverychev, "Trends," 37–47; using the example of the biography of the railway engineer Lomonosov, see Heywood, *Engineer of Revolutionary Russia*.

ployees. The state, having delegated care for the people to various administrations and private business, neither defined nor regulated it.[18] Until the social insurance laws of 1912, the provision of medical care and prevention to employees remained at the personal discretion of entrepreneurs who commonly considered the efforts required as acts of philanthropy.[19] Before the 1880s, most railways belonged to private companies, so in real terms no medical services existed prior to 1900.[20] The medical sections of local railway companies often consisted of a single physician, whose primary function was the medical assessment of new employees or of accident victims. His purpose was to minimize the risk of accidents and the associated costs for pensions and individual damage claims.[21] The railway physician was an employee in the company's service.

Toward the end of the nineteenth century, the multifarious processes facilitating the state's monopolization of the railways began. For one, the patterns in ownership changed. Around 1900, about two-thirds of the railway network was directly controlled by the state and, via shares and bonds, the state owned 90 percent of the private companies' total assets.[22] Furthermore, the state increasingly tried to centrally steer the administration, usage, and employment policies of the railways.[23] This process began with the reorganization of the Ministry of Transportation: in 1898, it established a Department of Railways with which the Ministry gained a dominant role in the operative control of state and private railway companies.[24] Within this

---

18 G. Zinin, "Fabričnaja medicina i rabočyj vopros," *Zavety* 5 (1912): 60–81.

19 Zinin, "Fabričnaja medicina," 60–81; D. Orlov, "Fabričnaja Medicina v Moskve," *Medicinskaja Beseda* 7–8 (1905): 140–42. Both authors discuss how entrepreneurs logged their duty to provide healthcare services as philanthropy in their bookkeeping.

20 On property ownerships patterns up to the 1880s, see Cvetkovski, *Modernisierung*, 227. For health provision at the state and private railway lines before 1900, see I. M. Puškareva, *Železnodorožniki v buržuazno-demokratičeskich revoljucijach* (Moscow: Nauka, 1975), 67f.; Reichman, *Railwaymen*, 99–102.

21 This function was shared between the railway physician and the factory physician. See Zinin, "Fabričnaja medicina," 60–81.

22 On finance policy, see Cvetkovski, *Modernisierung*, 225–230; V. V. Zhuravlyov, "Private Railway Companies in Russia in the Early Twentieth Century," *Journal of Transport History* 1.4 (1983): 51–65; Laverychev, "Trends," 37f. In 1913, twenty-three railway lines with a total track length of 46,684 kilometers belonged to the state. Fourteen railway lines with a total track length of 20,290 kilometers were owned by private companies. Bespalov and Eliseeva, *Železnye dorogi*, 72f.

23 Important here was that, around 1900, the directors of the private train lines were integrated into the state as civil servants. Laverychev, "Trends," 39f. On the state's role after 1905 from a Soviet perspective, see Puškareva, *Železnodorožniki*.

24 All financial matters remained in the Ministry of Finance's domain and that of the highest tsarist accountancy office (*gosudarstvennyj kontrol'*), which had representatives on the administrative boards of the local train lines. See RGIA, f. 273, op. 8, d. 6, l. 23–26, "O preobrazovanii central'nych učreždenii

department, a public health section was created to oversee the local medical services in its name.[25]

Four years after this reorganization, the Medical Decree of 1894 was the first to officially determine the organization and purpose of railway medicine. Until its revision in July 1913, the decree theoretically applied to state railways only.[26] However, since the turn of the century, the Department of Railways had steered the health policies of the local railway lines with temporary edicts and regulations, and did so with the purpose of controlling labor policy.[27] A decisive impetus for the state's governance of labor policies came with the 1905 Revolution, during which numerous train lines experienced strikes that brought the empire's communication and transportation arteries to a standstill.[28] The Ministry did not respond with repression alone, however.[29] It recognized that the railway workers' poor living and working conditions contained an explosive social force.[30] Health policies became increasingly relevant to the state in terms of cementing the political order as a means of social and economic control. In 1906, the Department of Railways invested about a million rubles in the expansion of medical provisions and the creation of institutions for preventive medicine.[31]

MPS i ob organizacii vračebno-sanitarnoj časti upravlenija železnych dorog, 1899–1901": "Vysočajse utverždennoe mnenie gosudarstvennago soveta. O preobrazovanii central'nych ustanovlenij MPS."

25 The 1894 decree established independent medical services: ibid., "Otčet o vračebno-sanitarnom sostojanii kazennych železnych dorog za 1898 god. SPb 1901" (l. 338–39).

26 The 1913 decree prescribed the organization, terms of use, and duties of medical personnel belonging to railway medicine for all railway services. "Pravila vračebno-sanitarnoj časti, otkrytych dlja obščestvennogo pol'zovanija," *VŽMiS* 10 (1913): 7–45.

27 RGIA, f. 273, op. 8, d. 183, "O porjadke predstovlenija železnodorožnye vrači vračebnoj otčetnosti, 1905–1912" (duty to report annually); "O mestnych soveščatel'nych s"ezdov železnodorožnych vračej, 1909–1915," f. 273, op. 8, d. 315 (duty to convene local congresses of railway physicians), or "Ob administrativnom delenii ž.d. po vračebnoj službe," f. 273, op. 8, d. 340 (on the normatization of the territorial organization of medical provision).

28 Regarding the strikes during the revolutionary year, see Reichman, *Railwaymen*; Reichman, "The 1905 Revolution on the Siberian Railroad"; Puškareva, *Železnodorožniki*; Schenk, "Imperiale Raumerschliessung: Die Beherrschung der russischen Weite."

29 See Reichman and Puškareva, who follow the contemporary socialist perspective, such as, for example, in Dmitriev, "Byt' služaščich i rabočich." In doing so, the creation of a railway police, the prohibition of the organization of labor unions, projects geared toward the militarization of labor through soldier brigades, and the membership of Minister of Transportation Ruchlov (1909–1915) in the right-wing nationalist League of the Russian Nation came to the fore.

30 Dmitriev, "Byt' služaščich i rabočich," 281–287, explained the dominance of the repressive side of this dual carrot stick strategy as being due to the state lacking the funds for an effective improvement in working and living conditions.

31 RGIA, f. 273, op. 8, d. 211, l. 1–9, "Ob ustanovlenii dolžnosti železnodorožnych sanitarnych vračej, 1906–1915": "Kopija. Žurnala Komiteta Upravlenija železnych dorog. Po vračebno-sanitarnoj časti. 4–14 fevralja/2–14 marta 1906 goda. No. 737." A total of 375 new jobs were created across the sixteen

The aims of the 1894 decree were now to be realized across the entire railway network.

In the expansion and homogenization of railway medicine, the Department of Railways and the railway physicians were guided by the public health system, institutionalized in the local self-government (*zemstvo*) of the empire's European provinces.[32] This system of medical care rested on a number of core principles. The entire population of the administrative area was to have access to free medical provisions funded by estate taxes and state subsidies. The territory, therefore, was divided into standardized medical precincts of equal size, population density, and institutions. Statistics and their analysis were supposed to provide empirical evidence of the costs, usage, and requirements of medical care. The *zemstvo* physicians and administrations were to collaborate on healthcare policies. And, finally, the overarching strategy of intertwining curative and preventive medicine (*sanitarija*) was significant. It expressed the ambition to statistically capture the population's current health in terms of its living and working conditions and to direct (preventive) medical practices according to these findings. Such a broad range of activities, as they emerged from the practice of *zemstvo* medicine pursued by public health statistics (*sanitarnaja statistika*), was peculiar to the Russian Empire.[33]

The adaptation of this medical system, which had evolved in the *zemstva* since the 1870s, generated specific problems and ambivalences for rail-

state railway services in 1906, of which a hundred were precincts physicians and sixteen were public health physicians (sanitary physicians). A precincts physician's annual salary was between 2,100 and 2,400 rubles.

32 The *zemstva* were established in 1864 in the European part of Russia as self-governing bodies of the provinces and districts. The Department of Railways—that is, its medical section—did not explicitly establish any links with *zemstvo* medicine. For the railway physicians, though, *zemstvo* medicine was the only point of reference with regards to medical provisions, health prevention, their own working conditions, or their professional identity. They declared railway medicine to be the partner of *zemstvo* medicine, or to function as its pioneer in relation to the Asian part of the Russian Empire. See, for example, Michajlov, "O pravil'noj postanovke," 298–304; A. A. Gryslov, "Obščestvennoe značenie železnodorožnoj medicinskoj organizacii," *VŽMiS* 9 (1915): 277–86; V. V. Krasnov, "O različnych trebovanijach k sostavleniju registracionnych i sanitarnych kartoček," *VŽMiS* 5 (1915): 49–55.

33 In contrast to medical statistics or vital statistics that captured demographic changes (births, deaths, marriages), the *zemstvo* medical statisticians also produced comprehensive statistics on diseases based on medical appointments and hospital stays as well as epidemiologic-topographic and socioeconomic research. See S. Novosel'skij, "Ob organizacii gosudarstvennoj sanitarnoj statistiki," *Obščestvennyj vrač* 9–10 (1917): 343–49. On this, as well as the principles of *zemstvo* medicine: P. I. Kurkin, *Zemskaja sanitarnaja statistika: Opyt' postroenija schemy raboty. Doklad soveščaniju sanitarnych vračej pri upravlenii o-va russkich vračej v Moskve* (Moscow, 1912); on organization and implementation, see for example Z. G. Frenkel, *Obščestvennaja medicina i social'naja gigiena* (Leningrad, 1926); and Z. G. Frenkel, *Očerki zemskogo vračebno-sanitarnogo dela* (St. Petersburg, 1913).

ways. True to the tradition of beneficent promises during the second half of the nineteenth century, the 1894 decree had also envisaged the free provision of medical care for railway employees and their families.[34] But it was only with the gradual implementation of the medical decree's objectives after 1906 that a multitude of unexpected confusions emerged. A chronic problem was that (legitimate) demand far outstripped supply.[35] Contrary to what had been the case with *zemstvo* medicine, railway medicine was not a care system for an equally entitled and sedentary population. Many railway employees, considering their line of work, were inherently mobile, and fluctuations in workloads were high. Following a series of temporary, locally distinct regulations, the Ministry of Transportation's 1913 Decree on Railway Medicine established a three-tier system of provisions for a total of ten social groups in their administrative area.[36] The organization of provisions and patient administration was similarly complicated.[37] Although norms for medical precincts emerged—they defined the territorial dimensions, personnel, and infrastructure along the track network—they did not spatially allocate people and patients per medical precincts.[38] But how was one to calculate budgets and requirements, regulate the tiered entitlements, or gain a view of the overall health situation if one was unfamiliar with the object of the care itself, namely the population and its spatial distribution?

The railways, profit-oriented and locally state-owned or private enterprises, were thoroughly intertwined with the hierarchical power structures of the autocratic state. Railway medicine, too, belonged to this administrative rank order and was itself organized according to this principle.[39] The adaptation of the *zemstvo* medicine's principle of collegiality—in the form of regular congresses—hence produced less innovation and collegial ex-

34 See RGIA, f. 273, op. 8, d. 6, l. 106–7, "Spravka," regarding the decree and the annual medical report for 1898 on the medical provisions for state railway lines (ibid., l. 338–39).

35 See, for example, Paškorskij, "O lečenij za sčet dorogi členov semejstv služaščich," *VŽMiS* 5 (1913): 61–63. The 1912 annual report counted five million medical visits (not including repeat visits). M.P.S. UŽD. VSČ, *Otčet o vračebno-sanitarnom sostojanii ėksploatiruemych železnych dorog za 1912-yj god* (Petrograd 1915), 29.

36 "Pravila vračebno-sanitarnoj časti," 25–32.

37 This organization was envisaged by the 1894 decree. See RGIA, f. 273, op. 8, d. 6, l. 106–7, "Spravka."

38 RGIA, f. 273, op. 8. d. 340, "Ob administrativnom delenii ž.d. po vračebnoj službe."

39 The precinct physicians were subordinated to the local medical services, themselves led by a medical official. He alone had access to the local railway administration, which for its part answered to the Department of Railways of the Ministry of Transportation. "Pravila vračebno-sanitarnoj časti," 11–22; Reichman, *Railwaymen*, 26–34 and 118f.

pertise.[40] The hierarchical relationships, in which the personal or structural dependencies of (individual) patronage were similarly important, also furthered competition and selfishness among physicians, railway officials, and the various services, and could hinder the process. These ambivalences, which resulted in the emergence of railway medicine, left their mark on administrative practices, the interest in statistics, and how the "railway population" was defined.

A Reference Book: The Annual Medical Report

In the administrative reality, these contradictions manifested themselves in the problem of heterogeneity, which appeared in relation to the importance of statistical information to a centralized leadership of railway medicine. The first report on railway medicine for the year 1898, published by the Department of Railways in 1901, stated that: "In the current report there is no route to presenting a general overview of the health conditions of the state railway lines, because the program [1898] for the accumulation of identical data among all of the local agencies, as worked out at the first Congress of Physicians and Delegates of the state railways, has been carried out by hardly anyone, which is why [...] it is almost impossible to integrate the various and insufficient information into any kind of system."[41]

This diversity was not only manifest in the quality and quantity of statistical material, but it also became an actual problem for the first time when the state's Department of Railways mobilized information techniques to create a modern social institution such as railway medicine.[42] The data, collected locally and patchily and entered into the reporting form, could not be subsumed into a coherent system. The statistical material was not a usable "instrument of cognition" in the invention of a rational railway medicine.

40 In 1909, the minister of transportation ordered the local railway lines to convene regular congresses. Individual services had already institutionalized these from 1900 onward. RGIA, f. 273, op. 8, d. 315. The railway's bureaucratic character, the hierarchical structures, and the railway physician as a "disinterested civil servant" was also discussed by the railway surgeons (*fel'dšer*) at the annual surgeons and midwives congresses. See D. Vetlugin, "Voprosy železnodorožnoj mediciny na 3-m fel'dšerskom s"ezde," *Fel'dšerskij vestnik* 45 (1912): 1392–1400.

41 RGIA, f. 273, op. 8, d. 6, l. 338–39, *Otčet o vračebno-sanitarnom sostojanii za 12-yj god.*

42 Don K. Rowney, "Imperial Russian Officialdom during Modernization," in *Russian Bureaucracy and the State*, 26–45. Rowney advances the thesis that the state administration had only become complex, unintelligible, and ungovernable through the modernization processes.

As a railway physician noted in 1907, the annual medical reports could not fulfill their purpose as "reference books of social reality" to guide and represent railway medicine; the information presented in the reports was becoming increasingly detailed, and even though it was well structured, there was so much data that it became impossible to draw any conclusions about the health condition of railway workers.[43] The heterogeneous numbers, which were filled in tabular forms, could not be interpreted. Hence, the Department of Railways found itself in a paradoxical situation, where it had an abundance of information about railway medicine that destabilized its understanding of public health conditions.

Neither railway physicians nor medical officials doubted that the creation and control of their healthcare system required comprehensible information. However, the problem of dissimilar datasets was interpreted in different ways. Railway physicians, overall, felt that the root of the problem was with the quality of the numeric data, which they considered to be the result of a lack of professionalism in the way the statistics were gathered and presented. They agreed that the statistical process had to follow a streamlined methodology and work pattern, and they demanded a congruent approach to recording data as well as professionally organized health statisticians (sanitary physicians).[44]

In doing so, the railway physicians took guidance from the public health statistics (*sanitarnaja statistika*) as practiced in the *zemstva*. There the emphasis was placed on an "as detailed as possible assessment of the object being studied, the population, [...] the knowledge of its most important so-

43 Michajlov, "O pravil'noj postanovke," 298. See Porter, "Statistical and Social Facts," 20, who considers the product of comparative suicide statistics by the Italian statistician Enrico Morselli to be a kind of catalogue. See the speech by the director of the medical section of the Department of Railways at the Fourth General Congress of Railway Medicine in 1911, in which he says that the annual report is necessary as a reference book (*spravočnik*) and hence must be an accurate reflection of reality. RGIA, f. 273, op. 8, d. 354, l. 166–73, "Forma otčetnosti po vračebno-sanitarnoj službe, 1910–1916": "4 Sovešč. s''ezd vračej. Vopros 31. O neobchodimosti novoj programmy dlja sostavlenija godovych vračebno-sanitarnych otčetov na ž.d. Doklad D. M. Uspenskago i G. I. Sodmana."

44 The sanitary physician was the new expert on public health matters. He typically had no special medical education, but had received practical training in laboratory research and statistics. Generally, his task was to observe and report on health conditions by presenting statistical and biochemical research. Michajlov, "O pravil'noj postanovke"; V. T. Kalita, "O mestnych soveščatel'nych s''ezdach železnodorožnych vračej na russkich železnych dorogach," *VŽMiS* 6 (1913): 215–30; "Kratkij obzor trudov mestnych soveščatel'nych s''ezdach železnodorožnych vračej, sostavil V. T. Kalita," *VŽMiS* 7 (1913): 238–78 and 8 (1913): 279–331 (*prodolženie*). In this series Kalita describes the most important themes of the local railway medicine congresses between 1900 and 1911, at which the topic of "professional" health statistics was also debated.

cial, natural, and biological categories, [and] its territorial distribution and mobility," as the *conditio sine qua non* of any statistics.[45] The sanitary statistics were grounded in a comparative methodology, and "the comparative process wants scales."[46] Changes in the health of this object of research over time were measured with a specific "observation device"—the "dense registration."[47] Every *zemstvo* physician registered his patients on special cards (*registracionnaja kartočka*) for each individual, including notes on social categories as well as a nomenclature of uniformly defined diseases.[48] This "parallelism of information" should allow the sanitary physicians working in the public health offices to deduce statistical laws and patterns from the raw material. Continuous registration, stringent formalization, and the division of labor between collecting and evaluating were to allow for a continuous updating of statistical facts as well as the constant control of the population's health, which was itself considered "a collective organism."

In contrast, the medical officers of the Department of Railways viewed the incompleteness of the data—that is, its quantity—as a hindrance to the production of homogeneity. According to their logic, the patchwork was the result of individual misconduct. This view also determined their course of action: detailed directives and individual reprimands appeared as adequate means in the creation of consistency and comparability.[49] This logic materialized in the new reporting scheme for the extensive annual medical report sent by the Department of Railways to state and private railway companies in the spring of 1910.[50]

45 Kurkin, *Zemskaja sanitarnaja statistika*, 14.

46 S. M. Bogoslovskij and P. I. Kurkin, "O metodach statističeskago izseldovanija professional'noj boleznennosti," *Obščestvennyj vrač* 6 (1911): 32. The railway physicians also made the case for the necessity of the census by invoking the correct proportionality. See N. N. Mjaznikov, "K voprosu ob organizacii odnodnevnoj perepisi naselenija na železnych dorogach," *VŽMiS* 7–8 (1912): 9.

47 The following quotes and observation are based on Kurkin, *Zemskaja sanitarnaja statistika*; and Bogoslovskij and Kurkin, "O metodach." On the registration as a statistical venture, see N. I. Miklaševskij, "Perepisi," in Ėnciklopedičeskij slovar' Brokgauz-Efron (St. Petersburg, 1898), 240.

48 A *zemstvo* physician spoke of the existence of a "sea of registration cards" in 1912. D. I. Vostrov, "Novyja tečenija v razvitii obščestvennoj mediciny v Rossii: okončanie," *Fel'dšerskij vestnik* 32 (1912): 983f.

49 See the diagnosis of deficiencies contained in the circular of the Department of Railways that accompanied the new reporting scheme. It speaks of the absence of important information and arbitrary deviations from the prescribed forms. RGIA, f. 273, op.8, d. 354, l. 54, "Forma otčetnosti po vračebno-sanitarnoj službe, 1910–1916": "O dostavlenii dorogami vračebno-sanitarnych godovych otčetov po novoj forme."

50 From 1903 onward, all local medical services of the state and private railways alike were obliged to submit the short annual report on March 1st, and the comprehensive annual report on May 1st. The short report included general information regarding the length of the railway track along with data on medical infrastructures, personnel, and expenses. The comprehensive report requested, among others, statistics on illnesses in relation to individual social and professional groups. See Michajlov, "O pravil'noj postanovke," 298f.

It consisted of a thirty-five-page-long form demanding the calculation of 70,000 entries across forty-seven tables.[51]

Subsequently, different interpretations of heterogeneity—and the conclusions drawn from them—collided during the negotiations between the Department of Railways, the railway physicians, and local management. They could not agree on how to implement the new reporting scheme. For their part, the chief physicians of the private companies appeared to have organized themselves. In identical letters, they declared that the new reporting scheme was impossible to implement.[52] They argued that it entailed an impossible workload for the chronically overburdened railway physicians. The necessary funds for further personnel, experts in statistics, and the swaths of new forms could not be raised, as the annual budget had been passed. What is more, the new annual report required statistical data from other railway services to which they themselves had no access, or dealt with matters wholly unrelated to healthcare.[53]

The state companies that apparently adhered to the central directive also failed, due to a lack of financial means, personnel, and cooperation from the other services.[54] As a sanitary physician put it at a local conference, the new scheme lacked comprehensive investment in the foundation of any public health statistics: a precise understanding of the railway's total population size via a census, a normatized and thorough recording of diseases and accidents, and the *zemstva*'s practice of dividing the labor between data collection and evaluation. The new scheme risked being useless at best, or promulgating incorrect results at worst.[55]

51 See RGIA, f. 273, op. 8, d. 354, l. 56–74, "Otčet o vračebno-sanitarnom sostojanii" (the new reporting scheme); "Pravlenie o-va Moskovsko-Kazanskoj ž.d. No. 7084/1. Dek. 22 dnja 1910. Moskva. V Upravlenie ž.d." (ibid., l. 169, complaint of a chief physician).

52 See the numerous replies in RGIA, f. 273, op. 8, d. 354, l. 125, l. 181, l. 156–58, l. 169, l. 164–65, l. 190. A private railway company, furthermore, pointed out that the circular had not been properly published through the official mouthpiece of the Ministry of Transportation, and were hence not binding for private companies (ibid., l. 156–58).

53 Ibid. In contrast to the state railways, many of the private companies did not yet have sanitary physicians at their disposal. The chief physicians of the medical services were bookkeepers and not statisticians. The information from other railway services included, for example, details about the living conditions in the workers' barracks. Information that, according to the chief physicians, lay beyond the realm of healthcare was related to religious/moral, cultural, and educational provisions for employees.

54 Ibid., l. 190, "M.P.S. Upravlenie Sibirskoj ž.d. Vračebnaja služba. 17. Oktjabrja 1911 g. No. 89962. Vo vračebno-sanitarnuju čast' upravl. ž.d." and l. 204–5, "MPS. Upravl. Zabajkal'skogo ž.d. Oktjabrja 5./9. Dnja 1912 g. No. 9710/3102. Irkutsk. V upravl. ž.d."

55 "Kratkij obzor trudov," 8 (1913): 288.

The conflict surrounding the new reporting scheme escalated during the Fourth General Congress of Railway Medicine in January 1911. The medical section of the Department of Railways swept objections aside with the argument that its demands had been decided upon in numerous previous congress resolutions and memoranda and which the new scheme had merely brought together. The main difference, namely the postulated knowing of a medical precinct's precise population size instead of average values, were not only in the interest of every railway physician, but also manageable without new recording techniques and in cooperation with other railway services.[56] This twin appeal to both the personal interest and professional eagerness of railway physicians did not work: the fourth General Congress spoke out against the introduction of the new reporting scheme. It decided to institutionalize the "necessary foundation" for it: every local railway management should now establish a health statistics bureau under the direction of a sanitary physician and replace the old recording procedures with the registration system. Furthermore, it was decided to conduct periodic population counts, and the organizing committee of the fifth General Congress of Railway Medicine in 1915 was tasked with its methodological and practical elaboration.[57]

The problem of heterogeneity was aggravated in unintended ways by the department's attempt to eradicate it through the postulate of quantitative completeness. Its actions not only evoked a collision of differing interpretations of the causes for the uneven data sets; the controversy surrounding the reporting scheme also revealed the tensions between a central state administration seeking to expand its sphere of influence and local (private) railway companies. It blatantly demonstrated the lack of cooperation between the individual railway services and their various administrative procedures. Homogenous, modern information technologies were not only unable to eliminate this heterogeneity of administrative structures; they were actually what first turned it into a problem.

The failure of the Department of Railways did not lead to a policy change, however. It persisted with the new scheme, although the institutionalization

56 RGIA, f. 273, op. 8, d. 354, l. 166–73, "O neobchodimosti novoj programmy." Lecture by the director of the medical section of the Department of Railways, D. M. Uspenskij, together with the sanitary physician G. I. Sodman (Perm).

57 Ibid., l. 171–2; S. E. Šrejber, "IV-yj vserossijskij soveščatel'nyj s"ezd železnodorožnych vračej," *Gigiena i sanitarija* 5 (1911): 261–3, and 6 (1911): 317–29.

of new recording practices cost local companies time and money. The eventual result was annual reports based on local reports, which either used the new or the old scheme.[58] The paradoxical reality, that a larger but more diffuse data set resulted in the reduction of knowledge, did not go away. The demands for a census of railway people—besides the organizing committee of the fifth General Congress—introduced further protagonists into the process. For instance, the minister of transportation tasked the statistical-cartographic department of his ministry with the organization of the census,[59] while at the same time the local medical services gathered similar data for their own purposes.

The "Railway Population": Questions of Belonging

The different census initiatives, designed or carried out by various actors following the fourth General Congress, widely perpetuated contradiction and heterogeneity. With the formation of the railway population, conflicts arose between the principle of territoriality, which became important to the development of a social infrastructure, and the differing employment and family law on the various local lines. In contrast to the *zemstva*, where all administrative realms related to the same object, i.e., the permanent residents of delimited administrative territories, its definition became more complicated in relation to the railways. Railway employees and their families were mobile and they could live on or away from the railway territory (*pole otčuždenija*).[60] What is more, belonging to the railway population was

58 RGIA, f. 273, op. 8, d. 354, the correspondence of l. 192, l. 193, l. 200, l. 204–5, local railway lines offer insights into the partial implementation of the new reporting form, that is, the new recording methodology. The annual report for 1912, though, was still in the old scheme. See M.P.S. UŽD. VSČ, *Otčet o vračebno-sanitarnom sostojanii za 1912-yj god.*

59 See M.P.S. UŽD. VSČ, *Otčet o vračebno-sanitarnom sostojanii za 1912-yj god*, 4, talks about a special commission chaired by the director of the Office of the Ministry of Transportation, which had created a census form accepted by the minister in July 1913. The statistical-cartographic department of the Ministry of Transportation was charged with the organization. See RGIA, f. 273, op. 8, d. 414, l. 272–7, "5-yj soveščatel'nyj s''ezd železnodorožnych vračej, 1912–1916": "5. S''ezd vračej. Vopros 17: O perepisjach naselenija na železnych dorogach," Doklad N. N. Mjaznikova.

60 The *pole otčuždenija*, literally "dispossessed land," was made available to the railways by the state or had, at times coercively, been purchased from private owners. "Kratkij obzor trudov" 7 (1913): 248 (lecture at the congress of the Rjazan-Ural'skaja line, 1902); N. N. Mjaznikov, "K voprosu ob organizacii," 14f.; on the lack of local rootedness in relation to questions of self-motivated action of the railway people, see G. I. Sodman, "Ob organizacii na železnych dorogach sanitarnych komissij i sanitarnych popečitel'stv soglasno par. 71–81 novych pravil vračebno-sanitarnoj časti," *VŽMiS* 3 (1914): 17–24.

not defined by a domicile, but by the legal and economic relationship between companies, employees, and family members.

These defining characteristics were extremely complex and varied. The difficulty began with the employees and their diverse labor rights and working conditions in the various local companies. They formed the base unit of the railway population.[61] Depending on the status of a particular employee, if they were financially dependent on him his relatives would also belong to the railway population. Equally important were legal and kinship relationships with the employee, but the local companies defined these differently. As the censuses demonstrated, railway medicine similarly displayed various legal interpretations and practices as to who belonged to the railway population. Furthermore, the family members were not recorded anywhere prior to the introduction of personal registration cards, which themselves were to serve both as a medical record and a legal form of identification. The sole source of information and verification for the family members of an employee was the employee himself.[62] Hence, the railway management only had a vague idea of the quantity of the relatives.[63]

This specific tension between different rights on the one hand and the increasing importance of territoriality on the other, expressed itself during seven local censuses carried out between 1910 and 1914, whose results became the subject of public controversies concerning railway physicians.[64]

61 Every railway service had, aside from the permanent employees, a set of various short-term and contract workers at their disposal whose legal status, although often given the same designation, varied from one service to the other. See para. 1, "The Invention of Railway Medicine."

62 See the lawsuit by a railway physician about malpractice due to lacking control at a local railway congress: "O lečenij za sčet dorogi členov zemejstv služaščich," *VŽMiS* 5 (1913): 61–63. See the order by a director of a state line in 1912 on the introduction of personal registration cards for employees and relatives, the "only documents for official/administrative queries." RGIA, f. 273, op. 8, d. 354, l. 208, "Prikaz načal'nika zabajkal'skoj z.d. 9. Janvarja 1912 goda. No. 14." See also V. V. Krasnov, "O različnych trebovanijach k sostalvelniju registracionnych i sanitarnych kartoček," *VŽMiS* 5 (1915): 49f. In contrast to the registrations in the *zemstva*, those of the railways pursued administrative/legal aims alongside health policy ones.

63 The medical services calculated the number of family members with a rigid coefficient for every employee. This coefficient was based on the family bulletin. These bulletins were only given to railway workers in the lower pay grades, because the family members economically dependent on them were entitled to free medical care. See Michajlov, "O pravil'noj postanovke," 302; Mjaznikov, "K voprosu ob organizacii," 9f. and 20; N. N. Mjaznikov, "Ešče ob odnodnevnoj perepisi naselenija na železnych dorogach: (otvet d-ru Zemblinovu)," *VŽMiS* 11 (1912): 64–73, especially 68 and 70.

64 Mjaznikov, "K voprosu ob organizacii"; V. I. Zemblinov, "Po povodu opyta odnodnevnoj perepisi naselenija Syzrano-Vjazemskoj dorogi," *VŽMiS* 9 (1912): 86–89; Mjaznikov, "Ešče ob odnodnevnoj perepisi"; S. A. Lebedinskij, "Dva slova v otvet d-ru Zemblinovu," *VŽMiS* (1912): 11, 74f.; V. I. Zemblinov, "K sporu odnodnevnych perepisjach železnodorožnogo naselenija i programmach ich," *VŽMiS* 2 (1913):

The core contention related to the function of the census. Some local companies and their medical services intended to use the census to determine a solely medical-administrative object; others claimed to define the entire railway population and therefore had exchangeable data for the whole of the railway administration.[65] The controversy also included questions of organization, counting method, inclusion and exclusion criteria, as well as the necessary information about the social differentiation of the railway population.

The proponents of a comprehensive census were interested in strengthening medical services within the Department of Railways and the Ministry of Transportation more broadly. They argued that physicians had always had a "natural" interest in demographic data, and that the management of the census ought to lie with the medical services and the sanitary physicians.[66] They asserted this claim with the methodology of the "one-day census," which relied on both the European censuses and the first population count conducted in the Russian Empire in 1897. It aimed to take a "snapshot" of the "reality" of any given moment and required a simultaneous and uniform execution of the census across the territory.[67] The fundamental condition of contemporaneousness was supposed to avoid the risk of duplications and omissions that resulted from the high level of mobility among railway workers.[68] To guarantee a simultaneous and uniform census required the division of the railway territory into registration districts that were organized coherently and whose work was directed centrally. One railway line tasked all railway services with counting their respective employees and kin. The result was spatially incongruent data that did not permit conclusions to be drawn on territorial distribution. Hence, railway physicians thought of it as an example of how not to conduct a census.[69]

43–49; N. N. Mjaznikov, "Novye dannye po voprosu odnodnevnoj perepisjach naselenija na železnych dorogach," *VŽMiS* 12 (1913): 37–43; N. M. Anastasiev, "O perepisi naselenija na Zabajkal'skoj dorogi," *VŽMiS* 10 (1915): 317–35.

65 See, for example, Mjaznikov, "Ešče ob odnodnevnoj perepisi," for the comprehensive, and Anastasiev, "O perepisi naselenija," for the medical function of the census.

66 RGIA, 273, op. 8, d. 414, l. 272–7, "5. S''ezd vračej. Vopros 17: O perepisjach naselenija."

67 See Miklaševskij, "Perepisi," 240–5. He distinguished between the census that takes a snapshot of reality and the continuous registration that would record changes in this reality over time.

68 Of the seven local population censuses, five used this method. Mjaznikov, "Novye dannye," 37–43.

69 RGIA, f. 273, op. 8, d. 414, l. 272, "5. S''ezd vračej. Vopros 17: O perepisjach naselenija." See also the self-criticism of a sanitary physician regarding the lack of precision in his data, as he had not conducted a one-day census: S. E. Šrejber, "O perepisi železnodorožnogo naselenija," *VŽMiS* 6 (1913): 67–88.

The core instrument of the "one-day census" was a counting card for every single employee—with the exception of day laborers and casual workers—on which his family members were also recorded.[70] Which relatives were recorded on the counting cards and thus belonged to the railway employee's family was dealt with differently by the local railway lines. Here, too, there were differing views on the function of the census and the fundamental definitional criteria that determined who did or did not belong to the "railway population." Railway physicians who had an interest in public health issues alone preferred to count only those individuals who could actually use the medical infrastructure. The person's home address or, more specifically, his presence on railway land—which is to say, the territorial principle—was more decisive than the theoretical entitlement to medical services. It is little surprising that physicians in a Siberian railway line would prefer this conception of the census, as the majority of its employees were recruited in European Russia, their wives and children were frequently thousands of kilometers away, and thus they were of no interest to the local railway management.[71]

A further point of contention between the proponents of a "railway population" for all administrative realms and the advocates of a medical object emerged in relation as to how to prioritize entitlements. The former group also took account of other employment rights—that is, in addition to the right to medical services—as well as the legal status of family members.[72] Parents and in-laws, widowed daughters and their children, unwed children, life partners, and nonadopted foster children, for example, were all excluded from this conceptualization of the railway community, even if they were financially dependent on the employee or lived with him, or even if the local practices and rights traditionally extended the entitlement to medical services to these types of family members.[73] In their opinion, a railway

70 The question of how long a temporary employee had to serve before starting to enjoy various employment rights was resolved by the local companies independently and in different ways. Most of the local counts considered all employees that had worked for the company for longer than six months. See Mjaznikov, "Ešče ob odnodnevnoj perepisi"; one of the counts set the bar at three months, see Anastasiev, "O perepisi naselenija."

71 Anastasiev, "O perepisi naselenija"; see also Zemblinov, "Po povodu opyta"; Zemblinov, "K sporu odnodnevnych perepisjach."

72 Further employment rights included, for example, room and board subsidies, the right to obtain identity documentation, free train travel, access to railway primary schools, and participation in pension funds. See Mjaznikov, "Ešče ob odnodnevnoj perepisi," 67f.

73 On local practices and rights, see, for example, Zemblinov, "Po povodu opyta," 86–89; Zemblinov,

family was comprised of a wife, sons and brothers that were minors, unwed daughters and sisters, and legally adopted children, as well as the maid, regardless of whether or not they lived with the employee or on railway land.[74] The controversy about taking local entitlements to medical services into account only abated when the revised medical decree of July 1913 made them mandatory for all railway lines.[75]

The categories on the counting cards were partially borrowed from those of the first census in the Russian Empire. They asked for the individual's age, gender, legal and educational status, religion, nationality, and profession. They also included categories that were of specific interest to railway medicine and railway administration: income and length of service, the population's distribution along stations, tracks and medical precincts, public or private accommodation, as well as individual services. As for family members, their relationship to the employee, the number of school children, and people in care (blind, deaf-mute, mentally ill, physically disabled) also had to be declared (see the figure of a counting card below).[76]

The local medical services were not the only ones planning or conducting censuses. They were in direct competition with the statistical-cartographic department of the ministry. Hence, railway medicine tried to prove that the department's method was insufficient for the healthcare system's needs; that is, that only railway medicine was in the position to produce a commensurable object for all administrative realms. Railway physicians criticized this method's underlying principle of selection that rested upon the criteria of bookkeeping (wage categories). Accordingly, the census program of the statistical-cartographic department worked with a definition of the railway family that predominantly considered the economic relationship between employees and family members, but not the legal relationships between relatives and employees, i.e., precisely those that also determined

"K sporu odnodnevnych perepisjach," 43–49; on their inclusion in two local censuses: Anastasiev, "O perepisi naselenija"; and Šrejber, "O perepisi železnodorožnogo naselenija," 67–88.

74 There were exceptions for maids: they were recorded according to their function without names and only counted if they lived with the employee. See Mjaznikov, "K voprosu ob organizacii," 9–22; Mjaznikov, "Novye dannye," 37–43.

75 See "Pravila vračebno-sanitarnoj časti," 22–25.

76 N. Ja. Chranilov, "Opyt razrabotki kartoček odnodnevnoj perepisi naselenija Syzrano-Vjazemskoj železnoj dorogi za 1911 god," *VŽMiS* 6 (1913): 7–13; Mjaznikov, "Novye dannye," 37–43; see the counting cards of the statistics section of the organizing committee of the Fifth General Congress of Railway Medicine, which were used during some local censuses. RGIA, f. 273, op. 8, d. 414, l. 280, "5. S''ezd vračej. Vopros 17: O perepisjach naselenija" (priloženie 3).

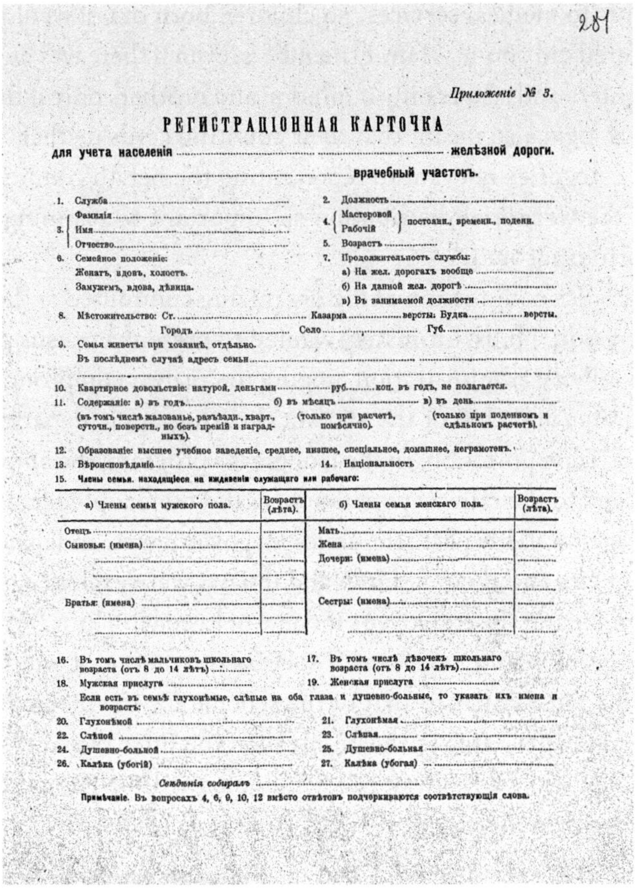

281

Приложеніе № 3.

РЕГИСТРАЦІОННАЯ КАРТОЧКА

для учета населенія ... желѣзной дороги.

... врачебный участокъ.

1. Служба ...
2. Должность ...
3. Фамилія ... Имя ... Отчество ...
4. Мастеровой / Рабочій — постоянн., времени., поденн.
5. Возрастъ ...
6. Семейное положеніе: Женатъ, вдовъ, холостъ. Замужемъ, вдова, дѣвица.
7. Продолжительность службы: а) На жел. дорогахъ вообще ... б) На данной жел. дорогѣ ... в) Въ занимаемой должности ...
8. Мѣстожительство: Ст. ... Казарма ... версты. Будка ... версты. Городъ ... Село ... Губ. ...
9. Семья живетъ: при хозяинѣ, отдѣльно. Въ послѣднемъ случаѣ адресъ семьи ...
10. Квартирное довольствіе: натурой, деньгами ... руб. ... коп. въ годъ, не полагается.
11. Содержаніе: а) въ годъ ... (въ томъ числѣ жалованье, разъѣздн., кварт., суточн., поверстн., но безъ премій и наградныхъ). б) въ мѣсяцъ ... (только при расчетѣ, помѣсячно). в) въ день ... (только при поденномъ и сдѣльномъ расчетѣ).
12. Образованіе: высшее учебное заведеніе, среднее, низшее, спеціальное, домашнее, неграмотенъ.
13. Вѣроисповѣданіе ...
14. Національность ...
15. Члены семьи, находящіеся на иждивеніи служащаго или рабочаго:

а) Члены семьи мужского пола.	Возрастъ (лѣта).	б) Члены семьи женскаго пола.	Возрастъ (лѣта).
Отецъ ...	...	Мать ...	...
Сыновья: (имена) ...	...	Жена ...	...
...	...	Дочери: (имена) ...	...
...	...	...	...
...	...	...	...
Братья: (имена) ...	...	Сестры: (имена) ...	...
...	...	...	...
...	...	...	...

16. Въ томъ числѣ мальчиковъ школьнаго возраста (отъ 8 до 14 лѣтъ) ...
17. Въ томъ числѣ дѣвочекъ школьнаго возраста (отъ 8 до 14 лѣтъ) ...
18. Мужская прислуга ...
19. Женская прислуга ...

Если есть въ семьѣ глухонѣмые, слѣпые на оба глаза и душевно-больные, то указать ихъ имена и возрастъ:

20. Глухонѣмой ...
21. Глухонѣмая ...
22. Слѣпой ...
23. Слѣпая ...
24. Душевно-больной ...
25. Душевно-больная ...
26. Калѣка (убогій) ...
27. Калѣка (убогая) ...

Свѣдѣнія собиралъ ...

Примѣчаніе. Въ вопросахъ 4, 6, 9, 10, 12 вмѣсто отвѣтовъ подчеркиваются соотвѣтствующія слова.

Figure 2.1: *A Counting Card for the Census of the Railway Population.* In: Mjaznikov, "About Census of the Railway Population" (paper for the Fifth Congress of Railway Medicine in September 1914, Tiflis), RGIA, f. 273, op. 8, d. 414, l. 284.

Explanation of Figure: 1) service, 2) work position, 3) name, 4) craftsman/worker: regular/temporary/under contract; 5) age; 6) civil status: married/widowed/unwed; 7) period of service: a) at the railways altogether, b) at this railway company, c) at this position; 8) residence: station/barracks/booth at which section of tracks; town/village/province; 9) family lives: at the head of the family/separate; in the last case: address of the family; 10) housing benefits: material/monetary/none; 11) wages: a) yearly (all incl. without awards), b) monthly, c) daily; 12) education: higher/medium/elementary/professional/home-school/illiterate; 13) confession; 14) nationality; 15) family members, who live from the salary of the serviceman or worker (with name and age): a) male: father, sons, brothers, b) female: mother, wife, daughters, sisters; 16) How many boys in school age (8–14); 17) How many girls in school age (8–14); 18) male servant; 19) female servant; 20) If there are deaf, blind, mentally ill, cripple, then write the name and age of this members.

entitlements to medical services. So children born out of wedlock or those being fostered did count as family members, even if there was no legal adoption; daughters and sisters only if minors; and brothers only if they were orphans. This logic also meant that their counting cards neither asked about the social categories relevant to representing the health condition, nor did they take the territorial distribution so important to planning healthcare provisions into account.[77]

The statistics commission of the organizing committee of the fifth General Congress in Tbilisi ultimately wanted to present a census program for the entire railway administration, hoping to create a compromise between local programs and that of the statistical-cartographic department of the Ministry of Transportation. In the Congress's program, the employee's parents belonged to the railway population, as did nonadopted foster children, apprentices, unwed life partners, children, governesses, and maids; but widowed daughters and their children and in-laws were excluded, even if they were dependant on the employee's income or lived with him.[78] Whether this census program would have been a success or whether it would have succumbed to a fate similar to that of the scheme for the medical annual reports, remains open. Due to the outbreak of the First World War, the Fifth General Congress of Railway Medicine, planned for September 1914 in Tbilisi, never convened.

Conclusion

The history of the formation of the "railway population" through the emergence of railway medicine illuminates what happened when the state's Ministry of Transportation mobilized statistics as a tool of governance and as a means of representation toward the institutionalization of a healthcare system. It served to promote a skewed strategy: the extension of state power into the railway sector and the adoption of health policies aimed to achieve social pacification following the strike by railway employees in 1905. The logic determining these actions was the homogenization of the healthcare system through the adaptation of *zemstvo* medicine—an already existing

77 RGIA, f. 273, op. 8, d. 414, l. 272–77, "5. S"ezd vračej. Vopros 17: O perepisjach naselenija."

78 Ibid., l. 280 and 281 (priloženie 2 i 3).

medical system in Imperial Russia whose object of care, the local *zemstvo* population, and their infrastructures were defined and managed through surveys and health statistics. Applied to the railways, this approach to rationalization led to ambivalences and paradoxes that could no longer be concealed: the statistical venture not only failed to represent a uniform order; it made differences visible, and therefore revealed a problem.

Locally collected numeric data used different theoretical assumptions and procedures, so that while figures were plugged into the homogenous format of an "annual report," they could not be interpreted. A paradox emerged whereby year after year, the central Department of Railways commanded ever more information, but its understanding of health conditions among railway workers became destabilized. The irony of the use of statistics as a technology of governance was that it did not allow for any insights into the object of health policies and a precise definition of the "railway population," but it certainly gave insight into the subject: the local railway managements that operated and functioned according to a different logic.

But this failure did not yield fundamental doubts about statistics as the only organizational and knowledge-producing tool for the rational planning and administration of railway medicine. Railway physicians and officials deemed the problem of nonhomogenous, and hence unintelligible data as entirely contingent upon the quantity and professionalism of its accumulation. Measures to rectify this, therefore, led not only to the statistical venture developing an independence all of its own; it perpetuated contradictions and fostered heterogeneity, in that creating an overlap between these different administrative procedures had far-reaching consequences.

The gap revealed by public health statistics—that there was a broad lack of knowledge about the "railway population"—could not be completely closed by the use of the census, a task that involved a multitude of actors each with their own agendas, local traditions, and experiences. Various administrative patterns of logic, legal interpretations, and practices collided both against each other as well as the principle of "territoriality." Territory became a new, important factor in the planning and management of healthcare provisions, as well as mapping out healthcare conditions of local objects in spatial terms. But territoriality did not work as the primary criterion of classification in the creation of a "homogenous railway population," because it could neither integrate nor neutralize local legal traditions and administrative procedures. To prioritize diverse rights over territory when considering issues of belonging appears to be specific to imperial states.[79]

Hence, the censuses and the individual registration of employees did not fashion a single "railway population," but produced several divergent social aggregates. Nevertheless, Russian railway medicine conducted an effective population policy. Toward the calculation, control, and assessment of medical provisions and their condition, the statistical practice recorded the railway employees and their family members in an increasingly closely meshed administrative net. In this way, railway medicine was part of the state-building process along the railway arteries up to the borders of the empire.

79 On this issue, see, for example, Benton and Ross (eds.), *Legal Pluralism and Empires.*

CHAPTER III

Mastering Troubling Borders: The Ambivalence of Medical Modernization in the Prussian Province of Posen[1]

Justyna A. Turkowska

In the spring of 1913, Posen, the capital of the Prussian province of the same name, witnessed the dedication of the new building for the Institute of Hygiene, founded in 1899. The institute's new home was one of the last new buildings designed for the Prussian cultural and governing authorities in the province. The new building, after fourteen long years of struggle, was the first facility to meet the hygienic, bacteriological, logistic, and infrastructural needs of an institute that had from its very inception been considered a focal point for medical expertise and diagnosis, and was also a driving force for the promotion of Germanness[2] in a region where only a minority considered themselves to be ethnic Germans. Around the same time, the city of Posen received a ministerial request from Berlin asking whether a further medical institution—the Academy of Applied Medicine, another center of medical training and the popularization of medical knowledge—would be welcome in the province, to what extent it would be able to support such an institution, and whether it was suitable for implementation.[3] In light of these efforts, and considering the fact that the political situation in the Prussian borderland was becoming increasingly vague as German hege-

1 This chapter was translated by Tudor Georgescu.

2 Letter from Richard Witting (Mayor of Posen) to Konrad von Studt (Ministry of Culture), June 30, 1900, in Geheimes Staatsarchiv Preußischer Kulturbesitz (GStA PK), I HA, Rep 76 VIII B, no. 3004, vol. 262.

3 See Archiwum Państwowe Poznania (APP), Akta Miasta Poznania (AMP), no. 2568. Documents concerning the creation of an Academy of Applied Medicine, 1912–1919.

monic aspirations faced an ever-growing resistance from the Polish national movement, 1913 marked a new Prussian attempt to strengthen its political authority by expanding its medical power and intensifying the medical impulse and its cultural presence in the province.[4]

With the introduction of hygienic institutions in the 1890s and the successive expansion of public health activity, the province of Posen experienced a new stage of Prussian hegemonic aspirations, as well as a new stage in the creation of a modern state and national loyalties. Medical mastery of the regional population—by virtue of its hygienic surveillance, improving its well-being, and by producing a homogeneous hygienic consciousness—was seen in Berlin as one of the main tools to take charge of the troubled borderland.[5] Such perceptions of the province were shaped by the fact that the otherwise largely homogeneous German Empire was confronted with a highly heterogeneous cultural setting, one in which non-German peoples, despite Prussian hegemonic policies, insisted on their cultural, linguistic, and confessional sovereignty.[6] Hence, the region was perceived as a warped edge of the empire, one that was not German enough and too strongly Polish, to be recovered and transformed into a culturally self-evident German borderland.

The attempt by Berlin to "medically master" the province was successful at first. However, it did not go as smoothly as expected. While the Institute of Hygiene celebrated the opening of its new building and the institute's reinvigoration, the debates concerning the founding of an Academy of Applied Medicine dissipated, and the academy was never established. Its purpose, the pros and cons regarding its creation, and the institution itself remained a topic of heated debate in the province, even after Berlin had dropped the idea. The request became nothing less than an invitation to the region to debate the possible routes to future development and power sharing between Berlin, Posen, and the regional elites. This was the case even

4 See Thum, "Imperialists in Panic," 137–62.

5 See, among others, GStA PK, I. HA Rep. 76 Vc, Sekt. 13, Tit. 23, no. 2, vol. 27: Richard Witting, Minutes of a meeting concerning "cultural elevation" on January 11, 1902; Application by the Society of Physicians of the Government District for the creation of an Institute of Hygiene in Posen, in GStA PK, Rep. 76 VIII B, no. 3004: Regarding the influence and administration of the (public) Institute of Hygiene in Posen, 1895–1900, vol. 15. See also Hüntelmann, *Hygiene im Namen des Staates*.

6 See Serrier, *Provinz Posen, Ostmark, Wielkopolska*; Belzyt, *Sprachliche Minderheiten im preußischen Staat*; Hagen, *Germans, Poles and Jews*.

though most of the participants agreed that "in the entire eastern part of the Prussian state [provisions] for improving the training of medical trainees were lacking"[7]; that new scientific advances were beneficial and desirable; and that the Institute of Hygiene was in itself not sufficient for the popularization of knowledge and the provision of continuing education on health matters. A common agreement could not be reached. What were the core differences? Why did jointly formulated desires for the region's medically directed enhancement fail? What, exactly, prevented the realization of the political-national desires for medical mastery of the province?

By looking closely at the debates around these questions, I outline how the medical impulses worked to change the image of the troubled province and the extent to which they stabilized the political and cultural situation in the borderland; that is, how they sought to produce regional/state/national loyalty by means of the public health system. I explore medical modernization as an instrument of imperial, regional, and national mastery, as well as the different visions of modernity resulting from medical impulses that were discussed and tried out (with varying success) in the Prussian borderland. The academy that had been abandoned before the First World War was one of the last attempts to achieve medical modernization pursued by Berlin, and the effort faced opposition, caused inconsistent reactions, and frequently yielded unintended side effects.

One of the main obstacles were the regional political interests of local elites that often differed from, and interfered with, the imperial visions of mastery of the empire and its borderlands. The centrally generated templates remained predominant, but the hegemonic attempts at homogenization partially broke down in the face of local opposition, because instead of supporting the congruence of medical actualization (understood as validation and upgrading), local elites attempted to steer it themselves. Local interests outweighed imperially concocted visions of Germanness. The resulting recurrent divergences led to tensions, further amplified by incoherent Prussian regional policies. The variations in regional politics were partially owed to changing political trends, but mainly to political indecision on how to homogeneously rule a heterogeneous borderland in such a way that the Polish population living there did not profit from the so-called "policy of

7 Municipal resolution from August 8, 1913, in APP, AMP, no. 2568, vol. 22.

elevation" (*Hebungsmaßnahmen*)[8] without being tangibly excluded from them, either. This inconsistent "Poland policy"[9] fed into a tense relationship that remained latently present until the end of the First World War and generated the second main set of obstacles to any attempt at gaining mastery: it led to the crystallization of the national interests of the Polish population, which faced a subtle but constant marginalization unto the point of exclusion, alleviated through the independent organization of hygiene provisions and the strengthening of indigenous medical power. Such a development was certainly not something the Prussian authorities welcomed, as it hampered all imperial homogenizing processes and spawned some in places that had not been considered by the state and only been sparsely influenced by these processes. State-sponsored medical modernization gained a highly ambivalent and problematic dimension. Unwanted and unintended, it was the result of a not entirely inclusive attitude toward some groups, causing homogenization attempts at the political periphery marked by Polish hygienists. The state-sponsored medical modernization and healthcare policy neglected them, but also viewed them with concern—and these worries became a self-imposed limitation. Nonetheless, as we shall see, it was precisely these societal margins that were the most receptive to the concepts emanating from the center. Both the state's central institutions and the Polish hygienists standing along the political system's periphery pursued the same goal, and did so despite proposing completely different perspectives and inherently highlighting a conflict of interests, namely population policies to master the troubled borderlands and their population. For Berlin, this mastery was to be advanced in the name of imperial nationalism;[10] for the Pol-

8 The "policy of elevation" (*Hebungspolitik*) was a government program to turn the province, by means of hygienic, economic, architectural, and cultural investments, into a "center for the display of the benefits of German material culture" (Blanke, *Prussian Poland in the German Empire [1871–1900]*, 201) to make it more attractive to the German-speaking population, more effectively linked to Berlin, more Prussian and, in that sense, to render the region modern. See, among others, Schutte, "Deutsche und Polen in der Provinz Posen."

9 See, among others, Wehler, "Polenpolitik im Deutschen Kaiserreich."

10 At the end of the nineteenth century, in the age of imperialism, both nationalizing the empire and imperializing the nation were intertwined. Nation-states tried to expand their power and territory by establishing a homogeneous national culture to be imposed on all people in its dominion. The empires, for their part, with few exceptions, tried to promote homogenous reference points with such tokens as a single state language, a culturally shaped educational system, and national symbols. There were exceptions (such as the Habsburg Empire) that did not build up its identity entirely in terms of a homogeneous national culture, but even they tried to establish a common reference system with specific national characteristics. For more on this, see for example, Miller and Rieber (eds.), *Imperial Rule*.

ish doctors, in the name of the Polish nation, which in Berlin's vision was to be Germanized or otherwise not exist at all. In contrast, for the local Posen elites, this imperial ambition marked a threat to their positions and, if at all, was to be realized in the name of regional (semi-feudal) interests. The introduction of medical institutions and public health issues was anything but a neutral approach to providing for the population's well-being. It produced a structure with highly divergent loyalties and interests that could not always be harnessed to the imperial desire for mastery.

Health as an Instrument of Imperial and National Mastery

The empire's creation ushered in a new political era in Prussia as well as the province of Posen, characterized by the state's intensified nationalizing and homogenizing tendencies. Both the loyalty-inducing betterment of the nation and the reformation of the state had the goal of creating a well-structured and transparent state apparatus reaching and regimenting as many jurisdictions as possible. The expectation was that the state could control all spheres of public as well as private life, in order to service and direct them in the name of the state's prosperity (however that may be defined). The focal point of these ambitions had been the creation of a homogeneously codified territory in which the reach of the state's monopoly on violence was to be secured along with the people's loyalty, and this monopoly was to be codified nationally. The empire's eastern provinces in general, but particularly the culturally extremely "foreign"—not only Prussian, but also Polish influenced—province of Posen was to be absorbed and branded with Prussian characteristics. One legacy of the three partitions of the Polish–Lithuanian state in 1772, 1793, and 1795 was that Prussia not only increased its territory, but also its population, which now became far more heterogeneous along its eastern peripheries in ethnic, linguistic, and confessional terms. The newly integrated territories registered a higher presence of especially Polish-speaking Catholic people who, with the rise of the Polish national movement, increasingly perceived themselves as ethnically Polish. Since the empire's founding, Prussia had succeeded neither in wholly integrating these people into the Prussian codified state, nor was the desire for a nationally construed state consistent or pervasive.[11] The creation of the empire, going hand in hand with the rise of national expansionism and the amplification of hegemonic aspirations, changed this.

The anti-Polish measures introduced in the 1870s, and their growing remits, were gradually being exacerbated by aggressive settlement, language, and school policies.[12] The desired results remained elusive. These results could not be gratuitously imposed due to the legal equality of all Prussian citizens, irrespective of whether they saw themselves as ethnically Polish or German, in other words, independently of how they were perceived statistically. The political gaze began to shift; that is, it gained a second focus: While the Germanizing idea based on the domestication of the Polish-speaking population was to be driven forward through specific, oppressive measures, the province and its inhabitants, especially the German-speaking inhabitants, were now to be advanced politically, economically, and culturally, and their Germanness strengthened. The region itself was to be culturally and visibly Prussian—through the densification of German-speaking associations, German symbols, Prussian architecture, etc.—and made recognizably modern. The creation of the Institute of Hygiene marked a beginning.[13] Among the Institute's core remits were disseminating and popularizing knowledge; providing further and continuous training for physicians, disinfectors, and to some extent midwives; assisting district physicians and all other medical officers; developing bacteriological and chemical expertise; and "supporting and scientifically stimulating the physicians as well as other participating districts from the province."[14] In particular, the Institute's work to popularize scientific knowledge and provide professional training were supposed to promote medical capacity and homogenization in the region, as well as cement the population's medical and hygienic understanding and, by doing so, encourage the "policy of elevation" that was meant to be realized by means of medical doctrines, among others. It be-

11 See Kleemann (ed.), *Niemiecki Wschód*.

12 See, among others, Witold Molik, *Inteligencja polska w Poznańskiem w XIX i początkach XX wieku* (Poznań: Wydawnictwo Poznańskie, 2009); Knabe, *Sprachliche Minderheiten und nationale Schulpolitik in Preußen zwischen 1871 und 1933*.

13 On the Institute of Hygiene's history, see, among others, Erich Wernicke, "Das neue Hygienische Institut in Posen," *Veröffentlichungen aus dem Gebiet der Medizinalverwaltung* 3 (1914), 21–34; Turkowska, "Im Namen der 'großen Kolonisationsaufgaben.'"

14 APP, Landrat zu Czarnikau, no. 207: Business instruction to the Institute of Hygiene in Posen, first paragraph.

lieved that medical and hygienic education, along with the subsequent assumption of responsibility for the "national body"[15] it was to enable, would serve to foster increased societal involvement in the national identity.

The role of the Institute meshed perfectly with the state's spheres of activity, which had prescribed the aims of medical and hygienic institutions to underpin nationally codified statehood.[16] On the back of an efficient and effective health policy, not only the health of the individual but that of the entire nation was to be improved and secured.[17] Medical welfare and enforcement across the board, which in itself made the regions governable, not only represented medical, technical, and administrative modernization, but also became the epitome of cultural progress and national distinction.[18] With the help of medical measures, national loyalty and homogenous nationally codified state territory were to be molded into shape.

This approach was to be followed in the province of Posen, too. There, however, it caused several problems. Representatives of the Berlin government did not always seem to be in agreement about how to define and realize imperial ambitions without compromising national German loyalties. Because the Polish population was to be integrated in an imperial sense but could hardly be disciplined in a national sense, over time it experienced an intensified political codification as an "other." In the context of imperial and especially Prussian regional politics, in Berlin the Polish population was increasingly seen as a foreign body that was difficult to integrate, problematic, and less deserving of consideration. The medical institutions were to be used, for example, to Germanize Polish physicians while simultaneously preventing them from profiting too much from the

15 The concept of a "national body" (*Volkskörper*), circulated in the nineteenth and early twentieth centuries as a (scientific) term in the fields of (national/social) hygiene, medicine, and population theory, among others, and was simultaneously a political metaphor for a biological understanding of people/nation/community. See, among others, Walkenhorst, *Nation-Volk-Rasse*; and Sarasin, *Reizbare Maschinen*. For the period of World War I, see Michl, *Im Dienste des "Volkskörpers"*.

16 With the extension of the medical and hygienic network, initiated, among others, by the creation of the first Chair in Hygiene in 1865 and the founding of the Reich Health Office [Reichsgesundheitsamt] in 1876, the Reich entered into a new "hygienic era." The transition to a rational population policy began. On this, see among others, Hüntelmann, *Hygiene im Namen des Staates*.

17 "Die Petition an den Reichstag, betreffend die Verwaltungsorganisation der öffentlichen Gesundheitspflege im Norddeutschen Bund" including motives and a short introduction, in *Deutsche Vierteljahrsschrift für öffentliche Gesundheitspflege* 2 (1870), 134, quoted in ibid., 44.

18 See, among others, Göckenjan, *Kurieren und Staat machen*; Nikolow, "Die Nation als statistisches Kollektiv"; Sachsse and Tennstedt, *Soziale Sicherheit und soziale Disziplinierung*; Labisch, *Homo Hygienicus Gesundheit und Medizin in der Neuzeit.*

medical initiatives. Similarly, it was similarly to involve the Polish population in the health measures, but only insofar as was necessary for them to see the benefits of such changes, without allowing them too much control over the process or the arrangements.[19] In this sense, mastering troubled borders with medical and hygienic institutions and a tighter healthcare system was anything but regionally and ethnically neutral, even if the ethnic-national component was stoked by the Prussian regional policy before it appeared on Berlin's imperial-political agenda. Its retranslation into the region, against all expectations, was certainly not uncomplicated. Local resistance and local political identities did not always go hand in hand with Prussian regional politics. In the end, where the political destabilization and accompanying ethnically codified exclusion were produced was less relevant to regional realities. The pursuit of mastery begot a process of political struggle and ethnic competition for regional power as well as regional and cultural belonging. The debate surrounding the Academy of Applied Medicine made this struggle more visible than ever. It exposed how the introduction of medical and hygienic institutions made the province more modern and comparable to other regions of the German Empire, but it also produced side effects that were difficult to foresee and, in their regional setting, even more difficult to manage.

What mattered in the regional application were the healthcare system's practices and real-life implications. These were, albeit subtle, often hardly inclusive of the Polish members of the population. For their part, Polish hygienists sought to counteract them with their own health-related measures. These efforts were not entirely pragmatic; nor did they claim to be. The creation of medical and hygienic institutions as public services, the growing interest in themes surrounding the politics of public health and social hygiene, and the concurrent conversion of many previously individual vices into urgent social questions contributed to the deprivatization of health and its transition into a public matter and a national resource. With the sharpening of national attributes and the promotion of the national body (*Volkskörper*), it gained strategic significance. As with the state, so did Polish hygien-

19 See GStA PK, I. HA Rep. 76 VIII B, no. 3004: Letter from Richard Witting to State Minister Konrad von Studt in the Ministry of Culture on June 30, 1900; Report on institute plans from the meeting on the topic of elevatory measures for the province of Posen on May 21, 1889, quotes according to: GStA PK, I. HA Rep. 76, VIII B, no. 3004, 26, and according to Schutte, *Die Königliche Akademie in Posen*, 85.

ists recognize it as a tool that could be used to master the population. While Polish hygienists welcomed the state's public health measures, used them, and sought to fill the gaps left by the state,[20] they also loaded the semantic triangle of health–statehood–modernization with their own nationally codified contents. Polish hygienists organized themselves in the context of the exclusionary stance of the state and the similarly exclusionary societal attitude[21] that typically confronted parts of the Polish population. By creating their own medical space, they, at least partially, made themselves independent of the state or urban impulses, and, moving on from a desire to take over the role of healthcare providers for the Polish population, sought to mobilize themselves in terms of national population policy. These hygienists, who deemed themselves to be national leaders, consisted of a group of reform-minded, socially engaged physicians who led the Polish Society of Social Hygiene (Towarzystwo Hygieny Społecznej)[22] and other Polish hygiene societies and were associated with the Polish medical journal *Nowiny Lekarskie*[23] (*Medical News*, notably the only medical journal in the province). They belonged to a German-characterized medical community and participated in German medical debates, but nonetheless experienced official discrimination and understood themselves as part of the Polish national movement.[24] While Berlin argued with Posen and the local elites about updating the medical system and establishing the Academy of Applied Medicine, they were already focused on their own modernization campaign; yet they remained, under the guise of addressing national-political concerns, present in the debate surrounding the academy.

20 The implementation of reforms, as well as the occupation of many social-hygienic/social spaces, stemmed from the initiative of public and semi-official actors. The state provided the impulse, but the implementation followed the suggestions that came from the bottom up, or only recognized specific social spaces years later and then declared them its own. See Hull, *Sexuality, State and Civil Society in Germany, 1700–1815*; Hähner-Rombach, *Sozialgeschichte der Tuberkulose.*

21 Compare the testimonies of a multitude of German and Polish physicians on the social fragmentation of Posen society: Otto Lubarsch, *Ein bewegtes Gelehrtenleben* (Berlin: J. Springer, 1931), 156–60; and Tadeusz Szulc, *W Poznaniu i wkoło niego: Wspomnienia poznańskiego lekarza* (Poznań: Wydawnictwo Miejskie, 1995).

22 See, among others: *Nowiny Lekarskie* 1–2 (1904), 108–10; *Dziennik Poznański* 5, March 5, 1910; *Dziennik Poznański*, 62, March 17, 1910; *Kurier Poznański*, 87, April 14, 1916.

23 *Nowiny Lekarskie* [Medical news] was a scientific journal founded and edited in Posen that tried to reach all three of the partitioned Polish lands.

24 See Paweł Gantkowski, "Opening Address to the Polish Hygiene-Congress in Lviv," quoted in *Kurier Poznański*, 166, July 23, 1914.

Regional Challenges and the Limits of Medical Integration

Without doubt, the ministerial request of 1913, which had sounded out the political and medical mood of the province and offered the city of Posen and therefore the whole region further medical support, caused several controversies about the public healthcare system and its constitution.[25] As mentioned earlier, the debate surrounding the academy in a way invited a self-determined update and appraisal of the already existing medical network. It offered the opportunity to discuss how a medically underpinned statehood could be realized from a provincial perspective, where the priorities were, who would participate in the modernization and who would profit from it. With the benefit of hindsight, it offered a chance to review the successes and failures of the medical system's trajectory, and hence to allow for a dialogue between the different views on how to localize medical and health-policy measures.

Apart from officials in the Ministry of the Interior in Berlin who addressed the request, the debate involved the governor of the province and the governing council (as provincial representatives of the state government), the magistrate, the Posen mayor and the city council (as provincial representatives of the city of Posen and—in their capacity as capital city—as representatives of the province), medical officers, as well as individual representatives of medical institutions,[26] such as Director Erich Wernicke of the Institute of Hygiene, the chief consultants at the Posen Hospital, and the chief consultants of the Deaconess Hospital. A short but vibrant debate primarily between German elites began.

Virtually from the outset, it became apparent that Berlin's modernization proposals would hardly chime with provincial (political) self-perceptions and local views on self-determination, and that the core ideas could not withstand local experiences and expectations. The academy was in part supposed to become an additional center of medical knowledge, along the

25 The debate concerned the creation of an Academy of Applied Medicine in 1913–1914, that is to say, from the period in which the province already had the Institute of Hygiene, the Medical Survey Office, the midwifery training college, the disinfectors' school, as well as the Royal Academy as core providers of continuous training. In relation to medical provision, the first two functioned as primary knowledge hubs and supervisory bodies for bacteriological and medical matters.

26 The physicians, in their respective institutions, offered further and continued education courses, taught medical trainees, and served as local experts and potential bearers of the process of the medical transformation.

lines of what had already been done in other parts of the empire.[27] It would provide support for the Institute of Hygiene in its goal to disseminate scientific knowledge and augment it by expanding local expertise. However, because the idea originated in Berlin, the improvement of medical practice in the region would serve Berlin's goal of homogenizing the regions medically and culturally and tying them to the central government. Finally, there was the issue of domesticating healthcare nationally in line with the Prussian template and to establish the province of Posen as a locus of health protection in the empire.[28] Without well-trained physicians familiar with new developments—that is, with individuals who had never come into contact with hygienic-bacteriological procedures and/or did not even believe they were necessary—it was possible neither to epidemiologically survey the region, nor to systematically introduce and enforce hygienic standards (ranging from individual disease prevention to the maintenance of public sewer systems). It was commonly accepted that the standards needed to be improved. However, what could not be determined was how they needed to be improved and who should be in charge of the changes to be made.

The brief correspondence between Berlin and Posen illustrated that a further communal institution in Posen was not advisable, because the models designed in Berlin that had been tried in other provincial settings would not easily translate into the eastern provinces, considering their national-political and financial situation. Furthermore, Posen's views were too contradictory to allow a fast and successful collaboration underpinned by a consensus. Hence, the ministerial request was simply filed away. As with most obstacles, especially those aggravated by national-political considerations, the troubling aspects came to outweigh the desire for mastery of a borderland that nobody knew exactly what to do with or how to render more German and more modern in such a way that investments would be profitable but not produce undesirable results.

27 The Academy of Applied Medicine already existed in Cologne and Dusseldorf. See: Max Greve, *Geleitwort zur Feier der Eröffnung der allgemeinen Krankenanstalten und der Akademie für praktische Medizin in Düsseldorf* (Düsseldorf: A. Bagel, 1907); Heinrich Hochhaus, "Die ersten zehn Jahre der Kölner Akademie für praktische Medizin," in *Festschrift zur Feier des zehnjährigen Bestehens der Akademie für praktische Medizin in Cöln* (Cöln: Akademie für Praktische Medizin, 1915), 1–43.

28 See "Ein hygienisches Institut für Posen" in *National-Zeitung*, July 19, 1898, in GStPK, Rep. 76 VIII B, no. 3004: Regarding the influence and administration of the (public) Institute of Hygiene in Posen, 1895–1900, 40; Letter by the district president (*Regierungspräsident*) of the province of Posen to the minister of the interior from 11.04.1913 in GStA PK, I Ha Rep 76 VIII B, no. 3020.

In Posen itself, the debate continued and was driven forward by the magistrate. It turned into a kind of resurrection and continuation of the old "University Debate"[29] at the communal level, becoming a debate about the (self-)direction of scientific life in the province along with the route to its future advancement. It focused on whether the adoption of existing templates was sensible, to what degree local (political) realities should actually be taken into account, what solutions promised the greatest success, and how to emancipate the region scientifically and thereby account for national-political concerns.[30] Among the greatest points of contention that arose as a result of the prospective creation of the academy (and that were mainly contested between the Posen magistrate and the city council) revolved around the centralization of expertise versus local expertise, the deployment of local resources and their administration, national-political concerns, and the question of costs and benefits.

The magistrate, whom the city council accused of not having consulted with them in advance and of having made decisions without them, strove to bring the Academy of Applied Medicine to Posen, albeit in such a form that was suitable to local conditions. Similar to Posen's governor, the magistrate wanted to attach the academy either to the existing Institute of Hygiene or to the Royal Academy,[31] which was founded in 1902 and also offered medical courses. The aim was to bring specialist expertise to Posen and extend it outward into other eastern regions, and to do so without having to pay for it or, should the academy threaten to become too autonomous, needing to submit to it.[32] The medical elevation of the province was desired but in a po-

29 The "University Debate," although laid to rest by the turn of the century, was repeatedly retopicized from the mid-1890s onward in the run-up to the founding of the Royal Academy in Posen in 1902. It concerned, on the one hand, the question of the province's cultural emancipation, as it, apart from West Prussia, was the only one not to have a university center. On the other, it concerned national-political thoughts rather than scientific-cultural ones, especially the degree to which a university would contribute to the undesired emancipation of the Polish-speaking population. They also debated the regional distribution of cultural resources (such as the constant competition between the two district capitals—Posen and Bromberg—and their role as strongholds of Germanness in the region), that is, the regional weighting of modernizing processes.

30 For more on the "University Debate" about the potential creation of a university in Posen, see Schutte, *Die Königliche Akademie*, 28–31.

31 The Royal Academy was an educational establishment founded in 1902 that had assumed a quasi-university role, but was unable to offer a university education and did not have the powers or renown of a university. It primarily offered popular science courses. For more on this, see Schutte, *Die Königliche Akademie*.

32 See Note in the files of the meeting between representatives of the state, the city, and medical staff on 15.06.1913, in APP, AMP, no. 2568, 20; Municipal resolution on 08.08.1913, in APP, AMP, no. 2568, 22.

litically and regionally controllable format, one in which the local authorities were not responsible to provide the means to achieve it.

After years of negotiations surrounding the reconstruction of the Institute of Hygiene,[33] which the Berlin government imposed on the province at Posen's expense, and having been much lauded but barely supported financially beyond the first few years, the city of Posen was no longer willing to shoulder further unplanned costs and to simply carry all public institutions. The medical, health-political improvement was to remain centralized with the Institute of Hygiene for Posen and guaranteed by the Medical Survey Center for Bromberg, and according to the provincial government did not require a further change, especially not an expensive and autonomous one. As it was, the situation may have not been ideal, but was deemed regionally solvable. The proposal to attach the academy to an already existing institution aimed to establish a stronger grip on it and to place it in the care of the local physicians and the city of Posen.[34] The desire to bring the academy to Posen owed more to the city's prestige and control over the province than it did to a realistically desired improvement to its medical infrastructure. The possible expansion of the Institute of Hygiene or, in particular, the Royal Academy, was seen to offer Posen as well as the deputies of the provincial government an opportunity to enlarge one of their institutions, take "the now dead organism […] [and] breathe new life into it through our involvement,"[35] and thereby bestow upon the province a university-esque prestige.[36]

In the city council, comprised of communally elected representatives of the German-speaking population,[37] this proposition—attaching the academy to an already existing institution—generated considerable discontent.

33 The negotiations on the new building for the Institute of Hygiene started in the early 1900s (around 1904–1905) and it took years until a mutually acceptable solution was found. The core issue was the division of costs between the state and the city of Posen and the new design of the Institute. See Schutte, *Die Königliche Akademie*, 328–331.

34 Note in the files from the meeting between representatives of the state, the city, and medical staff on 15.06.1913, in APP, AMP, no. 2568, 20.

35 City councillor Hartwig, Report of the debate on the Academy of Applied Medicine, in APP, AMP, no. 1109, 43.

36 Letter from the municipal authorities to the minister of cultural affairs on 12.08.1913, duplicate, in APP, AMP, no. 2568, 26–27.

37 Due to the electoral system that favored wealthy (home)owners, the city council had a particularly high number of representatives from the German-speaking (German and Jewish) population. See *Władze miasta Poznania, Wykaz członków władz miasta 1253–2003*, vol. II (Poznań, Wydawnictwo miejskie, 2003), 1–62.

For the city council, which was against any of the magistrate's proposals and hence against founding the academy, the academy was unnecessary and its possible attachment to already established structures would only weaken and diminish them.[38] The creation of an additional medical educational facility in the form of the academy would lead, so the city council believed, to the disadvantaging of Posen's established physicians. This would be the case especially if the planned academy was staffed with physicians from outside the region.[39] By being a conduit for the latest scientific developments, it would inevitably prefer its own graduates to the provincial physicians. "To peddle theory with the medical trainees here," it was said in the city council meeting, "is superfluous, and it is even far less necessary to create something for the provincial physicians."[40] "Please do not believe," said Dr. Max Landsberg, a city councilor and one of the most vehement opponents of the Academy, "that the Academy will bring the sense of reason that our magistrate so painfully misses in our hospital administrators."[41] In his view, the chief consultants lacked suitable teachers, but not so the local medical body that—and this was the true concern that lurked behind such arguments—did not want further centralization and did not need external medical instruction, but knew how to organize itself locally and how to gain further skills in the necessary and respective fields.[42] Louder than considerations about the uniformity of health and hygiene and improved standards, perhaps, were the medical profession's fears concerning their political involvement, as well as conflicts within the medical community itself.[43] Both limited their field of vision. Support for the very notion of the academy, Landsberg said, rather than being offered a medical upgrade, could lead to

38 See the discussion of a possible Academy of Applied Medicine in the city council in *Posener Neueste Nachrichten*, second supplement, no. 4362, September 26, 1913.

39 Note in the files of the meeting between representatives of the state, the city, and medical staff, 16.04.1913, in APP, AMP, no. 2568, 8. During the creation of the Academy of Applied Medicine in Cologne some physicians—in particular, those at the clinics in Bonn—also raised concerns that the academy could threaten their work by encroaching on their areas. See Hochhaus, "Die ersten zehn Jahre," 3.

40 Review of the city council's debate of the Academy of Applied Medicine, statement by city councillor Kirchner in *Posener Neueste Nachrichten*, second supplement, no. 4362, September 26, 1913.

41 Dr. Max Landsberg, Report of the debate about the Academy of Applied Medicine in *Posener Neueste Nachrichten*, second supplement, no. 4362, September 26, 1913.

42 Note in the files of the meeting between representatives of the state, the city and medical staff, 16.04.1913, in APP, AMP, no. 2568, vol. 8.

43 Regarding the professionalization of physicians, see, among others, Huerkamp, *Der Aufstieg der Ärzte im 19. Jahrhundert.*

Posen being accused of offering poor-quality education and as a result be stripped of its right to provide medical training. The Royal Academy would become even more of a patchwork than it already was. State support, professional accreditation, and the regional ability to "care for oneself" would be withdrawn. Although this rejectionist attitude among the majority of city councilors did incur the accusation that they lacked patriotism, it was countered with national-political considerations about German–Polish antagonisms. These surfaced with every imaginable change and were, as councilor Hugo Kindler emphasized, invariably controversial, even if one was a liberal and thought little of these fears.[44] In order to avoid having to discuss these concerns again in public, the councilors preferred to point out that the academy's role models—the academies in Cologne and Dusseldorf—did not fulfill their roles. So, either way, the Academy of Applied Medicine could not be relied upon to bring great—all reservations notwithstanding—changes.

This view was challenged by many of the discussants. However, it did steer the discussion back toward medical improvement, which seems to have been forgotten for a time. The actual architects of the medical challenge—the physicians, apart from the five chief consultants—were hardly being consulted, as though medical modernization could be driven and enforced entirely administratively and politically and did not need to be linked back to regional medical expertise and capabilities. The Posen elites seemed rather more concerned with their own influence and rights than with improving the medical welfare system. Medical modernization as concocted in Berlin appeared to be less important, and less relevant regionally, than the maintenance of their authority. It leads us to the question of whether the central government's effort to establish a modern population policy with the help of medical providers was going to work within the regional political agenda, and whether such efforts were valued at all. The local responses betrayed a provincial mindset that dismissed the value of any centrally generated improvements if it threatened local power arrangements.

While medical and health-related initiatives were seen as part of the "policy of elevation" by Berlin, their communal or even provincial implementation was met with little enthusiasm beyond the purely pragmatic dimension, their political façade, and the resultant prestige. They were desired

44 Hugo Kindler, report of the debate about the Academy of Applied Medicine, in APP, AMP, no. 1109, 31.

only in so far as they bore (political) benefit to the communal power brokers.[45] The main concern here was whether "something comes of this that will be of benefit to the city of Posen," and not whether it would result in something transcending local realities that would allow for a closer connection to Berlin and transregional processes of homogenization. Semi-feudal power interests and loyalties counted more and outweighed the national-political considerations and fears that were otherwise so pronounced in the region and that were projected onto it. This was because—aptly summarizing the national-political development of the region—"every now and then the bearers of knowledge and the ethos in the country decided that the folk have to 'hate' themselves, and that the [Polish] Stanislaus 'hates' the obedient [German] Wilhelm. Precisely such an era of enmity had been conjured up. People reflected on their nationality."[46] This notion, though, was often secondary to confessional differences[47] or internal government conflicts between Berlin and Posen. It was politically desirable and always present on the political-cum-national agenda, even if the regional implementation of this agenda mainly served to legitimize positions that operated via other bands of loyalty, rather than being a core argument.

Ethnic Challenges and the Limits of Medical Integration

Polish voices remained absent from the debate; Polish physicians, along with the entire Posen medical establishment, were not included.[48] The Polish representatives of the Polish Circle (Koło Polskie)[49] showed no interest in the process. Their disengagement could be attributed to their having less representation in the debate forums (the magistrate and the city council) than other regional groups, and to their not being the primary clientele of the planned academy, which was in the first place geared toward medi-

45 Magistrate resolution on August 8, 1913, in APP, AMP, no. 2568, 22.

46 Marianne Mewis, *Der große Pan* (Dresden: Reißner, 1908), 249.

47 Confessional identities were fundamental to national ones.

48 Similar criticisms had previously been raised by physicians regarding the creation of the academy in Cologne. In Posen, it was less about the physicians demanding their rights and rather more about communal politicians and city representatives. See Hochhaus, "Die ersten zehn Jahre," 31–4.

49 The Polish Party (Koło Polskie) was a Polish parliamentary faction, in both the Prussian House of Deputies as well as in the Reichstag, which represented the Polish people from the provinces of Posen, West Prussia, and Upper Silesia. See Heimann, *Der Preussische Landtag 1899–1947*, 52–3.

cal assistants and trainees of German origin. Supporting Polish physicians and representing their interests was undesirable. This was all the more true since Polish doctors were only conditionally interested in state-led improvement in the healthcare provisions. Despite the political directive from Berlin to not allow Polish physicians to profit from the state's health initiatives, there was professional cooperation between German and Polish doctors. They often shared the same views about medical and hygienic improvements and modernization[50] and they occasionally even worked together on their implementation,[51] but they always appeared separately in public. They were for the most part also separated institutionally[52]: despite frequent vacancies, hardly any Polish physicians worked for the Institute of Hygiene or the Medical Survey Center.[53] Most hygiene-focused societies defined themselves in national-linguistic terms.[54] While German-speaking physicians were favored and financially supported by the state, Polish physicians were continuously refused posts as district physicians (since 1904 at the latest),[55] and they could not hope for financial aid.[56] They were sporadically sus-

50 See Biblioteka UAM, Dział Zbiorów Specjalnych i Rękopisów, sign. 2803/2: Tadeusz Szulc, W Poznaniu i wokół niego (wspomnienia) vol. 2 (V) Część Piąta, Wolna Polska. 1918–1939; *Kronika Miasta Poznania z.T. Lekarze (dt. Ärzte)*, Heft 1, 2001; Reports in *Nowiny Lekarskie* (1871–1918).

51 This collaboration was context dependent and heavily reliant on individual people. Polish physicians' willingness to cooperate was characterized by pragmatism. They wanted to use the state infrastructure to enhance professional linkages through collaboration with German physicians and state medical-hygiene institutions while not entirely negating the state. Many of the Polish hygienists (such as, for example, Paweł Gantkowski or Tadeusz Schultz) were, due to their specialist knowledge and social-reformist and/or professional connections, respected and consulted by both German physicians as well as medical officers.

52 Polish, German, and Jewish doctors (these last ones were mostly perceived as German anyway) cooperated admittedly within the Posener Medical Council (established 1889) and organized joint medical courses for provincial doctors, though these activities had a purely professional and pragmatic context and were never conducted on a large scale. The tendency to focus on national-linguistic defined audience seemed to be stronger than the desire for professional cooperation. See Molik, *Inteligencja polska w Poznańskiem w XIX i początkach XX wieku*, 429–36.

53 See GStA PK, I. HA Rep. 76 VIII B, no. 3013: Letter from Erich Wernicke to the Ministry of Culture, May 16, 1907; APP, Hygiene-Institut, no. 4: Correspondence between Erich Wernicke and the Ministry of the Interior, especially 114–18.

54 An exception here is the Society for the Prevention of Tuberculosis, along with all activities combating tuberculosis. Joint German–Polish cooperation in this area owes to more than just cooperative will: tuberculosis was a social disease that transgressed categories of class (and not primarily the categories of gender or nation/race), which means that it pervaded all linguistic, national, and confessional communities alike. Furthermore, the battle against it was expensive and hence demanded a joined up effort by all communities.

55 The last Polish-speaking district physician, Dr. Walenty Panieński, held the post from 1894 to 1904. See Biblioteka PTPN, Rkps. 1860: Życiorysy Jana i Walentego Panieńskich.

56 See, among others, APP, Oberpäsidium, no. 9619.

pected of being engaged in political agitation among the rural population. The same was true of Polish midwives. Despite the need for Polish-speaking midwives, they were trained in ever fewer numbers, and courses taught in Polish were drastically reduced after 1900.[57] Furthermore, the Polish population was, if not explicitly excluded from many offerings—such as German-language hygienic exhibitions or the lecture series by the Institute of Hygiene—then certainly infrequently included and even then hardly welcome.[58] In some rare cases, the Institute of Hygiene even turned down inquires regarding bacteriological tests for Polish-speaking patients.[59]

Although the Polish population was never left entirely without access to medical health provisions, access was made more difficult through language barriers—especially in rural areas where the population was commonly less fluent in German—or complicated and less supported by state administration due to national-political considerations. This subtle marginalization led to a segmentation of healthcare. Polish hygienists remained excluded from parts of the official network as well as political debates, which were often held behind closed doors in ministerial or internal government circles. The publically discussed aspects of the debate, whose fragmentation city representatives also complained about, were too hermetic, so that, as with the case of the Academy of Applied Medicine, the city's Polish-language newspapers concluded with regret that "from the presentation we could not quite ascertain what the whole matter was about and it seemed as though there were something hidden in the whole matter, something one did not want to openly express."[60] Denied as bearers of the state's or the city's medical actualization, they became bearers of a medically induced education campaign, which they understood in a national manner as an invocation for national consolidation. Responding to an acute situation, they seized the initiative, guaranteeing them a strong political role in the Polish population on the one hand, and allowing for direct access to this population on the other. They did much—within the limits of available means—to offer consultations and treatment services and to reach as broad a spectrum of the Polish

57 I.HA. Rep 76 VIII B, no. 1480: Treatise on the "Hebammen-Lehranstalt in Posen während der Jahre 1811 bis 1911 von Prof. Dr. med. Lange," 1911 Bojanowo, 12.

58 See, among others, GStA PK, I. HA Rep. 76 VIII B, no. 3004: Letter from Richard Witting to State Minister Konrad von Studt in the Ministry of Culture, June 30, 1900.

59 See, GStA PK, I. HA Rep. 76 VIII B, no. 3006: Report by Erich Wernicke, September 9, 1906.

60 *Kurier Poznański*, no. 222, September 26, 1913.

population as they could. To achieve this, they organized a dense network of hygienic and medical courses, addressed mainly to professional but also to lay audiences. They offered private professional development courses, courses for community nurses,[61] lectures in individual district cities, popular science lectures for mothers, a lecture series on alcoholism, hygiene courses, etc. These lectures were published in the Polish-language press and via traditional Polish networks, such as the Catholic Church.[62] For example, courses for community nurses were addressed mainly to rural Polish Catholic women (announced via the Catholic Church) in order to offer them a community-certified service (away from the state) and to mobilize them for the cause of national solidarity, as well as to furnish them with knowledge of the treatment of venereal diseases and to help them avoid inevitable discrimination by German-speaking doctors (the Polish population was often considered morally lax and therefore more prone to contracting venereal diseases[63]). The Association of Social Hygiene founded a dedicated polyclinic[64] offering consultations to the poor within the Polish population. Through such medical services, Polish hygienists created a safe space for the Polish population and, simultaneously, a space in which a *healthy nation* could be honed and tended. In doing so, they focused on their own medically introduced and implemented societal and national mastery.[65]

With no financial or infrastructural means to challenge the state's health system, and because they spoke from a marginalized position, the medically induced policy was primarily understood as an education program with the aim to establish national loyalties. While Polish hygienists could not lay claim to the so-called *decision space*, they could claim *identity space*[66] through the locally conceived and organized assumption of responsibility

61 For such an announcement see, for example, *Kurier Poznański* 218, September 22, 1918.

62 All of these popular science lectures were announced in the local Polish-speaking newspapers—mostly in *Kurier Poznański* or *Dziennik Poznański* for Posen, in *Dziennik Bydgoski* for Bromberg, and in other local newspapers. For 1908 see, for example, *Kurier Poznański* 24, January 1, 1908: Information about open lectures for mothers on pedagogy; *Kurier Poznański* 73, March 28, 1908: Popular lectures in Pleszew on infectious diseases; *Kurier Poznański* 110, January 13, 1908: Open lectures on alcoholism in Posen.

63 Recording of a discussion about the spread of venereal diseases within the army, Berlin, March 3, 1915, in GStA PK, Kultusministerium I HA Rep 76 VIII B, no. 3798. Similar accusations of Polish people can be found in many other nonpublic statements.

64 For more information about the polyclinic see, for example, *Dziennik Poznański* 7, April 6, 1906; *Kurier Poznański* 10, January 14, 1908.

65 See *Kurier Poznański* 149, July 3, 1914.

66 Maier, "Transformations of Territoriality 1600–2000."

for strengthening the medical expertise available to the Polish population. Furthermore, they wanted to legitimize and formulate it as the foundation for a future, eventual state of their own. They gained their (financial) support through a close alliance with the Polish Catholic Church—one that not only gave them a financial and infrastructural base, but direct access to the Polish Catholic population, as well as the strength of its voice. The Church, for its part, was integrated into the national movement, its doctrines unthreatened, and declared it an aspect of modernization.

This hygiene movement was conceived of as a hallmark of the modern nation.[67] In order to take over the medical provision for those least catered to by the system (the poor, those disenfranchised for linguistic reasons, etc.), Polish reformers founded a hygiene movement informed by international scientific theories, in Polish, and addressed solely to a Polish audience.[68] They were far more active in their pursuits than the German medical community, as they could not rely on state support and had to mobilize a range of networks (churches, physicians, women's societies, the press, individual patrons, and so on).

This parallel hygiene-medical movement of Polish social reformers was not intimated by the subtle but noticeable national-political considerations of the sort found in the debate surrounding the Academy of Applied Medicine, about receiving state support in the form of new (uncontrollable) opportunities to augment professional development. Even if the healthcare space, functionally, was segmented, Polish hygienists only targeted the Polish population, and the fact that such encounters only concerned people and not problems, Polish initiatives did not go unnoticed by the state. Rather, they became a constant irritant to those who oversaw state policies because the actions of Polish reformers were viewed with concern by the state as the strengthening of a foreign body within the German totality. In order to safeguard it, state authorities managed to keep the state and communal investments in check. They made reformers address the medical recreation of the region in terms beyond the context of the homogenization of the state,

67 See Reports of the Polish Society of Social Hygiene that were published in the Polish-language press from 1907 to 1918, among others: *Dziennik Poznański* 62, March 14, 1908; *Dziennik Poznański* 59, March 13, 1910; *Kurier Poznański* 87, April 14, 1916.

68 See Adam Karwowski, *O seksualnem wychowaniu młodzieży* (Poznań: Drukarnia I Księgarnia Św. Wojciecha, 1908); and *Berichte der polnischen Gesellschaft der Sozialen Hygiene in Dziennik Poznański*, January–March, 1903–1918.

and thus included the context of power struggles and national spheres of influence as well as fears of Polish national agitation. While Polish social reformers sought to demonstrate the modernization designs by example and set them up in close alignment with hygiene-medical values, the state's arguments were hampered by national-political considerations, and were often circular.

Conflicting Loyalties: Troubling Borders and the Politicization of Medical Impact

The debate surrounding the Academy of Applied Medicine ended after a few months. The instruction of medical trainees, the extent of the hygiene-medical network, and the provision of medical services changed very little. The goal of making improvements was set aside with the outbreak of the First World War and subsequently occurred only selectively, the status quo being kept stable as required. The debate itself, though, had not yet been shrouded in the shadow of war and hence reflected the expectations and disappointments that the medically introduced provincial mastery had brought and about which initial conclusions could be drawn. Furthermore, it was apparent that all actors involved in any subsequent medical improvements would have their own interests, that they might have difficulty in finding common ground with other actors in the process, and that Berlin's ideas could not just simply be projected onto any given regional setting.

The homogenizing ambitions emanating from Berlin on how to cement statehood medically and thereby render the region and its peoples politically and culturally more malleable, may have been welcomed. At the regional governmental level, though, it soon met resistance when translated into policies and confronted with local ideas and regional attempts to control the direction of precisely these state homogenization efforts. While Berlin aspired to master the troubling borderland in a modern Prussian way through subordination and by adopting the latest standards (and in so doing also aspired to strengthen the modern state and national loyalty), the local political elites remained constrained by their regionalism. Berlin's attempts at homogenization were frequently feared in Posen, at both the provincial and communal level, as a threatening process of centralization and an infringement upon the right to self-determination. They were also felt to be an additional financial burden that seemed to be neither predictable nor profitable in the short term. The situation was further aggravated by institutional competition in the province (in particular during the debate surrounding the academy between the magistrate and city council). All this meant that local elites became torn between their own interests, regional loyalties, and the state's assertion of an imperially construed nationalization. The resulting tensions were hardly resolvable, all the more so as Berlin's "Polish and regional policy" itself was anything but consistent. The Berlin-initiated attempt to master the medical character of the region failed, meanwhile, in part due to a lack of local appreciation and cooperation. The Prussian population policy itself was ambivalent about how to coordinate the provincial space most effectively, both nationally and politically, who should benefit from what measures, and how the Polish population could be most effectively domesticated without becoming emancipated at the same time. It attempted to modernize and master the region, but was neither consistent enough nor engaged in their pursuit to succeed. This policy had always been shaped by Berlin's fear that these attempts at modernization, instead of having a purely Germanizing effect, could also have an unintended emancipatory affect on the Polish population. This was so because even if the Polish national movement had already begun to take shape and had created a partially parallel existing (medical) space independent from the state's initiatives, it remained a foreign body that was to be brought in line with the state's interest. Its otherness was to be mitigated through medical mastery, but, as a result of the political and structural fluctuations in medical practice, it was only solidified further.

While the regional space remained ambiguous, and from the state's perspective highly problematic and politically volatile, it became unidimensional to Polish hygienists. Their sole aim was to direct the Polish population in healthcare matters, to offer access to healthcare services, and mobilize it as a *Polish community* in a national, population-political sense. With their Polish identity fortified through the hygiene movement, Polish hygienists sought to connect to the supra-regional Polish movement. Their actions took their bearings from the state's measures and the German-language discourses in which they operated, using the state's framework, albeit without wanting to entrench their loyalties to it. Consequently, hegemonically concocted modernization processes were transported to the peripheries that eventually robbed them of the ability to modernize and that underscored their own ambivalence. As the attempts at homogenization were not inclusive enough, they succumbed to their own inability to configure the imperial ideas in a more open and flexible manner both regionally and nationally.

CHAPTER IV

The Material Side of Modernity: The Midwife's Bag in Bosnia and Herzegovina around the Turn of the Century[1]

Sara Bernasconi

When, after a three-month-long operation, the Austro-Hungarian army occupied Bosnia-Herzegovina in accordance with the Treaty of Berlin (1878), tens of thousands of soldiers found themselves on the territory.[2] They needed to be catered for, food had to be secured, accommodation found, and encampments built.[3] By the end of 1878, the military occupation formally became a bureaucratic administration, soldiers settled down, and sanitary services were created to care for them.[4] The flow of people and goods, though, continued. The newly built railway brought civil servants from the various corners of the Habsburg monarchy, along with their families and households, and in their wake workers, servants, and other personnel arrived, including midwives.[5] In these years, public health was not a main preoccupation of Habsburg rule in Bosnia-Herzegovina, as soldiers were treated by military surgeons, civil servants had their physicians, and locals had their own services. Over time encounters intensified, and polit-

1 This chapter was translated by Tudor Georgescu.

2 Bencze, *The Occupation of Bosnia and Herzegovina in 1878*, 99f.

3 Unrivalled for their descriptions of material culture are the works by Hamdija Kreševljaković, the most relevant being *Sarajevo za vrijeme austrougarske uprave (1878–1918)*, 11.

4 On combating prostitution, see Kasumović, "Prilog povijesti marginalnih skupina u Bosni i Hercegovini u doba austro-ugarske uprave: prostitutke," 162.

5 How expensive, exhausting, and costly such a removal was can be see through the example of midwife Marie Martinović's relocation from Slavonski Brod to Sarajevo in 1879. Historijski Archiv Sarajevo (HAS), Gradsko Poglavarstvo (GP)-1, k. 9, 5035.

ical pressure and tensions grew—the administration had to engage with the locals, although they were not formally citizens of the monarchy.[6] In regards to childbirth, the Habsburg monarchy's care for the "population" developed mainly through the actions of midwives and with the help of the midwife's bag.[7]

The point of departure of this chapter is the midwife's bag, which was introduced by the Habsburg administration, provided to midwives for free, and regularly inspected by medical officers. The bag was used by midwives, medical officers, political authorities, and those involved with pregnant women or women in childbirth.[8] Tracing the bag from the moment of its introduction in 1898, we can observe how state midwifery in Bosnia-Herzegovina evolved. The bag's objects were a manifestation of the contemporary knowledge of asepsis/antisepsis as applied in hospital birth and that was supposed to be taken out of the clinic and "into the field" by the female professionals.[9] Furthermore, the objects in the bag point us toward the ideal behavior of the "modern" midwife.[10] However, as soon as these things and objects were in the midwife's hands, they became independent and began to manifest a life of their own.[11] This is what I call the material side of modernity.

The Habsburg administration explained the takeover of Bosnia-Herzegovina as a "civilizing mission," thereby legitimizing state intervention by employing a discourse on modernity.[12] According to this logic, it was the Austro-Hungarian administration that, after four hundred years of Ottoman influence in the region, brought "modernity" to Bosnia-Herzegovina. Bosnia-Herzegovina's "backwardness" was expressed through medical met-

6 For the unusual constitutional construction for Bosnia-Herzegovina, see Okey, *Taming Balkan Nationalism*, 123f.

7 For a discussion of politics based on the model of the British Empire in India, see Löwy, "The Social History of Medicine: Beyond the Local," 471. For readability reasons, I refer to the midwife's bag as a "bag," even though it took different forms over time and, until 1906, was actually a hard case.

8 The notion of the "assembly" of human and nonhuman actants in networks is from Bruno Latour, *We Have Never Been Modern*.

9 I presume a circulation of knowledge following Kreuder-Sonnen, "Wie die Mikroben nach Warschau kamen"; "Zirkulationen," *Nach Feierabend, Zürcher Jahrbuch für Wissensgeschichte* 7 (2011).

10 Thévenot, "Die Pluralität kognitiver Formate und Engagements im Bereich zwischen dem Vertrauten und dem Öffentlichen," 260f.

11 For multiplying processes, see Akrich and Pasveer, "Multiplying Obstetrics: Techniques of Surveillance and Forms of Coordination."

12 Ruthner et al. (eds.), *WechselWirkungen: Austria-Hungary, Bosnia-Herzegovina and the Western Balkans, 1878–1918*.

aphors, which was particularly evident in the apparent lack of medical infrastructure in the region.[13] The central and contested figure in this discourse was the "Muslim woman," in which Islam's "backwardness" and Bosnia-Herzegovina's otherness culminated. A veiled figure, she had withdrawn herself from Habsburg male view and was orientalized as both dirty and desirable. Current historiographic research has shifted perspectives on Muslim women as actors, and questions the relationship between gender, religion, and empire.[14] Therein, ambivalent (social) spaces, practices of appropriation, and an expansion of the Ottoman gender norms become visible. Applied to the example of midwives—which were not Muslims—and using a symmetric anthropological approach, I inquire into the interplay of gender and modernity as a specific modern concept of an empire's population.[15]

The Midwife's Bag as a Tool of Administrative Rule

On May 26, 1902, the city council of Bijeljina debated the dismissal of the municipal midwife Aloisia Schwetz.[16] The medical officer, Dr. Chamoides, began litigation against the birth attendant after a wealthy family's newborn developed an eye infection at the end of 1901. The court sentenced her to pay a fine of ten Krone, because she had not immediately summoned the doctor and thereby violated "midwifery regulations."[17] The district leader approved the dismissal, as the midwife had previously refused to familiarize herself with the official "Guidelines for Midwives" introduced in 1898, and resisted the mandatory quarterly "inspection of midwifery utensils."

13 Fuchs, "Orientalizing Disease: Austro-Hungarian Policies of 'Race,' Gender and Hygiene in Bosnia and Herzegovina, 1874–1914," 58.

14 For example Giomi, "Forging Habsburg Muslim Girls: Gender, Education and Empire in Bosnia and Herzegovina (1878–1918)," 276; Demirci and Somel, "Women's Bodies, Demography, and Public Health."

15 My approach, beside to Latour's work, owes much to the publications of the sociology of conventions. See Boltanski, *Love and Justice as Competences*; Boltanski and Thévenot, *On Justification: Economies of Worth*. Equally important were the discussions with Caroline Arni's team at the University of Basel and with Mischa Suter, Magaly Tornay, and Niklaus Ingold.

16 All quotations in this section, unless otherwise noted, are taken from Archiv Bosne i Hercegovine (ABH), Zemaljska Vlada (ZV), 1903, 52-11/12. Regional office Bjelina concerning a call for applications for the role of midwife. See also: ABH, ZV, 1902, 52-11/9. Regional office D. Tuzla concerning disciplinary action against the midwife Aloisia Schwetz for violating the Midwife Decree.

17 The 1898 "Guidelines for Midwives" [Naputak za babice] were based on the Midwife Decree and had, in reality, the character of laws. Paragraph 10 prescribed the midwife's duty to prevent eye infections in newborns. Her behavior in this case was litigated as a contravention of paragraph 10: HAS, Biblioteka, Naputak za babice (primalje) u Bosni i Hercegovini, br. 67.637/I ex 1898, 10.

In the Ottoman Empire, to which the Bosnian provinces belonged for almost 400 years, until 1878, anyone had been free to work as a healer.[18] The types of medical training that were controlled related to doctors only, although the quality of the remedies was subject to regulations and checks.[19] The "population issue" had started to matter after the Tanzimat reforms, less for health than for economic reasons.[20] These measures included the politics of reproduction and a more severe and detailed regulation of the midwife's profession.[21] The Austro-Hungarian authorities augmented these regulations in the first year of civil rule, 1879, with a legal decree[22] that allowed for the first midwives to be hired. They were recruited for the newly arrived wives of Austro-Hungarian civil servants, who followed in their wake from the various regions of the Habsburg monarchy because the officials' families did not trust the local midwifery services.[23] These female professionals were nevertheless most commonly paid from municipal funds.

In 1898, after several serious childbirth accidents in Bosnia-Herzegovina,[24] the state-led organization and control of midwifery was set out in great detail. Henceforth, municipal midwives were to care for anyone giving birth, for a fee for the wealthy and for free for the poor. Detailed "Guidelines for Midwives"[25] were issued by the highest administrative echelons, along with a standardized instruments bag. The latter was to be given to all midwives for free. This second, successful, attempt at midwifery reform was led

18 Moulin and Ülman, *Perilous Modernity: History of Medicine in the Ottoman Empire and the Middle East from the 19th Century*; Shefer Mossensohn, *Ottoman Medicine: Healing and Medical Institutions, 1500–1700*; Đurčić and Elazar, *Pregled istorije farmacije Bosne i Hercegovine*, 144, 158.

19 Winterbottom, "Of the China Root: A Case Study of the Early Modern Circulation of *Materia Medica*." In reality, it was more complicated, because from the Tanzimat on there were many interactions between the Ottoman and the Habsburg Empires. See Chahrour, "'A Civilizing Mission'? Austrian Medicine and the Reform of Medical Structures in the Ottoman Empire, 1838–1850."

20 Dursun, "Procreation, Family and 'Progress': Administrative and Economic Aspects of Ottoman Population Policies in the 19th Century," 161.

21 Demirci and Somel, "Women's Bodies," 393f.; Balsoy, *The Politics of Reproduction in Ottoman Society, 1838–1900*.

22 "Decree 13791 from the 24. August 1879," in *Auszug aus der Sammlung der für Bosnien und die Hercegovina erlassenen Gesetze, Verordnungen und Normalweisungen: 1878–1880; I. Band, Allgemeiner Theil—politische Verwaltung* (Vienna: Landesdruckerei, 1880), 110–12.

23 ABH, ZV, 1900, 52-11/58. Report of the regional Office in Prozor.

24 ABH, Zajedničko Ministarstvo Finansija (ZMF), 1888, k. 53, 9092. File with the request by the provincial government and two drafts.

25 HAS, Naputak za babice. It is a variant of the 1897 official regulations for midwives decreed for the Austrian half of the monarchy: "216. Verordnung des Ministeriums des Innern im Einvernehmen mit dem Ministerium für Cultus und Unterricht vom 10. September 1897" with which the new guidelines are decreed, in *RGB*, 1897, 11. September 1897, 1287.

by Otto von Weiss (1857–1901), the chief physician for midwifery and gynecology at Landesspital, the main hospital in Sarajevo, and the man who had developed the "Guidelines for Midwives."[26] It was a ten-year project that required Weiss to engage in an active correspondence between Vienna and Sarajevo, as well as to personally travel from the Bosnia-Herzegovina capital to Vienna to present his case to the Bureau of Bosnian Affairs of the Joint Finance Ministry, which controlled Bosnia-Herzegovina rather than the provincial government.[27]

Across Europe, in the closing decades of the nineteenth century, there had been feverish efforts to find new ways to improve obstetrics.[28] Medical and political expertise coalesced into an increasingly state-led attempt to "care for the mother" and, soon, for the infant as well. Childbirth was made more accessible to the rule of the state, with its linear logic, as the "area of reproduction."[29] The discovery of germs as the cause of the dangerous puerperal fever—particularly in hospital labor wards and the maternity homes of large cities like Vienna, Budapest, or Prague—ultimately led, following detours and early difficulties in its wider reception, to a preventative hygienic body of knowledge on aseptic/antiseptics.[30] Its aim was to preemptively prevent the "fever," as contemporary medical treatments hardly had any effect once it had spread from the woman's uterus to her abdomen and through her entire body. These infections, following some forty horrifically painful days, were mostly fatal for women. In Bosnia-Herzegovina, however, as was the case in most "peripheral" regions of Europe, the overwhelming majority of births were delivered not in a clinic but at home.[31] There, the specter of puerperal fever was somewhat less frightening, albeit concerns about the

26 A first attempt was made in 1888, but did not pass at the Bureau of Bosnian Affairs of the Joint Finance Ministry: ABH, ZMF, 1888, k. 53, 9092. See also: ABH, ZMF, 1898, k. 53, 8241. Report of the provincial government concerning the publication of the "Guidelines for Midwives."

27 ABH, ZMF, 1896, k. 3, 288. Promemoria Dr. Otto von Weiss'; ABH, ZMF, 1897, k. 60, 9018. Neumann's approval and data collection; ABH, ZMF, 1897, k. 52, 7660. Report by the provincial government on midwifery.

28 See, for example, the annual publication *Jahresbericht über die Fortschritte auf dem Gebiete der Geburtshilfe und Gynäkologie,* which started appearing in 1888; Buklijaš and Lafferton, "Introduction: Science, Medicine and Nationalism in the Habsburg Empire from the 1840s to 1918," 680.

29 On the conception of reproduction as a male-linear genealogy, see Meyer, "Zum Phantasma der Selbstgeburt."

30 Loudon, *Death in Childbirth: An International Study of Maternal Care and Maternal Mortality, 1800–1950.* Recognition of the discoveries was a long way off. See also Maria Zarifi's chapter about the discovery of cholera.

31 McIntosh, *A Social History of Maternity and Childbirth: Key Themes in Maternity Care,* 39.

mother were nonetheless substantial, because it took considerable time for an effective (operative) intervention to materialize locally, should an emergency arise.[32]

Hence, the midwifery reform also had to consider these new scientific insights gained in Europe's clinics and to simultaneously guarantee their "translation" into the poorly understood realities of Bosnia-Herzegovina.[33] Academic knowledge of asepsis/antisepsis, should it have an impact, had to be conveyed to the midwives. Reciprocally, locally collected data were to flow back into academia—for which the spread of puerperal fever among the indigenous population of Bosnia-Herzegovina was of particular interest.[34] The midwife's bag appeared to be the right tool for achieving this. The challenge was to determine precisely what was needed to facilitate aseptic work practices across Bosnia-Herzegovina, which almost exclusively practiced home births. How would it be possible, far removed from a clinic, to ensure a sterile environment during birth—for the women in labor, her surroundings, the attendants, as well as the instruments? Similarly, how could birthing assistants[35] trained in "preaseptic times" be moved, if at all, to supplement their tried and tested experiences with new expertise and methods in battling germs?

To practice using the midwife's bag's equipment aseptically, Chief Physician for Midwifery and Gynecology Weiss considered the creation of "taster courses" he wanted all midwives in his department of the state hospital in Sarajevo to complete.[36] He imagined they ought to spend two weeks in the clinic to gain a theoretical understanding of aseptic conduct, practice it, and familiarize themselves with the instruments and the new legal regulations. However, providing instruction to the hospital's maternity ward, midwives

32 See the report of the Regional Office in Prozor from 1900: ABH, ZV, 1900, 52-11/58. See also Löwy, "The Social History of Medicine: Beyond the Local," 465–81.

33 There were no medical statistics to provide information until 1894, when the statistical Department was founded in Bosnia-Herzegovina. See Leopold Glück, "Über die Sanitätsverhältnisse unseres 'Okkupationsgebietes,' insbesondere über einige daselbst beobachtete Infektionskrankheiten," offprint from the Vienna Medical Press, 17, 19, 21, 22, 23, 24 (1884), 2. For statistics, see Angelika Strobel.

34 ABH, ZV, 1900, 52-11/58. Report of the Regional Office in Prozor.

35 In particular, I distinguish between "birth assistants" for companions of women giving birth of all stripes, and the officially legitimized "midwife" as the professional women.

36 ABH, ZMF, 1897, k. 52, 7660. Report by the provincial government on midwifery; Otto von Weiss, *Mittheilungen aus der Abtheilung für Geburtshilfe und Gynäkologie des bosn.-herceg. Landesspitals in Sarajevo (1. Juli 1894 bis 31. December 1896)* (Vienna: Safar, 1898), 32; ABH, ZMF, 1898, k. 70, 10641. The provincial government applied for the preferential treatment of premature births and miscarriages.

could not be guaranteed since there were too few suitable births to use as teaching cases. The paying patients from among the civil servant class and local elites, the primary users of the hospital's maternity services, were not inclined to allow their treatment to be used for educational purposes.[37] Similarly, the costs of hosting all the midwives in Sarajevo for two weeks would be too high, resulting in the agreement that only those midwives living in Sarajevo or those moving to Bosnia-Herzegovina should attend it. Others had to be trained locally by medical officers. It became the physicians' "earnest duty" to "personally introduce [midwifes], to appropriately explain to them the individual provisions [of the guidelines], and to awaken and actively maintain in them an appreciation of the nature and importance of antisepsis and asepsis."[38] From then on, midwives were subject to the local political offices with regards to staffing and disciplinary matters, and to the medical officer in professional ones.[39] The doctor was supposed to make it clear that permission to continue working as a midwife depended on how well she managed to adopt and implement the new guidelines, the outcomes of her bag's quarterly inspection, and how, more broadly, the relationship between midwife and medical officer developed.[40] Until then, it had been sufficient for the midwife to register at the local registry office, if she was a citizen of the Habsburg monarchy or of Bosnia-Herzegovina and could present qualifications issued by an authorized educational institution of the dual monarchy.[41] Acceptance of this registration by the administration was at the same time the permission to practice the profession. That changed decisively in 1898.

The medical officer in Bijeljina followed these regulations when he tried to summon the municipal midwife Aloisia Schwetz, with the support of the

37 ABH, ZMF, 1897, k. 52, 7660. Report by the provincial government on midwifery. The common practice of accepting poor women in labor in exchange for using them as "material" for midwives or medical students was widespread across all of nineteenth-century Europe. Maternity homes also often had foundling homes attached to them, where illegitimate children could be taken after being born. See Pawlowsky, *Mutter ledig—Vater Staat: das Gebär- und Findelhaus in Wien 1784–1910*; Scheutz, "Demand and Charitable Supply: Poverty and Poor Relief in Austria in the 18th and 19th Centuries," 52–95.

38 See for the quotations in this section: ABH, ZMF, 1898, k. 53, 8241. Report by the provincial government on the publication of the "Guidelines for Midwives."

39 HAS, Naputak za babice, 3–4.

40 ABH, ZMF, 1898, k. 53, 8241. Report by the provincial government on the publication of the "Guidelines for Midwives."

41 Decree 13791 from August 24, 1879, 110–12.

political authorities.[42] Aloisia Schwetz did not understand why she had to suddenly subject herself to repeated questionings by a physician, especially a doctor who had moved to Bijeljina after her. According to the official minutes, she responded that: "I have been here for ten years and have always done my duty." Her view was that the conflict with the doctor was caused by professional jealousy and competition. The medical officer, she testified, felt insulted because she would not recommend him to the wealthy households to which only she had entry; this is why he tried to take revenge on her with a lawsuit. In response, she submitted a countersuit against him to the same department.[43]

Similarly, the midwifery reform's implementation was taken very seriously by the local administration in other towns. Apparently, it directly established the future closer ties between political office, medical officer, and midwife. The officer was obliged to only hand a midwife a bag after her successful instruction and examination.[44] An archival box full of correspondence and non-standardized reports by various doctors and local officials document these encounters in the new constellation through which midwives had been more deeply integrated into state administration: a few doctors subjected the midwives to veritable exams, while others reported on the exemplary conduct of midwives during difficult births they had been brought in to assist with.[45]

Often, these reports also revealed tensions between midwife and physician or problems relating to material-practical, communication, and financial matters. For instance, some birth assistants who lacked writing skills were criticized. In this uncertain situation, in which the authorities had to judge midwives without having clear criteria to do so, literacy mutated into a means of differentiation. In two of about sixty documented cases, the relevant doctors or the political offices decided against giving "their" midwife the bag.[46] Both women were over sixty years old and, according to the report, could either not read or write, or only do so poorly. Because they had

42 All quotations in this section, unless otherwise noted, are taken from: ABH, ZV, 1903, 52-11/12.

43 She was not the only one issuing a countersuit: ABH, ZV, 1908, 105–45. Court trial.

44 ABH, ZMF, 1898, k. 53, 8241.

45 ABH, ZV, 1899, 52. Primalje.

46 See for the following examples: ABH, ZV, 1899, 52-9/15. Regional office Brčko to the D. Tuzla Kreis office; ABH, ZV, 1899. 52-9/30. Regarding the bag of midwife Gjurgja Jeftić: ABH, ZV, 1899, 52-9/45. District doctor to the district office in Konjic.

done so for a long time and enjoyed substantial support within the community, they were allowed to continue practicing their trade, but without the bag they became something like hybrid "half-midwives."

Once established through the conferral of the bag and the guidelines upon the midwife by the medical officer, their relationship was regularly refreshed through a repetitive administrative routine. Because the bag remained state property and its instruments were only being loaned to the midwife, she was subject to periodic surveillance.[47] The doctor was to take this opportunity to fortify the midwife's knowledge through repeated testing and passing on new scientific findings. The guidelines of 1898 consequently prescribed that medical officers should inspect the bag every three months (or even more frequently) and report complaints.[48] The midwife was summoned along with her bag and had to present it.[49] The doctor opened the tin box, untied the white parcels piece by piece, and removed the instruments and remedies from the tin clasps that held them. He inspected each one to determine whether the instruments were clean and the vials filled, and immediately returned them to their rightful place in the bag.

Most importantly, the medical officer had to be certain that the midwife had been using the disinfectants provided in the bag, as this was taken to be a confirmation that she was working aseptically. The medical officer questioned the midwife about the regulations and the births that had taken place. Based on the birth diary and the midwife's recollections, data were transcribed onto the birth tables for the quarter (or semester). At the end, the doctor refilled the consumables, which were provided free of charge.

The reports of these encounters, which were sent to Sarajevo, became increasingly homogenous over time. They were condensed down to tabular directories of all midwives in a given district: "Cleanliness of utensils found to be painstakingly maintained according to guidelines," "Bag's condition, tidy." The administrative methodology found its concrete, efficient, and rational linguistic expression, attuned to the column width of the directory of midwives. If a midwife refused to line up, this, too, was reported.[50]

47 See for the next sentence: ABH, ZMF, 1896, k. 3, 288. Promemoria Dr. Otto von Weiss.

48 ABH, ZMF, 1898, k. 53, 8241. Report by the provincial government on the publication of the "Guidelines for Midwives"; HAS, Naputak za babice, 3–4.

49 I imagined the following encounter based on the surviving administrative records.

50 ABH, ZV, 1912, k. 347, 105-2. Summative birth register of the Bihać district.

The appended birth tables and later the summative district birth registers up to 1917, often in the physician's handwriting, prove that the encounters between midwife and physician continued until the end of the period of Habsburg rule, and perhaps even beyond that.[51]

The condition of the bag was also the centerpiece of the argument put forward by the district judge as to why the dismissal of municipal midwife Aloisia Schwetz in Bijeljina in 1902 was appropriate.[52] He wrote that she apparently prioritized her personal needs over her duties as a midwife and, moreover, was a wholly unclean person. Furthermore, "her midwife's bag and its contents, despite years of ownership, today still look like new, and she herself admits that she does not take the bag to every birth because it is too heavy for her. She does not even know how to use the bag, for example, to boil the instruments, and similar [tasks]." The conclusions the judge drew following an inspection of the bag by the medical officer were apparent: a midwife that did not use the prescribed instruments, even admitted herself that she did not take them to every birth because the bag was too heavy for her, was not working aseptically, which means not according to the guidelines. The bag appears to be equated with the midwife. This could be a negative relationship, as it was for Aloisia Schwetz, but, in other situations, it could be a positive one. For instance, the Zvornik district physician Leopold Bauer began his reference for the midwife Therese Fischer Frauenglas, who had applied for the post vacated in Bijeljina, by saying that "the midwife [...] keeps her midwifery instruments perfectly clean and tidy."[53]

The relationship between the medical officer, the state institution, and the midwife was organized around the use of the midwife's bag. The use of the bag also served to stabilize the relationships among the midwives, who could now be seen as equal members in a profession and who carried out

51 The administrative praxis, that is, the reports, remained the same after 1906, when the second bag was introduced. After the First World War, when Habsburg rule in Bosnia-Herzegovina ended and Bosnia-Herzegovina became part of the Kingdom of Serbs, Croats, and Slovenes, printing was hampered by a paper shortage. Medical officers had to cut off the upper part of the old reports and glue them on to a new piece of paper to create new forms. See, for example, ABH, Zdravstveni odsjek ministarstva narodne zdravlje (ZOMNZ), 1923, k.89, 18.279. Antonia Savić, Prnjavor; ABH, ZV, 1906, K 85, 47-1 to 67. Midwives.

52 All quotations in this section, unless otherwise noted, are taken from: ABH, ZV, 1903, 52-11/12.

53 ABH, ZV, 1903, 52-11/12. The applicant was given the job on July 31, 1902, by the municipal council, but only worked there for half a year (officially, she resigned for family reasons). During that time, Aloisia Schwetz had continued to work as an independent midwife and was then rehabilitated by the district leader before being rehired by the municipal council on May 27, 1903, albeit with a lower salary.

their tasks in a consistent and regulated way.[54] The professionalization of the midwives as a group was a significant improvement in the healthcare situation as far as the administrators were concerned, because the birth attendants practicing in Bosnia-Herzegovina around 1900 had differed greatly from one another. The differences related to their social and cultural backgrounds, language skills, and religion, as well as their personal circumstances. About twelve percent of the midwives had been born in Bosnia-Herzegovina, with the majority of migrant midwives having been born in the neighboring Habsburg or Hungarian territories in Dalmatia, Croatia, and Slavonia.[55] None of them was Muslim, although Muslims formed about 40 percent of the residents. Almost twenty percent of all midwives came from Hungarian territories and were raised in Danube-Swabian settlements, where they spoke German and not Hungarian or the local language. Another twelve percent of the women who moved to Bosnia-Herzegovina had been born in a state structure that did not exist anymore in 1900: the former military borderlands. From there, they moved across the Sava River into the Bosnian borderlands, the Bosanska Krajina, where a similar "frontier" identity was common.[56] Formally, Serbian citizens did not fulfill the requirements to carry a work permit as a midwife, although Orthodox people made up more than 40 percent of the residents. The Austrian-Hungarian rulers' fear of Serbia led to a formally strict policy against everything and everyone "Serbian."[57] But reality was more complicated, as the college founded in Belgrade in 1899 was nonetheless still considered a legitimate educational institution and Serb-Orthodox–raised midwives who married Catholics in Bosnia-Herzegovina (and had converted to do so) were particularly popular with the Serb-Orthodox merchant elite.[58] Formally, they were attributed a religious affiliation that enabled them to work, whereas in reality they were being called upon for their previous religious denomination. This complex diversity of attributes, similarities, and boundaries faded

54 Crucial for this concept of professionalization is Labouvie, *Beistand in Kindsnöten: Hebammen und weibliche Kultur auf dem Land (1550–1910).*

55 ABH, ZV, 1900, k. 239. 52-11. Midwives; ABH, ZV, 1901, k. 237, 52-11. Midwives; ABH, ZV, 1902, 52-11. Midwives; ABH, ZV, 1903, k. 137, 52-11. Midwives; ABH, ZV, 1904, k. 39/40, 47. Midwives.

56 Smajić, *Bosanska krajina: Historija, legende i mitovi*; Matanović, *Grad na granici: slobodni vojni komunitet Brod na Savi od sredine 18. do sredine 19. stoljeća.*

57 Okey, *Taming Balkan Nationalism*, 74f.

58 For example Jelka Stojčić in Bosanski Petrovac. ABH, ZV, 1900, k. 239, 52-11/52 to 52-11/56. Birth tables of Jelka Stojčić. For the topic of conversion, see Gelez, "Se convertir en Bosnie-Herzégovine."

away with the seductive simplicity of what the bag offered: to contain everything that defined the professional midwife.

Leaning on established Austrian supranational concepts of belonging, the administration's ideal midwife was a neutral, professional woman whose allegiances lay with her profession and the bag, rather than her linguistic, cultural, and religious communities and background. This ideal also expressed itself in the fact that midwives were recorded in the administrative files without data on their religious denomination or ethnicity. This, though, did not address the needs of women giving birth and their families, neither those of the Habsburg civil servant families who had moved there, nor those of the upper classes in Bosnia-Herzegovina who preferred birth assistants they were close to.[59] An important exception consisted of the wealthy Muslim families which were loyal to the Habsburg elites and who were among the first to summon Habsburg midwives. Hence, in this latent conflict the bag could turn into the opposite: an expletive. It was a central component of the disparaging label for civil servants around 1900, *kuferaš*, which had two overlapping meanings.[60] The word derived from the term *kufer* borrowed from the German *Koffer*, that is, bag or suitcase, and so *kuferaš* denotes the "bag's bearer." But the Arabic word *kufr* resonates in it, too, which in Islam is the term for the "non-religion" of followers of the other book religions, Christians and Jews. The "unbelieving bag bearer" is, from a Bosnian perspective, therefore reduced to the bag they serve, as well as its contents, which represent their only property and signify their origin and "beliefs."[61] Such a life was not appealing to many Bosnian or Herzegovinian women or to many other citizens of the Habsburg monarchy at the end of the nineteenth century. Nonetheless, the midwives' services were in demand during emergencies, regardless of the bag, even if they were rather poorly equipped for extreme cases.

59 They insisted on their right of free choice, as we can see in the conflict between the two midwives Katharina Tautner and Agnes Kučer in Bosanski Brod in 1901. Wealthy women "effectively demonstrated their right of a free choice" by calling on the midwife of the neighboring town, Slavonski Brod, after the hiring of a municipal midwife in their own town, Bosanski Brod. See: ABH, ZV, 1902, 52-11/17.

60 Thank you to Prof. Dr. Carl Bethke and his students for the 2014 invitation to Tübingen to lecture in their seminar about the Habsburg monarchy and their helpful questions in the discussion.

61 A pretty description thereof can be found in Dževad Karahasan, *Sara i Serafina* (Sarajevo: Dobra knjiga, 2007), 98.

From the Bag's Tools to the Midwife's Modern Actions

If we look beyond its administrative function, the midwife's bag was, materially and in the first instance, a "vessel" that contained a range of objects. These objects were supposed to enable the midwife to realize her role as defined by the administration. Everything the bag contained was supposed to guide the midwife—from form to information—toward a "modern" mode of working.[62] Taking each object from the bag one at a time, I will use them to identify and explicate the "modern" duties of the midwife, starting with the description of each object as found in the 1898 "Guidelines for Midwives," which grouped them according to purpose.[63] The "bag" itself was not a soft container made of leather, but a hard case. If all the equipment was removed from the base and the lid, half of it could be filled with water or a soda water solution in which the objects could be boiled (and sterilized) on a spirit heat lamp or an oven. The tin case was covered with a dark, waterproof sheet in whose cavity (between bowl and sheet) one was supposed to store the prescribed apron and textbook.[64] A suitable handle was riveted to the case, and the bag could be carried over long distances. As we learned from the aforementioned Aloisia Schwetz, the midwife dismissed from Bijeljina in 1902, the bag was too heavy for her and she had to leave it at home sometimes. She was not the only midwife to do so; the bag's weight was one of the main reasons a new and lighter bag was introduced in 1906, the Nowakowski bag.[65] By 1908, the bag was being used across the monarchy (see Figure 4.1).[66] That the bag was also thought to be intimidatingly large can be seen from a 1898 report from Stolac: "In particular, people are startled by the bag's size."[67] The bag substantially changed the midwife's appearance.

62 Thévenot, "Die Pluralität kognitiver Formate," 260f.

63 HAS, Naputak za babice, 4–7. How the items were to be used, and what their precise purpose was, was explained in detail in the appendix to the "Guidelines," the "Instructions" (*pouka*). See ibid., 16–38. I also consulted the teaching materials for midwives used at the Midwife College in Zagreb: Antun Lobmayer, *Primaljstvo: učevna knjiga za primalje* (Zagreb: Kraljevska zemaljska naklada, 1898). I thank Salome Stauffer, a historically well-versed midwife in Zurich, for helping me imagine what the instruments and substances were used for. Thank you also to Kristin Hammer, lecturer at the College for Applied Sciences in Zurich, Department for Midwives, for the critical review of the description of the objects.

64 Beside the textbook, the bag contained a "diary" and the "Guidelines for Midwives": HAS, Naputak za babice, 4–7, 15.

65 ABH, ZV, 1906, k. 85, 47-1. New midwife's bag.

66 Image from Rüb et al., *Aller Anfang*, 253.

67 ABH, ZV, 1899, 52-9/45. Mostar Kreis office to the provincial government (reports of the districts of Mostar, Nevesinje, Konjica, Ljubinje, Ljubuški, Trebinje, Stolac, and Bilek).

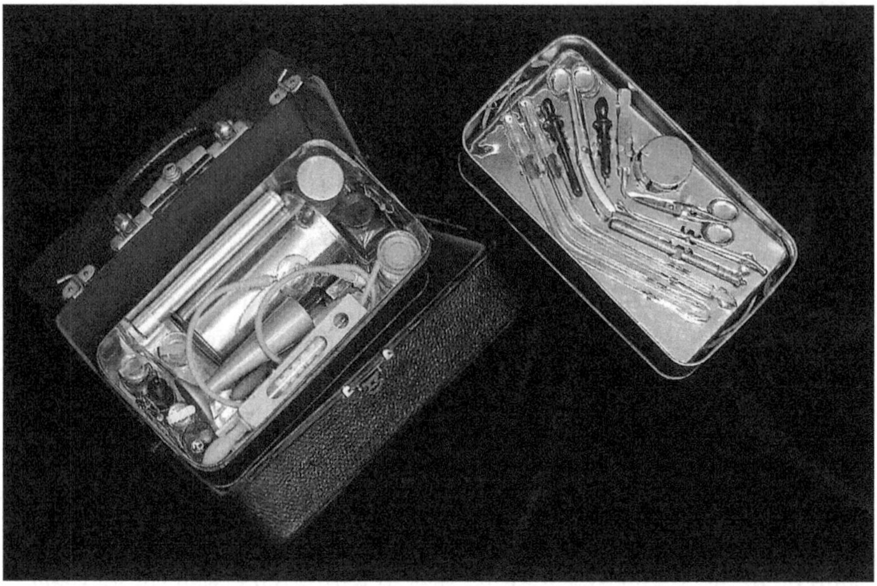

Figure 4.1: *The Nowakowski Bag*, introduced for midwives in Bosnia-Herzegovina in 1906. Scan of the photo by Ernst Reinberger, "Hebammentasche nach Nowakowski," printed in Dorothea Rüb et al., *Aller Anfang* (Vienna: Österreichisches Museum für Volkskunde, 2002), 253. Copyright by Anton Schaller.[68]

The most conspicuous and largest component in the Nowakowski bag was a piece of irrigation equipment. This irrigator came with attachments that enabled the midwife to perform vaginal douching and enemas on mother and child.[69] One of the tubes had a small hole that could be used in an emergency to inject hot water, which would stop heavy bleeding,[70] but generally the main purpose of the apparatus was to "purify" the mother before and after birth, as well as the newborn. This procedure was the modern equivalent of an ancient custom—purification through irrigation, suction, and other methods designed to release or balance humors in the body. This practice was part of a broader understanding of bodily equilibrium that had emerged from antiquity (starting with Galen), been handed down

68 I would like to thank the Prof. Dr. Anton Schaller as well as the Österreichische Museum für Volkskund in Vienna for the permission to reprint the above images. Despite thorough investigations not all possible copyright owners could be identified. In case I have by any chance and involuntarily infringed on any copyright, I hereby declare that the use of the images is entirely non-commercial and solely serves educational purposes. Therefore, I claim that the use of the images meets the requirements of the fair use statute.

69 HAS, Naputak za babice, 4–7.

70 HAS, Naputak za babice, 29–31.

through Arabic translations of ancient Greek medical texts, and was very much alive in Bosnia-Herzegovina.[71] The concrete action of purifying the mother through irrigation before giving birth was in essence the same, but the ways of doing it and their interpretation changed. The new irrigation equipment introduced in 1898 replaced the simple enema syringes that the midwives had been using only a few years previously.[72] Therefore, these new objects, through a retrospective extension of their use and the knowledge to describe and interpret the actions, speak to a continuity in practice while they experienced a change in form and knowledge. What is "modern" in this example is the mode, the shape, and the interpretation of the action—the attributes become the essence.

A similar example can be seen in the cord bands. One of the most ancient responsibilities of the midwife was to cut the umbilical cord between newborn and mother. For this purpose, in 1898 the bag contained simple cord bands to tie the cord and a pair of cord scissors to cut it.[73] These bands can be compared with contemporary cord bands that have been preserved in the State Museum, which was founded in 1888. The bands in the museum were embroidered with congratulatory messages from members of the local elites and were part of collections of objects relating to national culture and medicine designed to represent different birthing traditions.[74] The material used to make the bands was a strong fabric not too different from those in the museum. The key difference between the two types of bands is the decoration (congratulations and dedications) on the museum bands. In 1898, such embellishments were considered by medical authorities as expressions of a "backward" folk culture rooted in a mix of religion and tradition. The new, unadorned bands were thus part of the move toward the spread of "modern" and "clean" medical practices.

The modern ritual of cleaning involved other tools in the bag and was also designed to replace the traditional and religious actions accompanying birthing. In the "Guidelines for Midwives,"[75] the process of cleansing was imagined as follows: first, the midwife had to clean herself and her en-

71 Mašić, *Korjeni medicine i zdravstva u Bosni i Hercegovini.*

72 ABH, ZMF, 1888, k. 53, 9092.

73 HAS, Naputak za babice, 4–7.

74 Zemaljski Muzej (ZM), Odjeljenje za etnologiju, Zbirka narodne medicine i narodnih vjerovanja. Danijela Križanec-Beganović compiled an inventory of this collection in 2008.

75 HAS, Naputak za babice, 7–8, 16f.

vironment. Her personal hygiene was important, because her body was seen as the main source of dirt and germs, which could be transmitted to the parturient. The guidelines placed great emphasis on the midwives' nail care, because dirt could easily gather underneath nails and also because sharp or long nails could injure the mother during internal examinations. For this purpose the bag contained a metal emery board, nail scissors, and a nailbrush.[76] The apron protected the midwives' clothes from serious staining. Second, the midwife had to disinfect the instruments, boil water, and mix sufficient disinfectant liquids. The delicate cleaning materials served to combat germs and consisted of a piece of good white soap or 50 grams of soft soap housed in a glass or tin container in the bag.[77] For disinfection purposes there were 100 grams of Lysol in a dark bottle along with the corresponding glass stoppers as seals. Ensuring the correct solution was in itself a problem, because if the Lysol was not diluted enough it could cause severe burning, and if it was overdiluted it would be less effective. A small glass measuring tube with engraved markings helped the midwife measure the precise amounts that, diluted with boiled water, made the correct disinfectant solution. The bottle was to be labeled either "Lysol" or "poison" as it was a dangerous substance, and yet clinical trials on women had—for various reasons—showed it to be the most appropriate option.[78]

In the third part of the imagined ideal ritual, it was the pregnant woman's turn to be cleaned.[79] If the stage of labor she was at permitted it, she could be bathed, her whole body washed, and subsequently dressed in clean clothes. In any case there should be enough time to clean her stomach and abdomen with sterile water and disinfecting fluids. At this point an external examination could be carried out, during which the midwife (according to the textbook of the Zagreb Midwifery College) was supposed to take note of the size of the belly, the shape of the womb, the contractions, the movements of the baby and its position, the size of the pelvis, waist, and genitals, as well as the birthing woman's strength.[80] Following a repeated, complete

76 HAS, Naputak za babice, 20–21, 25.

77 Compare the passage: HAS, Naputak za babice, 5, 19, 26.

78 Lobmayer, *Primaljstvo*, III; "Bericht über das Jahr 1891," *Jahresbericht über die Fortschritte auf dem Gebiete der Geburtshilfe und Gynäkologie* 5 (1892): 303. Lysol was first introduced in Germany in 1889 by Dr. Gustav Raupenstrauch.

79 HAS, Naputak za babice, 23f.

80 Lobmayer, *Primaljstvo*, 87–9.

cleansing of her hands, the midwife was to conduct an internal examination by feeling the cervix and uterus, determining whether labor had set in, how far along it had progressed, and whether the baby had reached the pelvis. Before this period, internal examination was not a common part of the birthing process, which explains why this stage of the process is covered in such detail in the textbook and guidelines.[81] If the midwife found serious irregularities, she was supposed to verify her findings. The main preoccupation of the authorities was to prevent puerperal fever, even though it does not seem to have been widespread in Bosnia-Herzegovina in this period. In some regions of Bosnia-Herzegovina it was even unknown, according to reports by women physicians.[82] To help evaluate whether there were disease-causing germs at play, the bag contained a thermometer, the single entirely new addition to the midwife's basic equipment. If the thermometer showed the women's body temperature to be over 38 degrees Celsius, the midwife was to tell the woman's husband or another family member to summon a doctor, who would have the additional instruments and expertise to hand a problematic birth. In essence, the thermometer was the midwife's yardstick in differentiating a physiologically healthy from a pathological confinement.[83]

The reconstruction of the administrations' ideal conception revealed a gap: the midwife's bag lacked operative instruments, which included not only forceps but also a scalpel or even a simple needle.[84] The training given to many midwives in Bosnia-Herzegovina at the Zagreb Midwifery College taught them that they were only responsible for "orderly" or "normal" births, that is, "if the women can give birth without help and without danger to her health or the baby's health."[85] In the case of "extraordinary" births, "when she [the woman giving birth] needs to be supported with hands, or with instruments or when mother and child [might] die during labor," midwives had to call upon the physician. The midwife's role in childbirth was limited

81 Ibid; HAS, Naputak za babice, 7–8, 16f.

82 See various reports by female physicians, for example: ABH, ZV, 1900, 52-11/51 and ABH, ZV, 1907, k. 51, 38–9. Reports Olszewska; Das Sanitätswesen in Bosnien und der Hercegovina, 1878–1918, mit 2 Abbildungen und 2 Karten, herausgegeben von der Landesregierung für Bosnien und die Hercegovina. (Sarajevo: Landesdruckerei 1903), 26.

83 *Jahresbericht über die Fortschritte auf dem Gebiete der Geburtshilfe und Gynäkologie* 2 (1889): 82.

84 This was not the case across all of Europe. For example, midwives in Scandinavian countries around this time carried short forceps alongside knives and scissors in their bag. *Jahresbericht über die Fortschritte auf dem Gebiete der Geburtshilfe und Gynäkologie* 4 (1891): 351–4.

85 Lobmayer, *Primaljstvo*, 71–2.

to patiently waiting with the pregnant woman under the assumption that a woman could manage a natural birth by herself. In her bag, the midwife had two stimulants and no means of pain control. In case of weakness Hoffmann's Drops could be administered,[86] and a cinnamon tincture was presumably administered to induce and amplify contractions. So the midwife was to ensure clean conditions before and after birth, between which the spontaneous and "natural" birth could take its course. The midwife was supposed to merely observe the birth attentively and not intervene. We might assume that experienced birth attendants had the means and techniques to assist births, but this is not the story the normative sources are telling us.

This meant that a birth attendant working as a midwife in Bosnia-Herzegovina around 1900 had no equipment to use in the case of an extraordinary or difficult birth, no instruments to support an intervention, as they were all held by the doctor. "[I]f such an emergency arose, such where one cannot wait for the doctor to come, as commonly happens in rural areas—then the midwife must do the work herself and conduct even such midwifery tasks that the doctor would do manually under the circumstances, but only of the kind that she has been taught at the institution, without using any kind of instruments."[87] This contradictory situation arose in Bosnia-Herzegovina as there were relatively few obstetrically trained physicians, and even these were poorly trained. Midwives were also called with the hope of not having to summon the doctor, that is, not only in the case of emergency, but also when the expectant mother was worried (she was young or of an advanced age, she was having her first child, she had had a high number of births, she had a history of miscarriages or other bad experiences of birthing, etc.) or was socially isolated and in need.[88]

The lack of real instruments in case of a childbirth emergency was not the only ambiguity regarding midwives and their bags. The introduction and free provision of Lysol as the main disinfectant in the 1898 incarnation of the bag soon resulted in several court cases, in which midwives were accused of having aided or carried out an abortion. The first known trial

86 This was derived from "liquor anodynus mineralis" (also called "spiritus aetherus") by Friedrich Hoffmann, and was composed of sulfuric acid and a small amount of ether. See for the passage: ABH, ZMF, 1888, k. 53, 9092; Müller-Jahncke, "Hoffmannstropfen."

87 Lobmayer, *Primaljstvo*, 1.

88 ABH, ZV, 1900, k. 239, 52-11/52 bis 52-11/56. Birth tables.

known dates from 1902, when a midwife from Prijedor and another in Banja Luka were taken into custody and accused of complicity in providing abortions.[89] In another case from Sarajevo from 1906, a fifty-seven-year-old midwife was convicted of having carried out an abortion on an unmarried cook using Lysol.[90] The accused cook explained that she had asked the midwife for help because her period ("her time") had stopped and "there had been no washing" for three months. The inquiry appeared undecided until the hospital's physician confirmed "that a hot liquid with Lysol was injected into the belly." Lysol had been injected into the uterus, where it provoked an abortion. This method was safer than others, but the use of an incorrectly mixed Lysol solution caused severe internal burning. The cook, as the doctor expounded in court, had been in hospital for thirty days with a serious internal injury, probably caused by the disinfectant, which had been injected by the midwife, the only person legally having access to the substance. Thus, the most potent cleaning agent in the bag of the midwife reversed its purpose and was used to carry out an abortion.

Conclusion

In this chapter, I approached the modern Austrian-Hungarian regulation of midwifery in Bosnia-Herzegovina symmetrically through the midwife and her bag, shedding light onto the material side of modernity. The development of midwifery followed the professionalization of all medical activities, but what was unique about Bosnia-Herzegovina was the way it was adopted. The intensity of colonial demands and top-down implementation opened up a large gap between imperial claims and the local response. From the moment of its introduction in 1898, the midwife's bag played a key role in creating a concrete, material management system for midwives. These women, who came to Bosnia-Herzegovina mostly from the Habsburg monarchy, first needed to be integrated into the Habsburg administrative system, so that the state could guarantee a framework of midwifery to care for women in childbirth. Beyond this, the midwife's bag worked as a unifying tool, turning the birth assistants from diverse social and cultural back-

89 ABH, ZV, 1902, 52-11/53. Inquest into abortion.
90 For the rest of the section: ABH, ZV, 1906, 47–67. Withdrawal of the midwife's license.

grounds into professionals—modern midwives. In accordance with the requirements of the administration, the midwife's bag contained everything a midwife needed to perform her task in a modern, "clean" way. Ideally, she had to be a neutral bag bearer, a professional whose allegiances lay with the bag and were not determined by her background or her personal affiliations. The use and application of the midwife's bag worked to establish a professional class of midwives under the direction of a central administration and to provide them with a tool to monitor births. Finally, a repetitive administrative routine was used to establish the relationships between the main medical actors around childbirth, which continued after the First World War and the end of Habsburg rule in Bosnia-Herzegovina.

Tracing the introduction of the midwife's bag reveals the ideal of the neutral midwife and the function of material culture in providing a new "modern" meaning to well-known actions. The technical features of the Nowakowski bag sustained the modern ritual of a "clean birth." This concept can easily be located as an element in the contemporary cleanliness dispositive.[91] It is via these practices in creating cleanliness and health that the midwife was assigned her role by the state and her purpose in establishing and tending to the health of mothers and newborns. The midwife's bag with its corresponding instruments supported and shaped the birth assistant far more in her role as the "cleaner" than any guidelines, textbooks, or birth registers.[92] The embodiment of the modern professional midwife could succeed only with the help of the bag. The lack of real instruments in cases of emergency is one of the gaps caused by modernity, and these ambiguities, like the possible use of Lysol as an abortifacient, show us the path to modernity.

91 Burschel and Marx (eds.), *Reinheit*; Fayet (ed.), *Verlangen nach Reinheit oder Lust auf Schmutz?*; see also Douglas, *Purity and Danger: An Analysis of the Concepts of Pollution and Taboo*; Sarasin, *Reizbare Maszchinen: eine Geschichte des Körpers 1765–1914*.

92 Dodier, "Konventionen als Stützen der Handlung," 75.

PART II
Public Health After Europe's World Wars

CHAPTER V

Who Belongs to the Healthy Body of the Nation? Health and National Integration in Poland and the Polish Army after the First World War

Katrin Steffen

Introduction

Following the First World War the formation of new states in Central and Eastern Europe, including Poland, coincided on the one hand with the necessity to cope with the huge devastation the war had left and the legacy of the fallen empires, and on the other hand with a phase of rapid change and high social mobility. Large segments of society were affected by the war, be it by disease, the loss of family members, or the reordering of family and gender relations during the years following the war. The period between 1918 and 1939 was a potentially unstable period of transition, in which an exemplary and contentious transformation of those lands that had formerly been divided among Prussia, Austria-Hungary, and Russia were combined into a new Polish state. The Poland that emerged was the result of the war, of the peace treaties of Versailles, as well as of the Polish-Russian War. Rather than think of it as constituting a "nation-state"—indeed, 30 percent of the population belonged to a national minority—it would be more accurate to call it a "nationalizing state."[1] Nevertheless, for many people—especially those on the political right—and increasingly after the assassination of President Gabriel Narutowicz in 1922, who was accused of being a president elected by the minorities, the state was mainly conceptualized as an ethnic nation-

1 Brubaker, "Nationalizing States in the 'Old New' Europe—and the New."

state; the kind of nation-state that the elite of the country, the *inteligencja*, had desired for a long time.[2] Hence, from 1918 on, this nation-state as well as the others in the region constantly had to prove their superiority against the former empires as a form of political organization of society; there was also a strong need of those almost always contested states of the region to prove their legitimacy. Therefore, the pressure for this undertaking to be a success was high. At the same time, this constellation also created a space of possibilities, full of opportunities and challenges, in which established social, political, economical, ethnic, and gender relations were ordered anew. In this way, Poland became "a living laboratory" for experiments in modern life, producing new models of politics, self-help, culture, and identification.[3]

This holds true also for the fields of public health and public hygiene, which will be further highlighted in this chapter.[4] After a long period of being a nation without being a state, concern over the national existence in a biological sense played an important role in discourses about modernization—matters of health went along with striving for modernization in Poland. Consequently, the first minister of health in Poland, the physician, hygienist, and eugenicist Tomasz Janiszewski, wrote in a letter to the president of the United States that his ministry was intended to produce a "new breed of men."[5] But who was to form this "new breed of men" in a country where 30 percent of the inhabitants were members of the minority groups of Jews, Germans, Ukrainians, Lithuanians, and Belorussians? The question arises if and how those minority groups were to be included into the national program to create the "new men." In this chapter, I will explore how the system of public health in Poland emerged out of the necessities the war created, and how the minorities (especially the Jewish population) were regarded. I will also delve into the close interaction between health policy and the defense of the country. This means asking how institutions such as the Polish Army conceptualized the "healthy bodies" of soldiers of different ethnicities, since it was a declared goal of the army to absorb the

2 Sdvižkov, *Das Zeitalter der Intelligenz. Zur vergleichenden Geschichte der Gebildeten in Europa bis zum Ersten Weltkrieg*, 135–6.

3 Kassow, 'On the Jewish Street 1918–1939,' in *Polin: 1000 Year History of Polish Jews*. Kassow states this for Jewish life in Poland, but this can be applied to the whole of Poland as well.

4 For a more detailed analysis of the public health sector, see Steffen, "Experts and the Modernization of the Nation: The Arena of Public Health in Poland in the First Half of the 20th Century."

5 Tomasz Janiszewski, "The Versailles Treaty and the Question of Public Health," *International Journal of Public Health* 2 (1921): 140–51.

national minorities for the Polish state, to educate them to become loyal citizens of the state and—primarily in the case of the Slavic minorities—to Polonize them.[6]

Public Health in Poland: The Hour of the Experts

In 1918, public health in Poland first and foremost had the functional role of preventing epidemic infectious diseases and providing a hygienic infrastructure for a country that until 1920 had to deal with six armed conflicts at its borders. Poland was largely materially destroyed and economically devastated. It had suffered huge human losses and the population was seriously undernourished and poor.[7] Migration from east to west and from west to east during and after the war also accounted for the spread of contagious diseases.[8] In contrast to many soldiers, who had been vaccinated while serving in the armies of the partition powers, Poland's civilian population had not enjoyed this "privilege" and was affected more often by diseases than servicemen. Especially in the countryside—and 70 percent of the Polish population lived in rural areas—hygienic conditions were described as highly dissatisfying.[9]

Besides the functional role public health had to play in the fight against diseases and in the development of a national administration and a social infrastructure, it also served ideological ends by enhancing social and ethnic cohesion and setting normative values in terms of behavior, consumption, physical fitness, gender relations, and relations of the majority toward minority groups. Public health was an arena in which meaning and relevance were produced for and in complex interaction with an audience for which precisely this meaning had to be understandable—or else be made understandable. Some voices in Poland went so far as to call for the establishment of a kind of biological order of the state. These people viewed the nation as an "organization based on a biogenetic community"[10] and in this

6 Wierzbicki, "Białorusini w Wojsku Polskim (1921–1939)."

7 Balińska, "The National Institute of Hygiene and Public Health in Poland, 1918–1939."

8 On international (mainly US) help and relief programs for Poland during this period, see Rodogno, Piana, and Gauthier, "Shaping Poland: Relief and Rehabilitation Programmes Undertaken by Foreign Organizations, 1918–1922."

9 See, for example, Posłuszna, "Stan sanitarno-higieniczny wsi polskiej w okresie II Rzeczypospolitej."

10 Adam Paszewski, "Znaczenie biologji dla społeczeństwa," *Odbitka z Czasopisma Przyrodniczego* 7–8 (1931): 1–8.

way wanted to discipline bodies and regulate the (seemingly excessive) population. Such concerns are typical issues in biopolitics. Medical expertise and public health were therefore used to develop political stability, a productive industry, and military manpower. During the interwar period the care for physical education, and in a broader sense for the body culture of the entire society, became an important element of the defense policy of the country.[11] Health turned out to be of immediate importance to the new state.[12]

The dynamic development of public health and hygiene in Poland first arose from the necessity to fight large epidemic diseases following the First World War, especially typhus, which quickly spread from Russia and Ukraine. Poland fulfilled her responsibility to act as a cordon sanitaire to protect the rest of Europe from diseases that were perceived to be "oriental" or "bolshevik" plagues.[13] International, especially American, aid programs and American experts in the region (for example, the American Red Cross) played a significant role in providing financial aid, fighting typhus, creating a cordon sanitaire on the eastern border, and enforcing strict quarantine rules.[14] The Rockefeller Foundation took an interest in Poland and its role in improving health conditions in Europe and the advancement of American models of public health and hygiene in the region. The synthetic American idea of "public health" corresponded well with the ideas formulated by Polish health experts and was supposed to limit German medical influence in the region.[15] Experts from abroad interacted with domestic experts in establishing national politics and organizations. For example, the Cracow professor Emil Godlewski assumed control over all typhus relief operations, while Ludwik Rajchman, a member of the League of Nations Epidemic Commission, developed a much-praised operational plan to prevent further outbreaks of the disease by creating sanitary zones in key areas.[16]

11 Jan Kęsik, *Naród pod bronią. Społeczeństwo w programie polskiej polityki wojskowej 1918–1939* (Wrocław: Wydawnictwo Uniwersytetu Wrocławskiego, 1998), 155.

12 For a similar approach in neighboring Russia, see Sparks, *The Body Soviet: Propaganda, Hygiene and the Revolutionary State.*

13 Balińska, "The Rockefeller Foundation and the National Institute of Hygiene, Poland, 1918–1945," 422.

14 Rodogno, Piana, and Gauthier, "Shaping Poland," 270–1.

15 See Weindling, "From Disease Prevention to Population Control: The Realignment of Rockefeller Foundation Policies in the 1920s to 1950s," in *American Foundations and the Coproduction of World Order in the Twentieth Century*, 127–8.

16 Ibid.

The dynamics of development were reassembled on an institutional level after 1918, when a preliminary Polish administration was built which included health matters. In February 1917, the Department of the Interior instituted a subdivision for public health, which later grew into a "department," then a "section" and a "direction," and finally a "ministry" in April 1918. The above-mentioned Tomasz Janiszewski was appointed as the first minister of health in Poland. A university professor in Cracow, Janiszewski had received his scientific training in medicine and bacteriology at universities in Freiburg, Vienna, and Zurich. He had already played a prominent role in advocating for the independent state administration of health matters headed by a medical expert before Polish independence.[17] The foundation of the ministry took place in an overall difficult situation, since regulations in legislation, the economy, and administration were different in the partitioned lands and had to be unified, a highly complex process that did not fully come to an end until 1939. In addition, Poland had to struggle with a notorious lack of capital during most of the interwar period. Central planning and state subsidies, therefore, played a decisive role not only in the development of science, but also in regards to innovations in technology or medicine and their implementation in various branches of industry or health institutions. Furthermore, in the health sector the country lacked a highly differentiated landscape of private or state research institutions and universities. But this, however, also provided the advantage of making a relatively coherent and unified system possible. This complex situation provided health and hygiene experts with unique challenges and opportunities of the kind they would not have had in the more "established" states of Western Europe.[18]

In addition to the Ministry of Health, the Central Institute of Epidemiology was established in 1918 in Warsaw to act as a governmental agency to deal with the epidemic crisis in Poland following the First World War. The aim of the institute was to gather scientific knowledge in the field of epidemics, regarding both diagnosis and prevention, and to coordinate antiepidemic measures on a nationwide scale. The institute came into being following the initiative of Rajchman, who served as its first head. It later became the State Institute of Hygiene and dealt with all aspects of public health in

17 Tomasz Janiszewski, *O wymogach zdrowotnych przy odbudowie kraju* (Kraków, 1916).

18 See Steffen and Kohlrausch, "The Limits and Merits of Internationalism: Experts, the State and the International Community in Poland in the First Half of the Twentieth Century," 717.

Poland. Its effects were recognized on a worldwide scale, as was stated by experts on the International Health Board of the Rockefeller Foundation: "Dr. Rajchman, despite the difficulties of war conditions, has developed perhaps the best public health laboratory service in Continental Europe with the exception of Denmark—a central laboratory in Warsaw; branches at Lemberg, Cracov, Lodz, Thorn and Lublin; all in one administrative system under [the] health service."[19]

Rajchman, later the head of the Health Organization of the League of Nations and the founder of UNICEF, had received his medical training at the Jagiellonian University in Habsburg Cracow and had studied in Paris at the Institute Pasteur and in London at the Royal Institute of Public Health. As soon as independence had become possible, Rajchman came back to Poland and brought with him medical knowledge from the Habsburg Empire and from abroad, especially from London. To deal with the epidemic and the postwar health situation in Poland, he established the institute and to staff it gathered the most talented researchers and medical practitioners he could find. This was not an easy task since many of them had left the country before 1918 and had not yet returned (or did not want to return) to Poland. Despite this difficulty, Rajchman managed to persuade some outstanding scientists, among them his cousin, the well-known serologist and physician Ludwik Hirszfeld, to join the institute.[20] Hirszfeld had spent his years of education and research mainly in Germany and Switzerland and was very well known for his work in the field of serology. Since he spent the years of the First World War in Serbia and at Saloniki, where he encountered large epidemics of typhus, typhoid, and malaria, he was also very experienced in fighting epidemics and in epidemiology. When Rajchman left Warsaw in the early 1920s to become director of the Health Organization of the League of Nations, Hirszfeld unofficially replaced him as director of the State Institute of Hygiene (Rajchman retained the title of director of the institute until 1932). Rajchman, Hirszfeld, and many other researchers at the institute, such as Kazimierz Funk (who formulated the concept of the "vitamin") had all spent part of their life abroad, mainly for educational reasons, but some,

19 Rockefeller Foundation, RG 1.1, 789, Box 1, Folder 1, Minutes of the International Health Board, May 1922.

20 See Gromulska, "Ludwik Hirszfeld in the National Institute of Hygiene 1920–1941"; Steffen, "Migration, Transfer und Nation: Die Wissensräume polnischer Naturwissenschaftler im 20. Jahrhundert," in *Europäische Wissenschaftskulturen und politische Ordnungen in der Moderne (1890–1970)*.

like Hirszfeld, were already very well established in the scientific circles of their host country.

The constellation of a "homecoming" elite was not unusual. Since the newly formed state felt a strong need for expert knowledge in the building and reorganizing of its administration and institutions—a desire that was central to its self-conception as a "modern" successor state of the former empires—many researchers and academics who had been trained abroad during the time of partition were requested to return home. Some worked in the humanities, but even more worked in the natural and technical sciences. A strong motive to come back to Poland, whose structures were often not as well developed as in the countries the scientists came from, was likely that they expected to advance quickly in the newly built universities of Warsaw, Vilna, and Poznan. Indeed, the reestablishment of Poland offered chances (especially for younger scientists) they would have not had in the established countries from which they came. One-third of the university professors in the newly formed Poland had studied outside Polish structures of higher learning, while this proportion in the technical sciences was as high as 50 percent.[21]

As a result, many multifaceted processes of knowledge transfer from and into different directions took place in Poland. These new elites had gained a wide variety of experiences in three state traditions (not counting those who had been outside of the partitioned lands), experiences that now had to be incorporated into the structures of the new state.[22] These processes of knowledge transfer and the appropriation by national elites who were mainly trained at foreign universities constitute an important factor for Polish science and its institutions after 1918. Intense and continuous interaction between local and international agencies also continued during the interwar period. For example, the Rockefeller Foundation provided its Polish fellows with grants that were much higher than those coming from Germany.[23] These processes were not always free of conflict, since the elites coming

21 Dorota Mycielska, "Drogi życiowe profesorów przed objęciem katedr akademickich w niepodległej Polsce," in *Inteligencja Polska XIX i XX wieku*, ed. Ryszard Czepulis-Rastenis (Warsaw: Polska Akademia Nauk. Instytut Historii, 1981), vol. 2, 263.

22 This holds true for experts from many fields—Morgane Labbé, for example, makes this claim in relation to population experts. See "'Reproduction' as a New Demographic Issue in Interwar Poland," 37.

23 Weindling, "Public Health and Political Stabilisation: The Rockefeller Foundation in Central and Eastern Europe between the Two World Wars."

from abroad were sometimes met with caution by those who had stayed in Poland, especially when they came from countries perceived as potentially hostile toward Poland, such as Germany or Russia.[24] On the whole, however, this constellation of talent resulted in the outstanding ability of numerous Eastern European scholars to move and communicate in a multilingual and multiconfessional environment.[25]

This outlines a transnational space not only for the formation of sciences that was absent in most Western countries, but also for the emerging institutions of the new state. It should also be asked, however, how much the transnational space during this period was subsequently "nationalized" and adapted to the specific needs of the Polish state or the Polish nation? This was a more or less double-sided process: between scientists and the nation-state a complex structure and relationship arose which does not equal simple dichotomies—on the one hand an innocent, universal, and internationally oriented expert or scientist, and on the other hand an increasingly authoritarian state thinking only in state-oriented categories.[26] Rather, we find an entanglement in which both politics and sciences constituted "resources for each other."[27] Scientists wanted not only to profit from state funding—they also wanted to make their knowledge available for the modernization of the Polish nation and Polish society. "Modernization" was as topical as "backwardness," and crises resulting from the country's presumed backwardness were heatedly debated. Scientists and experts wanted Poland to catch up with supposedly "modern" Western developments, with modern European culture, but not just in a superficial way.

Modernization was to be achieved through the development of one's own institutions and individuals. Experts in the health sector were eager to develop their structures, in order to secure Poland a substantial role within global health politics (which they did quite successfully). Rajchman, for example, was an internationally admired figure, and as such was able to organize support from the Rockefeller Foundation for Poland on a large scale.

24 Marta A. Balińska, for example, asks whether Ludwik Hirszfeld's research did receive less financial aid than that of Kazimierz Funk, who came from the United States to Poland, while Hirszfeld's networks were mainly German-speaking ones. See Balińska, "The Rockefeller Foundation and the National Institute of Hygiene," 428.

25 See Kohlrausch, Steffen, and Wiederkehr (eds.), *Expert Cultures in Central Eastern Europe.*

26 See Steffen and Kohlrausch, "The Limits and Merits of Internationalism," 737.

27 Ash, "Wissenschaft und Politik als Ressourcen füreinander," in *Wissenschaften und Wissenschaftspolitik. Bestandsaufnahmen zu Formationen, Brüche und Kontinuitäten im Deutschland des 20. Jahrhunderts.*

One of the officers of the Rockefeller Foundation in Europe and a member of its International Health Division, Selskar M. Gunn, attested that he was "a very energetic and clever man who has done a wonderful piece of work in Poland during and since the war in the creation of the Central Institute of Hygiene at Warsaw. [...] There is a certain British flavor to his ideas, which is of course due to his contact of years with the Royal Sanitary Institute."[28] At the time Gunn wrote this, Rajchman had started an initiative to build a school of hygiene in Warsaw as a complementary educational institution to the State Institute of Hygiene. Gunn approved of the plan: "I think it must be conceded that in general his plan is a good one. [...] I think that Rajchman feels that Poland is entitled to consideration particularly on account of the fact that she did so much herself unaided during and since the war in public health work both in laboratory and field. In justice to Poland, I think this must be conceded. It was largely however because of the energy of Rajchman, who despite an enormous prejudice against him on account of his being a Jew was able to put the thing over."[29] Although both Rajchman and Hirszfeld came from assimilated families and identified mainly as Polish patriots, they frequently were considered as Jews—a situation many people with a Jewish background faced, not only in Poland. And just like Rajchman and Hirszfeld, many Poles with a Jewish background had chosen a medical profession, since those professions had long provided a unique possibility for upward mobility for everyone and everywhere in Europe. In 1931, 46 percent of all doctors in Poland were Jews, and 55 percent of all practicing physicians. In Lwów their number reached 65 percent.[30] Many non-Jewish doctors, students, and journalists made a veritable problem out of this situation. They called vehemently for a *numerus clausus* for Jewish medical students and inserted a so-called Aryan paragraph into the Union of Doctors of the Polish State in 1937.[31] Although Hirszfeld and Rajchman were also affected by this situation, they successfully used their personal and professional networks during the early years of the interwar period to make Warsaw a scientific center for public hygiene and public health and for research on epidemics and infectious diseases. Poland hosted many inter-

28 Rockefeller Archives RG 1.1, Series 789, Box1, Folder 1, Selskar M. Gunn to Wickliffe Rose, July 8, 1921.

29 Ibid.

30 Polonsky, *The Jews in Poland and Russia, Vol. III: 1914–2008*, 61; Ignacy Einhorn, *Towarzystwo Ochrony Zdrowia Ludności Żydowskiej w Polsce w latach 1921–1950* (Toruń: Adam Marszałek 2008), 60.

31 Einhorn, *Towarzystwo*, 58.

national conferences, such as a large sanitary conference in Warsaw in 1922, organized by the League of Nations Epidemics Commission. In addition, in 1927, the International Congress for Military Medicine and Pharmacy was held in Warsaw with the participation of about 150 military surgeons and physicians from thirty countries.[32] The State Institute for Hygiene gained a high international reputation as a world-renowned scientific center.

Figures like Ludwik Hirszfeld were not only enthusiastic scientists, they very also proud to be able to "adapt the development of our departments to the needs of the state."[33] He wrote numerous texts and leaflets in favor of the modernization of the state and his inhabitants, which necessarily had to go hand in hand with an active fight against bacteria. He gave public talks at the meetings of the Warsaw Hygienic Society and wanted to contribute to the development of a higher medical and sanitary culture in Poland, both interpreted as a fight for a healthy national body—including a "healthy soldier," which was seen as especially important.[34] Hirszfeld was convinced that contagious diseases eroded Poland's strength.[35]

The Polish Army and a Healthy Population

Poland's strength also stood in the center of interest of the Polish Army, which, comparable to the fields of science, was composed of many officers and soldiers who had received their military training and gained their knowledge within the armies of the three partition powers, mainly from the Habsburg lands, but also from Russia and Prussia.[36] The army constituted one of the most important institutions in the newly formed independent state. Not only because in Poland many people felt a permanent threat from at least two of the former partition powers, Germany and Russia—a perception that was not entirely unfounded—the state showed a great in-

32 International Congress of Military Medicine and Pharmacy and meetings of the Permanent Committee, Washington, DC, 1927.

33 Ludwik Hirszfeld, *Obsługa bakteriologiczna i epidemiologiczna Państwa. Przeszłość, teraźniejszość, przyszłość* (Warsaw, 1937), 6.

34 Ibid., 17; Ludwik Hirszfeld, "Nasi niewidzialni wrogowie i przyjaciele," in *Biblioteka Odczytowa Polskiego Towarzystwa Higienicznego* (Warsaw, 1937).

35 Ludwik Hirzsfeld, "W sprawie ostrych chorób zakaźnych w Polsce, jako najpilniejsze zagadnienia naukowego, dydatkycznego i sanitarnego," *Lekarz Polski* 5 (1938): 101.

36 For an example of this constellation of knowledge transfer, see the biographical approach by Boysen, "Gezeiten nationaler Identität: Josef von Unruh/Józef Unrug (1884–1973) als Offizier der deutschen und polnischen Marine (1907–1919 bzw. 1919–1947)."

terest in building up and maintaining a strong Polish army. The size of the army had been reduced by demobilization after the war, but it quickly expanded again, and along with it the amount of money the Polish government needed to spend to maintain it. The Rockefeller Foundation's Selskar M. Gunn observed in 1922: "With the enormous expense of maintaining a huge Polish Army it is really remarkable what the government is attempting to do for other departments of the government."[37] So questions of national defense and security played a significant role in interwar Poland—the ability to conduct a war counted as important evidence of the modernity of the nation-state and its society. This was, of course, not only relevant to Poland.[38]

As elsewhere, the army aspired to serve as one of the primary agents of modernization.[39] This modernization took the form of an intense fight against illiteracy among soldiers as well as a focus on questions of health and physical fitness. Adam Koc, an experienced officer and influential politician from the camp of Józef Piłsudski, put it like this in 1921: "A successful contemporary war can be conducted only when the whole society takes part it in, morally and physically."[40] General Gustaw Orlicz-Dreszer from the Polish Army postulated that the army had to be a "national school, a school from which the youth will emerge physically strong, skilled and trained to handle weapons, but also morally strong."[41]

Besides politicians or military specialists, health experts in Poland also appreciated army service as a "school of life."[42] In this vein, minister of health Janiszewski claimed that serving in the army "created physical vitality, toughened [people] up, and taught systematic thinking, order, punctuality, obedience, and rigor."[43] Military service was seen by many as the last step in the education of the citizens of a state, coming right after the fam-

37 Rockefeller Archives RG 1.1, Series 789, Box 1 Folder 2, Selskar M. Gunn to Wickliffe Rose, June 19, 1922. One example Gunn mentioned was the universities.

38 Langewiesche, "Das Jahrhundert Europas. Eine Annäherung in globalhistorischer Perspektive," 42. Langewiesche states this mainly for nineteenth-century Western Europe, especially around 1900, but this constellation seems to be applicable also for early twentieth-century Poland, where many norms, values, and structures from the nineteenth century were still valid.

39 Petrovsky-Stern, *Jews in the Russian Army 1827–1917: Drafted into Modernity.*

40 Cited in Kęsik, *Naród pod bronią*, 12.

41 Cited in Piotr Stawecki, "Kilka uwag o roli wojska w procesach integracyjnych i dezintegracyjnych II Rzeczypospolitej," in *Drogi integracji społeczeństwa w Polsce XIX-XXw*, ed. Henryk Zieliński (Warsaw: Polska Akademia Nauk, 1976), 194.

42 Tomasz Janiszewski, *Wojna obronna ze stanowiska eugeniki* (Warsaw, 1932), 8.

43 Ibid.

ily and school. Its effect on the development of the body was described as a very positive one, and physical education was directly linked to the fate of the nation.[44] In an article entitled "The Mobilization of Medicine for the Defense of the Country," venereologist and dermatologist Franciszek Walter expressed his conviction that "every step we take to lead this country into the future has to be firmly connected to the thought of the defense of the country and the state." To reach this goal, the state needed the healthiest possible population.[45]

In this context, and since socially connoted diseases such as tuberculosis or alcoholism turned out to be far greater killers than the spectacular epidemics of the postwar years,[46] the topic of eugenics was broadly discussed in Poland in general and in army circles in particular. Eugenics promised to deliver a scientifically substantiated solution to problems of health and the almost proverbial problem of agrarian "overpopulation" and poverty in the countryside. Eugenicists from the health sector met with other scientists from the economic sciences or from anthropology, who were also eager to solve these "problems" and to make the work of humans more efficient. Janiszewski incessantly stressed his wish for an "improvement of the people," the physical strengthening and hardening of the individual, a change of man himself. At the same time, as a rather unconditional eugenicist, he wanted to reduce the number of "vagabonds," the "unneeded," the "delinquents"—nobody was to hinder the country in its development.[47] To achieve this goal, he placed the purported link between demography and degeneration at the center of his ideas about the "quality" of the population.

Army physicians, such as Mieszysław Naramowski from Lublin, who served as a military doctor, embraced Janiszewski's ideas. In one of Naramowski's numerous scientific articles, he argued that Poland's ability to defend itself relied on its people in a more significant way than was the case for other countries, because of its geopolitical location between Germany and Russia. To enable Poland to withstand the anticipated threat he wanted to strengthen above all the ethnic Polish population, to create "fully valuable

44 Wincenty Czech, "Wpływ służby wojskowej na rozwój fizyczny żołnierzy," *Lekarz wojskowy* 27.1 (1936): 33–41.

45 Franciszek Walter, "Mobilizacja medycny dla obrony państwa," *Nauka a obrona Państwa, Kraków* (1937): 107.

46 Balińska, "The National Institute of Hygiene and Public Health in Poland," 442.

47 Janiszewski, *O wymogach zdrowotnych*, 64–5.

people in regard to physical and psychological fitness."[48] Naramowski was convinced that Poland desperately needed eugenic laws in order to raise the "quality" of its people and to eliminate "negative elements" with genetic diseases (for example by excluding them from the reproduction process). Experts from the army like Naramowski tended to be opposed to any ideas or suggestions aimed at lowering the birth rate in Poland—although Naramowski did complain about the size of Poland's agrarian population of eight million—especially measures that would affect ethnic Poles. Naramowski was convinced that physicians in the military in particular had to know everything about eugenics, since they had to work with the physically and mentally most vital parts of the Polish population.[49]

Eugenic ideas were well-known in military and health circles. In Poland, though, they differed from those in other countries, especially from the "racial hygiene" notion that was promulgated in Germany during this time. The connection between "race" and eugenics never gained a strong position in Poland, although some of its supporters argued in favor of it, but they were not a majority. Eugenic ideas in Poland appeared rather among liberals and in circles of progressive social reformers, who called for more education and enlightenment in all questions of health, hygiene, and birth control.[50] Consequently, state institutes taught many classes on hygiene for Polish soldiers. Ludwik Hirszfeld was a member of the Polish Eugenic Society and directed its scientific section from 1931 onward. Together with the School of Hygiene, Hirszfeld organized classes in eugenics for physicians interested in topics like population politics, the inheritance of mental illness, and the prevention of venereal disease. The close partnership between the military and this institution intensified in the 1930s, when Gustaw Szulc, who held the military rank of colonel, took over the position of director of the State Institute of Hygiene. The decision to remove Ludwik Rajchman as the director of the institution at the beginning of the 1930s, and also the decision not to replace him by Ludwik Hirszfeld, Rajchman's long-time deputy and scientific director de facto, was due to an ever more hostile atmosphere of discrimination and anti-Semitism in Poland. The official motivation for the appointment of Gustaw Schulz was the government's desire to use the insti-

48 Mieczysław Naramowski, "Eugenika i obronność kraju," *Lekarz wojskowy* 27.7 (1936): 401–13.

49 Ibid.

50 Magdalena Gawin, *Rasa i nowoczesność* (Warsaw: Neriton. Instytut Historii PAN, 2003), 210–40.

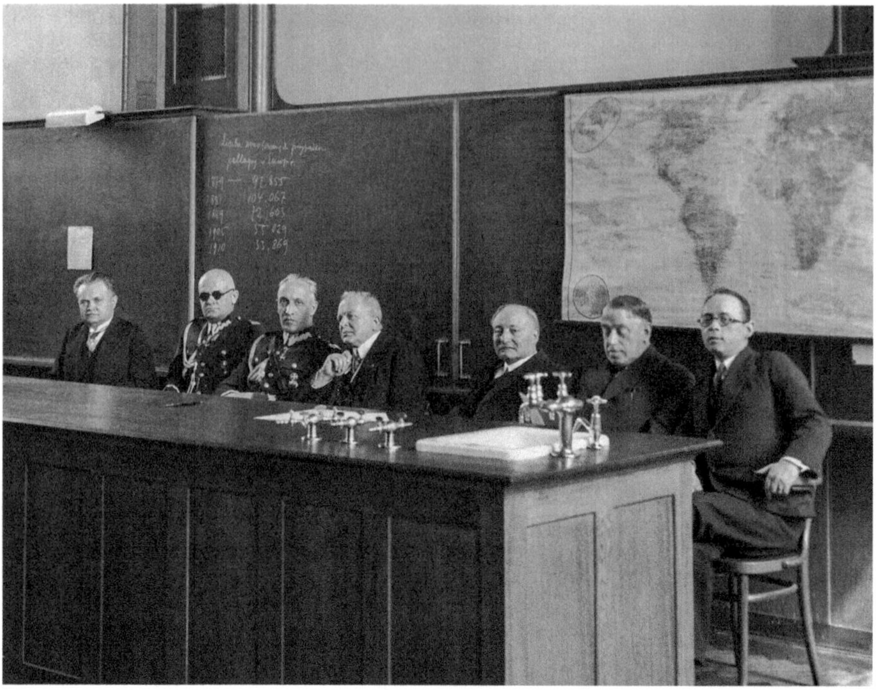

Figure 5.1: *Opening session for a class on tropical medicine in the State Institute of Hygiene*. Next to Director Gustaw Szulc on the left are two generals in the Polish Army, Stanisław Rouppert and Gustaw Orlicz-Dreszer, Warsaw 1930s. Narodowe Archiwum Cyfrowe/National Digital Archive Warsaw, sign. 1-C-969-1.

tute for military purposes.[51] The fact that the government appointed Szulc rather than Hirszfeld was a clear sign of the change in direction. Szulc was another supporter of eugenic laws to prevent the reproduction of "undesirable elements" in Poland, although he also warned of the danger of eroding the strength of the nation by eugenic measures that would reduce the birth rate in Poland. If that was to happen, he anticipated a fatal impact on the military strength of the country.[52]

Government and army plans to improve the physical fitness of the citizens of Poland and their ability to be able to fight a war were ambitious. The army wanted to reach more people, including women, than could be achieved by simply delivering classes in hygiene and eugenics to represen-

51 Hirszfeld, *The Story of One Life*, 86.

52 Gustaw Szulc, "Lekarz wojskowy jako eugenista," *Lekarz wojskowy* 27.4 (1936): 193–9.

tatives of the army or physicians. Military education was intended to reach the broad masses, especially members of the younger generation, and this became the focus from 1926 onward.[53] The army intensified the state's activities in this field, based on cooperation with civil departments, especially with the Ministry of Religion and Public Education. Under the slogan "A Nation under Arms" (*Naród pod bronią*), leading members of the government and especially the minister of military affairs himself, Józef Piłsudski, positively encouraged a close connection between society at large and the army. The program was based on two principles: promoting physical fitness and providing civic education.[54] The physical preparation of society was broadly approached, and this included addressing the personal hygiene and housing conditions of the people. An improvement of the health status was thought to bring about a positive relation to the state. One of the documents of the "Nation under Arms" program states: "It is easier to instill patriotism into people who recognize the advantages brought about by the state than into those poor fellows who only remember that they were better off under the rule of the Russian or the Austrian."[55]

From 1926 on, after the coup d'état by Józef Piłsudski, when the influence of representatives of the army on politics increased and the army became more dominant in society, the Ministry of Military Affairs, headed by Piłsudski from 1926 until 1935, was responsible for the coordination and implementation of the "Nation under Arms" program. Piłsudski showed a great personal interest in the fitness of society and sports for the masses.[56] The program also fostered social associations associated with scouting and sports. With the establishment of the State Agency for Physical Education and Military Training (Państwowy Urząd Wychowania Fizycznego i Przysposobienia Wojskowego, PUWFiPW) in 1927, the military became a fully independent player in sports policies and strove to control and centralize all sporting activities under its aegis.[57]

53 See Lech Wyszszelski, *Społeczeństwo a obronność w Polsce (1918–1939)* (Toruń: Wydawnictwo Adam Marszałek, 2007), 336–7.

54 Kęsik, *Naród pod bronią*, 187.

55 Kęsik, *Naród pod bronią*, 30, citing a memorandum entitled "Naród pod bronią" [Nation under arms] from the military archive collection of the paramilitary organization "Związek Strzelecki."

56 Ibid., 164–5.

57 Piotr Rozwadowski, *Państwowy Urząd Wychowania Fizycznego i Przysposobienia Wojskowego* (Warsaw: Bellona, 2000).

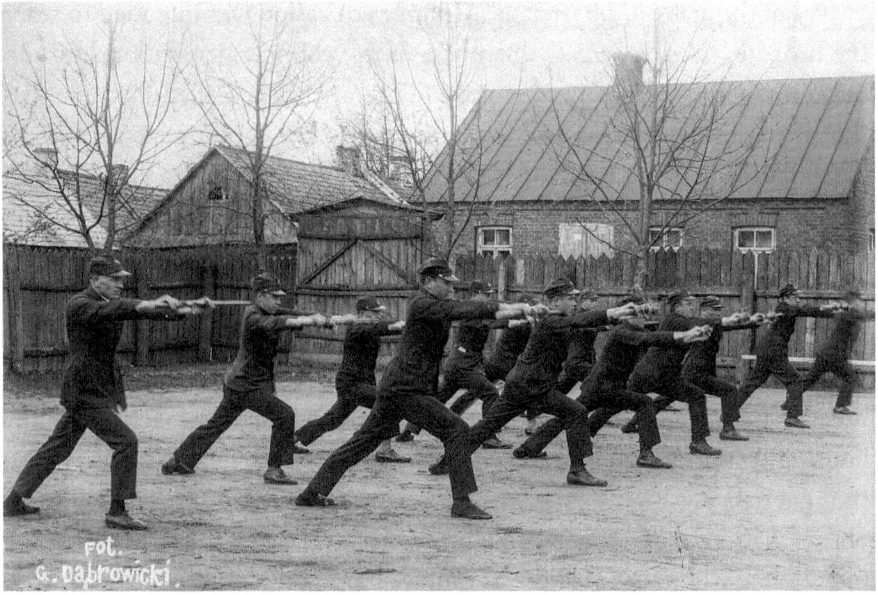

Figure 5.2: *Military training and physical education in a public high school in Pruschany in eastern Poland (today Belorussia)*, undated. Narodowe Archiwum Cyfrowe/National Digital Archive Warsaw, sign. 1-W-2466-3.

The PUWFiPW coordinated all activities relating to civic education, which was considered to be equally important as physical education.[58] Paramilitary organizations like the Riflemen's Association "Rifleman" (Związek Strzelecki "Strzelec") actively promulgated the idea that the defense of the state required all of its citizens to take action to ensure their physical fitness.[59] The association, which had about 500,000 members during the interwar period and was organized under the supervision of the Ministry of Military Affairs, concentrated its efforts in the countryside and among poor urban youth. It organized gymnastics classes, reading courses in its own libraries, and paramilitary courses on its own sports fields. A large number of citizens earned the national sports badge that was issued starting in 1930. From 1931 to 1938, more than 780,000 people earned this badge, and the Polish Army was among the leading organizations in the fields where the

58 Jan Kęsik, *Wojsko polskie wobec tężyzny fizycznej społeczeństwa 1918–1939* (Wrocław: AWF Wrocław, 1996); Kęsik, *Naród pod bronią*, 155–68.

59 "Miesiąc propagandy W. F" [A month of propaganda for physical education], *Strzelec. Tygodnik. Organ Związku Strzeleckiego* 14 (1937).

badge could be earned. In 1931, for example, 38 percent of all badges went to soldiers.[60] After the death of Piłsudski in 1935, the militarization of Polish society accelerated even more.[61]

The Army and the Physical Fitness of the National Minorities in Poland

During the first years of Polish independence, when the country was still involved in several armed conflicts concerning its future borders, practically no minorities served in the Polish Army. From 1921 on, however, once the wars had ended, a new dynamic emerged. The minorities were included in compulsory military service—the new Polish constitution of 1921 codified military service for all citizens of Poland and stated: "All citizens are obligated to [perform] military service."[62] This development was not a small change, since from then on one-third of all potential conscripts would come from one of the non-Polish national groups living within the Polish state. Many observers had questions about how this would affect the nature of the Polish Army. Olivier d'Etchegoyen, the French general staff officer and military observer in Poland, wondered: "If a crisis occurred, how would the soldiers conscripted in the border regions behave, the Galicians, White Russians, Lithuanians, so-called Little Russians and Silesians—these Poles against their will, who actually belong to nations that are hostile to Poland? How would the Jewish soldiers behave?"[63]

Even if these questions might imply that all members of the mentioned groups were equally and consequently opposed to Polish statehood, which was not the case, even if many of those groups would have preferred to live within the borders of a different state, it is likely that these concerns worried the Polish military leadership. After all, they had to change the character of the army because it was no longer possible to maintain the army as an ethnically homogeneous institution. It had to change from a national army into an army of the state, in whose structures equal rights and equal opportunities

60 Kęsik, *Naród pod bronią*, 168.

61 Wyszszelski, *Społeczeństwo a obronność*, 336.

62 Chodorowski and Konieczny (eds.), *Wybór tekstów źródłowych z historii ustroju Polski 1916–1939*, 55–77.

63 Olivier d'Etchegoyen, *Polens wahres Gesicht. Persönliche Erlebnisse aus der Gegenwart* (Berlin, 1927), 148. Quoted in Christhardt Hentschel, unpublished dissertation manuscript, 217–18; published as *Jeder Bürger Soldat. Militär, Juden und die Zweite Polnische Republik zwischen Geschichte und Gegenwart.*

should be granted to all soldiers, irrespective of their nationality. This was mirrored in an instruction by the minister for military affairs and the head of the general staff in 1921: "Our constitutive army was called national, and it was de facto like that in 1918, 1919, and 1920; today, however, in the time of drafting foreign elements to the ranks, the army will be a state army."[64]

Consequently, from 1921 onward the number of soldiers of a different ethnic origin than Polish began to rise. By the end of the year, 16.5 percent of all soldiers came from minority groups, and a couple of years later the figure was 34 percent.[65] The Ministry of Military Affairs perceived those figures to be a problem because certain minorities were believed to be unqualified for military service and mistrust remained a strong force. As a consequence, the officer corps was kept ethnically monolithic and was composed only of ethnic Poles. Soldiers who held the rank of corporal were also predominantly Polish.[66] Despite the misgivings of the military leadership, the Polish constitution, a fairly progressive document, required the integration of minority groups in the army. In any case, in order for the army to survive as an institution the drafting of soldiers from all minority groups had to take place. Under these terms, the civic status of minority groups altered. The state offered the opportunity for civic participation to these citizens, but it expected a certain behavior in return—mainly unconditional loyalty to the state. The goal was for minorities to be transformed into physically capable soldiers and enlightened citizens. Despite the continued presence of nationalizing forces in Poland, the state—dating from Piłsudski's coup d'état in 1926—felt committed to the concept of "state assimilation," to a pragmatic alliance with the minorities, and therefore to a civic conception of the Polish nation that demanded this unconditional loyalty to the state.[67] Piłsudski's vision of the state had little in common with ethnicity or language, but it seems that it was never fully accepted by Polish society. The "ethnic" vision of the country, represented by Roman Dmowski, continued to win new adherents among the Polish masses during the interwar period and was translated into a chauvinistic and anti-Semitic nationalism. This was characterized by Czesław Miłosz in the fol-

64 Cited in Kowalski, *Mniejszości narodowe w siłach zbrojnych Drugiej Rzeczypospolitej Polskiej (1918–1939)*, 154.

65 Kęsik, *Naród pod bronią*, 169.

66 Krotofil, "Ukraińcy w Wojsku Polskim w okresie międzywojennym," 139.

67 See Brykczynski, "A Poland for the Poles? Józef Piłsudski and the Ambiguities of Polish Nationalism," 13.

lowing way: "The Polish anti-Semitic obsessions took on the character of a psychosis, and in the late 1930s almost of insanity, obstructing thus a clear view on the quite real danger of war."[68] In this context the question arises: What did the civic and military leaders think of the minority soldiers in the army? The state wanted to create a "new breed of men," but while it propagated "state assimilation" it also tolerated nationalistic and anti-Semitic tendencies within society. Could the minorities meet the expectations?

In army circles, where descriptions of minority groups were not always differentiated but rather general, often not taking into account multiple forms of identification, members of German minority groups counted as good "physical material" and as valuable soldiers, but their attitude to the Polish state was perceived as being unfavorable and sometimes even hostile. The army saw little chance to change this, so the goal was to concentrate on encouraging them to do their duty as citizens of the Polish state without trying to Polonize them.[69] While in 1922, 1,834 young Germans served in the Polish Army, in 1923 this number had risen to 2,667.[70] During the interwar period, approximately 47,000 to 50,000 German speakers passed through the Polish Army.[71] Soldiers who were identified as Ukrainians also counted as "excellent physical material"—but as having little awareness of citizenship. They were seen as good soldiers, although at times they were under suspicion because of their national consciousness, but in the end they made valuable and disciplined soldiers, just like the Germans, but only if they did not come under the influence of the political parties of the Ukrainian minority.[72] They were to be Polonized, but this goal could have never been achieved. Soldiers of Belorussians descent were also seen as "good material." Much appreciated was their presumed ability to get along under difficult circumstances (such as, for example, a poor diet), so it was assumed that they possessed a great physical resistance against hunger and other challenging conditions.[73] It was appreciated that their national ambitions were marginal, so overall they were perceived to be suitable as soldiers and also for the goals of state assimilation.[74]

68 Miłosz, *Wyprawa w Dwudziestolecie*, 273.
69 Kowalski, "Mniejszości narodowe," 157.
70 Rezmer, "Służba wojskowa Żydów w siłach zbrojnych Drugiej Rzeczypospolitej," 114.
71 Ibid., 115.
72 Krotofil, "Ukraińcy w Wojsku Polskim," 145–7, Kowalski, "Mniejszości narodowe," 155.
73 Wierzbicki, "Białorusini w Wojsku Polskim (1921–1939)," 174.
74 Kowalski, "Mniejszości narodowe," 159.

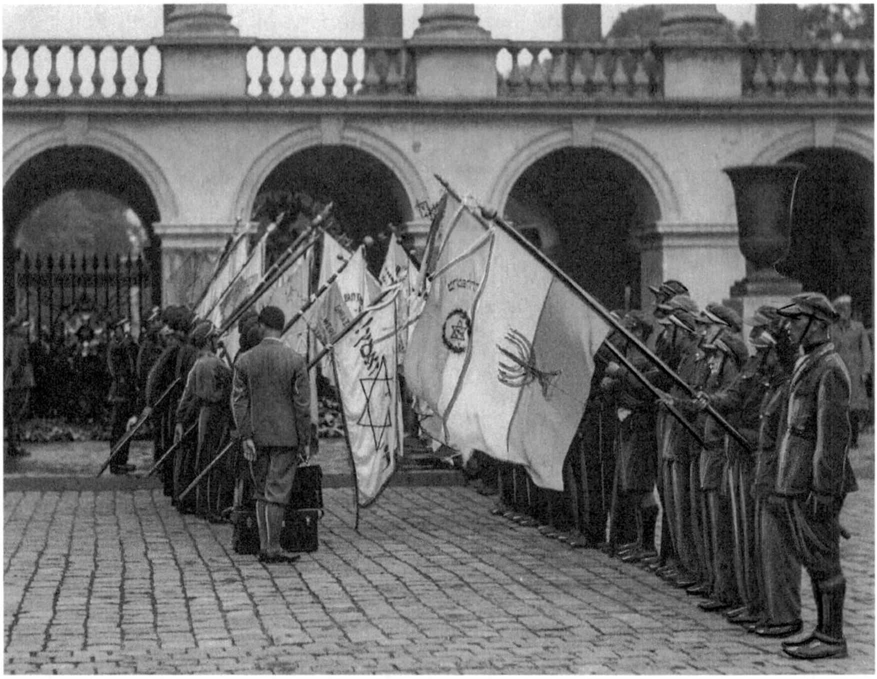

Figure 5.3: *Jewish military training organizations in front of the Tomb of the Unknown Soldier*, Warsaw 1930. Narodowe Archiwum Cyfrowe/National Digital Archive Warsaw, Sign. 1-W-2389.

Jews were held to be lousy, physically weak, and constantly threatened by illnesses. In military reports this view is shown in the following observations: "The Jews are the worst single element in the army. Unwilling to truly serve and dissembling, they constitute the most miserable raw material for recruits to the ranks."[75] Or: "The Jewish soldier, ever ready to desert, physically a weakling, fearful and lacking in obedience, is poor raw material for a strong, fighting soldier."[76] Physical constitution and character were combined in a number of reports from the barracks, merging into a totally negative image, such as when Jews were described in a single breath as "dishonest slobs."[77]

75 CAW, Oddz. II SG, sygn. I.303.4.2683, DOK VII SRI L.dz. 2254, [October] 1924 an Oddz. II Szt, for July–Sept 1924, 528, quoted in Hentschel, *Jeder Bürger Soldat*.

76 CAW, Oddz. II SG, sygn. I.303.4.2687, Żydzi (DOK IV. 3. Februar 1926), quoted in Hentschel, *Jeder Bürger Soldat*.

77 CAW, Oddz. II SG, sygn. I.303.4.2684, Raport narodowościowy DOK II Lublin za kwartał I-szy 1926, 17. April 1926, DOK II, SRI, L. 528/Inf 26, 90, quoted in Hentschel, *Jeder Bürger Soldat*.

In order to substantiate reports "scientifically," the state financed several anthropological examinations of Polish soldiers. From 1921 until the mid-1920s, some 80,000 soldiers were examined, and by 1939, 150,000 individuals had been examined and anthropologically classified. This examination was carried out by the Anthropological Division at the Department for the Individualization of the Soldiers at the Military Sanitary Institute, under the leadership of anthropologist Jan Mydlarski, a former officer who had served in the Habsburg Army and been educated at the University of Lwów. Mydlarski worked together with several colleagues, among them Wanda Halber, an assistant to Ludwik Hirszfeld at the State Institute of Hygiene. Again, we find a close cooperation between the army and the State Institute of Hygiene. The researcher measured noses, skulls, and the shape of faces and took blood samples from the soldiers. The findings suggested a link between popular racial physiognomic stereotypes and "East" and "West" serological types following the so-called "biochemical race index" that Ludwik and Hanna Hirszfeld had created during the First World War at the Macedonian front. There, they conducted over 8,000 blood tests among soldiers and civilians from sixteen different ethnic groups and came to the conclusion that blood group "A" was more frequent in the western parts of the world, while the percentage of blood group "B" increased while moving farther east. To articulate this pattern and to quantify their results, the Hirszfelds established the so-called "biochemical race-index," an equation which compared the incidence of blood types A and B within a group. With this research, they established the new research field of seroanthropology, combining serology and anthropology.[78] Later in his life, Ludwik Hirszfeld found himself being accused of holding "racist" views, because he and his wife had claimed to identify "racial types" associated with the western and the eastern parts of the world. However, the Hirszfelds' findings did more to challenge prevailing notions of race than to sustain them, since they insisted that their "biochemical index" did not correspond to race in the usual sense of the word, and also by the fact that all populations are mixed in regard to blood type. They undermined the idea that human races could be separated from each other sci-

78 Jan Mydlarski, "Sprawozdanie z wojskowego zdjęcia antropologicznego Polski," in *Kosmos. Czasopismo Polskiego Towarzystwa Przyrodników im. Kopernika* 50 (1925): 530–83; Wanda Halber and Jan Mydlarski, "Untersuchungen über die Blutgruppen in Polen," *Zeitschrift für Immunitätsforschung und experimentelle Therapie* 43 (1925): 470–84; and Mazumdar, "Blood and Soil: The Serology of the Aryan Racial State," 191.

entifically, since their results did not suggest the existence of race markers for a certain race, but a certain distribution of those markers among all races. This approach was quite innovative and provocative at the same time, because it replaced old definitions of race and ethnicity based on ideal anatomical types with ones based on the statistical evaluation of genetic data. Indeed, the Hirszfelds used—as many researchers have done since—conventional racial categories in their research design, and in this way their results seemed to confirm the organization of human diversity in races. Just like numerous Jewish and non-Jewish scientists who engaged with the "race question" during the 1920s and 1930s, the Hirszfelds also took it as a matter of course that humanity is divided into different races. Nevertheless, the Hirzsfelds' research marked the beginning of a profound shift in the anthropological understanding of racial categories.[79]

Following the seroanthropological research design established by the Hirzsfelds, Halber and Mydlarski reported that individuals with type A blood tended to have "longer skulls," "smaller noses, and narrower faces," which led them to express "no doubt" that type A blood corresponded with the so-called Nordic race. By contrast, those with blood type B tended to be "Slavic" (Laponoidal). Type O was identified with a Mediterranean type. It was also shown that blood type A appeared more often in the western parts of Poland than in the eastern parts.[80] Later, in 1956, Mydlarski admitted that the "matter was more complicated" because it could not have been proven that blood group B really was the most common blood group for the Slavic type.[81] But, for the time being, Halber and Mydlarski's research marked the beginning of a trend in the early 1920s to supplement seroanthropological studies with other traits, in the hope that this would lend some insight where blood alone could not. Because of the study's respective association between type A and B blood and Nordic and Slavic physiognomies, other blood scientists, especially from Germany, subsequently often cited it.

The official justification for this research had been that the Polish Army wanted to tailor new uniforms for their soldiers, which might have been a pretext, although in 1925 Poland's most famous anthropologist, Jan Cze-

79 Mikanowski, "Dr. Hirszfeld's War: Tropical Medicine and the Invention of Sero-Anthropology on the Macedonian Front," 115. See also Steffen, "Ludwik Hirszfeld, the Great War, and Seroanthropology: Expectations and Unfulfilled Promises."

80 Mydlarski, "Seroantropologia," 67.

81 Ibid., 65–8.

kanowski, came to the conclusion that in fact the anthropometric measurements had generated high savings for the army—savings used to finance this research—which made Poland in Czekanowski's eyes a leading nation in the field of anthropology.[82] But the editor of the journal *Anthropological Review*, the anthropologist and physician Adam Wrzosek, summarized its task rather as "an orientation in the racial diversification in all regions of the republic with the goal of reaching conclusions to serve practical military purposes."[83] After all, the results went further than that—maps were generated where the spatial distribution of different "race types" all over Poland was shown. Czekanowski, who argued against the (in his opinion) "outdated" notion that all humans "are the same," was convinced that the "main relevance of anthropology lies in its indirect impact on pedagogy, medicine, social sciences, and even military sciences by stating and researching the fact that mankind is composed of different races."[84] He commented on the findings of the anthropological survey as follows: "Our experience allows us to state that particular racial components of the people are not suitable for military service, and that the value of a soldier depends above all on his physical fitness. We all know that the Jews are physically inferior and that they are the worst soldiers. And we also know that the Nordic blond type constitutes the best material for the army, physically as well as mentally."[85] He also stated that Mydlarski's research had shown that the recruiting boards in the eastern parts of Poland often rejected the brachycephalic type found there, which led him to the decision not to locate military schools in those regions, where "mediocre" material was to be found.[86]

Anthropologist Karol Stojanowski, a student of Czekanowski, studied the writings on eugenics by German anthropologists as well as Polish thinking on the subject, before writing *The Racial Foundations of Eugenics* (1927). In it he concludes: "By the way, it is not without good reason that German science interprets Jews as a threat to the Nordic-European type. [...] [Y]ou do not have to persuade anyone in Poland that the Germans are totally correct in their findings." He continued: "From a eugenic standpoint the assimi-

82 Jan Czekanowski, "Nauki antropologiczne," *Nauka Polska* 5 (1925): 146.
83 Adam Wrzosek, "Review of Mydlarski. Sprawozdanie z wojskowego zdjęcia antropologicznego Polski," *Przeglad Antropologiczny* 1 (1926): 36.
84 Czekanowski, "Nauki antropologiczne," 146.
85 Ibid., 156.
86 Ibid., 157.

lation of the Jews is not desired. They either have to emigrate or restrict their natural growth or simply die out."[87] He accused Jews of demoralizing the Poles and hindering the progress of the anthropological types in Poland that constituted the best material for the development and expansion of a strong nation. Stojanowski wrote that Jews in other countries in Europe might well constitute a "problem," but in Poland it was all about the very existence of the country. Stojanowski's views as a scientist might have been extreme, but his arguments fitted very well into the contemporary form of biopolitical Jew hatred in Poland, and they connected most certainly to a global discourse on the construction of a social, national, or "racial" other, excluded from a supposedly "clean" and "healthy" national body. The conclusions of Mydlarski, Stojanowski, and Czekanowski were based on Hirszfeld's findings, but it is not clear what Hirszfeld thought about their work, even though he met them at anthropological conferences and they were members of the same Polish anthropological and eugenic societies. Once, Hirszfeld observed that Mydlarski "had drawn very far-reaching conclusions about the junction between serological groups and anthropological characteristics and about races living in Poland in prehistorical times," which sounds at least ambivalent.[88]

Under Stojanowski's supervision, students at the University in Poznań conducted research on Jews in the Polish Army. The subjects came from different parts of Poland but were serving their time in the Poznań area. They were all born between 1901 and 1906. Initially, forty-one soldiers were selected for the study, but only eighteen were participating regularly in exercises and were therefore eligible to be studied. The project aimed to compare their level of physical fitness to that of Polish sports instructors. When the results were published, the author came to the conclusion that the physical fitness of the Jewish soldiers did not equal that of the instructors, and was in fact far beneath their level. This was explained, on the one hand, by the fact that the instructors had access to special training and engaged in more exercise, but on the other hand, the results were taken to be a "confirmation of the popular and in the army well-known opinion that the Jewish material in the physical respect is less valuable than the Polish." It was also argued that the poor results of the Jewish soldiers were caused by faked ill-

87 Karol Stojanowski, *Rasowe podstawy eugeniki* (Poznań: Księgarnia M. Arcta, 1927), 68.

88 Ludwik Hirszfeld, *Sprawozdanie z dzialalności naukowej Państwowego Zakładu Higjeny i Państwowego Zakładu Badania Surowic w Warszawie. Z okazji 5-cioletniej rocznicy ich powstania* (Warsaw: PZH, 1924), 16.

nesses and dissimulation among the soldiers to avoid exerting themselves during their service (this constituted a common accusation made against Jewish servicemen during the interwar period).[89] Even if this was taken into consideration, the article concluded, the level of physical fitness of the Jewish soldier in the Polish Army was very low.

In order to enforce a better degree of fitness among Jewish youth in Poland, Jewish sports clubs (like Makkabi) received funds from the PUWFiPW. This happened not only as a part of the usual support provided for sports clubs, but also out of a desire to bring minority organizations, which were always suspected of being potentially hostile to Poland, under state influence. While German sport clubs showed a tendency to isolate themselves from Polish society, this was not the case with the Jewish ones, which actively took part in Polish sports life. Some parts of Ukrainian organizations also cooperated with Polish associations—for example, the "Welykij Luh" movement.[90] These contacts were also intended to reduce tensions between minority groups and the Polish majority in the army, which indicates the government's pragmatic approach to the treatment of minority groups.

Conclusion

The Polish state emerged in 1918 from three former powers. From then onward, many Poles found the opportunity to experience the nation as one territory, a territory where "identity space" was tantamount with "decision space,"[91] a territory where technological progress and industrialization could be experienced within the frame of sovereignty.[92] This does not mean that there was no legacy inherited from the former empires—on the contrary. In many fields of science like medicine, and in institutions like the State Institute of Hygiene and the Polish Army, knowledge from those empires or from different places abroad were transferred into the new state and adapted to national necessities. As a result, there was no simple dichotomy between a national and an international space—they were closely intertwined and

89 Zofja Walicka, "Przyczynek do sprawności fizycznej Żydów żołnierzy W.P.," *Wychowanie fizyczne* 7–8 (1929): 217f.

90 CAW Oddz. II SG, sygn. I.300.69.236, 20.4.1934.

91 Maier, "Transformations of Territoriality 1600–2000," 48.

92 To what degree this constituted a particular experience of modernity in Poland would be another question worth discussing; see Eisenstadt, *Multiple Modernities*.

overlapped. From international contacts and an international standing, the health sector and health experts gained legitimacy. They were able to build a highly complex, innovative, and dynamic system that was not a passive recipient of Western models. International competition also served to demonstrate national accomplishments. Within the laboratory that emerged after 1918, Poland tried to be a modernizing state.

This included thinking in categories of social engineering, meaning that actors tried to influence and change individuals and society in a technocratic and purposeful way, backed up by scientific research and knowledge and a sometimes exuberant belief in the power of science and the control of social processes by scientists. We find this kind of thinking also in the economic sciences, in ideas of scientific management and technocracy, and most certainly in the health sector.[93]

The health sector was thought to be closely connected to the security of the country—experiences from previous military conflicts, especially from the First World War and the battles fought during the years 1918–1920 on the Polish borders, contributed heavily to this constellation. For pragmatic and constitutional reasons, the national minorities had to have their share in the new nation, which was not an easy task to accomplish. As a result, the ethnonational and civic shape of the army fluctuated, which led its leadership to approach the handling of the ethnic diversity of the country with pragmatism.[94] Ethnic cataloguing was part of the modernization and civilizing project of the new nation-state. These efforts fed into a program of "state assimilation" intended to forge a pragmatic alliance between ethnic Poles and the national minorities in the country. Such efforts, however, still took place in an atmosphere of mistrust between Poles and the national minorities. Due to the overall political and economic development that headed toward increasing nationalism (not only in Poland, but in many European states) during the interwar period, this mistrust increased. When it came to the Jewish minority in particular, a certain biopolitically motivated anti-Semitism prevailed, whose representatives tried to convince themselves and others that Jewish bodies were unfit to serve the country and constituted a supposed threat to an envisioned ideal anthropological development.

93 See, for example, Rohdewald, "Mimicry in a Multiple Postcolonial Setting: Networks of Technocracy and Scientific Management in Piłsudksi's Poland," 63–84.

94 Hentschel, "Einführung. Der Militärdienst für Juden und die Verheißung der Emanzipation," 99.

CHAPTER VI

Transatlantic Humanitarianism: Jewish Child Relief in Budapest after the Great War

Friederike Kind-Kovács

Introduction

The First World War and its troubled aftermath not only radically changed the ethnic, linguistic, and national composition of Central and Eastern Europe, but also fundamentally affected the everyday lives and the health of its civilian population. The difficult "aftermath" found its perfect illustration in the challenging urban living conditions and the critical food situation that altered not only people's morale but also their health. The civil population of postwar Hungary, and especially of its capital, which is at the center of this chapter, can be seen as one local laboratory of Europe's postwar transformation process. It is here that the making of a new nation-state brought about geographic displacement, social uprootedness, and ethnic violence. When looking at the impact on family life, the collapse of the Austro-Hungarian Empire caused abrupt unemployment, homelessness, and impoverishment, which affected especially children's everyday lives and physiological development. The suffering of children—from neglect, malnutrition, and inappropriate housing to a lack of hygiene, diseases, and absence from school—was inscribed into their bodies and health. Postwar local health and welfare systems, however, were not prepared to meet this new scale of neediness and the requirement for instant material, nutritional, and medical relief. Yet the Great War, as an international disaster, "enabled" the internationalization of humanitarian relief that was needed to handle this "transition from war to peace."[1] A system of transnational health and food intervention came into being that complemented local and national health and welfare systems. In this context, the relief of children turned into a prime humanitarian undertaking in the 1920s, as children were considered the least guilty and the most needy of people requiring assistance.

Simultaneously, as the war and its troubled aftermath gave rise to ethnic conflicts throughout the region, certain ethnic groups suffered from discrimination and persecution. Various local Jewish communities throughout Central and Eastern Europe turned into prime targets of fierce and violent attacks and were thus exposed to additional challenges during the postwar period. Although in Hungary "Jewish assimilation had become a reality," among the "ultimate victims of the dissolution of the Habsburg monarchy have undoubtedly been the Jews."[2] In Budapest, the "wartime suffering" triggered a "great reversal of the favorable conditions" Jews had been living in up to 1914.[3] The delicate situation of the local Jewish communities did not, however, remain unnoticed. Local and international Jewish relief organizations called for their immediate relief and helped alleviate the everyday life of local Jewish communities. From the beginning of the war, the American Jewish Joint Distribution Committee (JDC) invested millions of dollars into the reconstruction and rehabilitation of Jewish communities and individuals in Eastern Europe.[4] The JDC was originally established in 1914 as the Joint Distribution Committee of American Funds for the Relief of Jewish War Sufferers, aiming to relieve the suffering of war invalids and to provide relief to Jewish communities in Central and Eastern Europe.[5]

In the case of Hungary, however, it was not primarily the war but rather the war's aftermath that exacerbated local neediness. While Hoover's American Relief Administration (ARA) or the American Red Cross (ARC) responded to the nondenominational call for child relief, the JDC raised funds to meet the special needs of Jewish children. Against this background, this chapter seeks to examine the relationship between postwar health chal-

1 Cabanes, *The Great War and the Origins of Humanitarianism, 1918–1924*, 5.

2 Deák, "The Habsburg Empire," 135.

3 McCagg, "On Habsburg Jewry and Its Disappearance," 91.

4 Zola and Dollinger, *American Jewish History: A Primary Source Reader*, 235.

5 Karlinksy, "Jewish Philanthropy and Jewish Credit Cooperatives in Eastern Europe and Palestine up to 1939: A Transnational Phenomenon?" On the work of the Joint in Russia, see Beizer and Mitsel, *The American Brother: The "Joint" in Russia, the USSR and the CIS*. On the general overseas work of the Joint, see Szajkowski, "Private and Organized American Jewish Overseas Relief, 1914–1938."

lenges, rising anti-Semitism, and (local and transatlantic) Jewish child relief in order to better understand the ethnic dimension of the needs of children and how they were met. Furthermore, it suggests approaching humanitarianism not solely as an arena of Western relief to a presumably backward Eastern Europe, but rather as a space of transatlantic interaction. In this space, local Hungarian agents, delegates, refugees, and émigrés who were temporarily or permanently settled in the United States and who were familiar with the "receiving" end of relief back in Hungary, were actively shaping American humanitarianism. In this way, as this chapter would like to suggest, local health agents affected global history and vice versa.

Local Anti-Semitism and Jewish Displacement

As the war on the Eastern Front between Russia and the Central Powers took place in the "heartland of East European Jewry,"[6] meaning territories that were largely populated by Jews such as Galicia, the war severely impacted local Jewish communities.[7] Anti-Jewish pogroms by the Imperial Russian army in Galicia resulted in the massive flight of Jews westward, especially to large cities like Vienna and Budapest.[8] The situation in Budapest became "complicated by the enormous numbers of refugees," who in most cases were "Jews from Galicia" and who were "in many instances absolutely without resources" when they fled to Budapest during the war.[9] An appeal to the League of Nations in Geneva "on behalf of the Jewish populations in Central Europe" from 1920 speaks of a "tragedy" for Eastern Europe's Jews, who arrived to Budapest and Vienna entirely "exhausted by hunger and rendered desperate by privations."[10] Beyond the tragedy for the adult population, the report details the "thousands of orphan children" who were "wandering along the roads and among the ruins" and whose "only hope of salvation from death and ha-

6 Over four million Jews lived in the region. Engel, "World War I."

7 On anti-Jewish violence in Galicia, see Prusin, *Nationalizing a Borderland*.

8 Rechter, "Galicia in Vienna: Jewish Refugees in the First World War"; Walter Pietsch, "A zsidók bevándorlása Galíciából és a magyarországi zsidóság," *Valóság* 1988. 11. Kötetben: U. ő.: Reform és ortodoxia (Budapest, 1999), 18–35; Dezső Kosztolányi, "Mi, huszonötezren," *Egyenlőség*, August 26, 1916.

9 *American Relief Administration Bulletin* 10, March 1, 1921.

10 Sylvain Levy, "II Appeals on Behalf of the Jewish Populations in Central Europe. I. Appeal from the Jewish Central Committee in Paris," to the President of the Council of the League of Nations in Geneva, Paris, December 8, 1920, *Journal of the First Assembly of the League of Nations Geneva* 1920, 289. National Archives London, Political, Western, League of Nations 4–22, TO P.P.3368, 1921, 7033.

tred" would lie in an intervention by the League of Nations.[11] The stream of Galician Jewish refugees had also brought many of these Jewish orphans to the capital city of Budapest who had to be cared for.[12] The more urban Jewish population of Budapest called these Eastern Jews from Galicia, pejoratively, "Galitzianers" and treated them "with suspicion" and dislike.[13] Nonetheless Budapest's Jewish communities provided emergency relief to their Galician brethren. Yet they expected them to either return home once the situation in Galicia had calmed down, or to move on. For this reason, it did not take long for Budapest, together with Vienna and Prague, to vigorously attempt "to send their Galician refugees back 'home.'"[14]

The Galician refugees, however, were unable to return to their homes and thus were struggling, side by side with their better-off Hungarian Jewish refugee fellows, with their integration into Hungarian society. In addition to the massive influx of Jewish refugees from Galicia, many Hungarian Jews (as well as non-Jews) also left their homes in the other former Hungarian territories, Transylvania and Vojvodina, "voluntarily," as they were unwilling to give up their Hungarian nationality in exchange for Serbian, Romanian, or Czechoslovak citizenship. Their displacement often went hand in hand with abrupt social decline and ethnic marginalization in the new Hungarian state. Many of them, together with other Hungarian refugees, were housed in abandoned cattle cars in the main train stations in Budapest, and lived there for several months or even years in terrible conditions.[15] It was not just in Budapest that the severe "housing problems, crowded conditions, hunger, and unreliable hygienic situation" resulted in particularly "high mortality rates, especially for Jewish infants" and the spreading of infection diseases, which they were accused of carrying.[16] When visiting a Jewish family in a poor dwelling, a Jewish relief worker encountered not only a sick mother and was informed about the father's paralysis, but also listened to the mother's everyday struggle to keep their three daughters, thirteen-year-old Erzsike, four-year-old Etelka, and

11 Ibid.

12 The Joint provided much of the relief to Jewish orphans from Galicia. "The American Joint Distribution Committee," *Egyenlőség*, April 20, 1929, 32.

13 Frojimovics and Komoróczy, *Jewish Budapest: Monuments, Rites, History*, 263–4.

14 McCagg: *A History of Habsburg Jews*, 204.

15 "A zsidó vaggonlakók," *Egyenlőség*, December 18, 1920, 2.

16 Zalshik and Davidovitch, "Taking and Giving: The Case of the JDC and OZE in Lithuania, 1919–1926," 61.

six-year-old Elemér, alive. While witnessing this intimate moment of physical suffering, the social worker heard three young soldiers complaining outside on the street: "Christian Hungary is starving, while the Jews are collecting all the money."[17] Openly blaming Jews for the starvation of Hungary's Christian population was part of the rapidly increasing social marginalization of Hungary's Jews as the scapegoat of postwar suffering. Lajos Szabolcsi observed in his "Childhood Memory" in 1920, how "[a]nti-Semitism currently flourishes."[18] He felt that it "fills the street, gets on the tram, and shows up in the press, the theater, the coffeehouse."[19]

The political upheavals that resulted from the war and the end of the empires had led to ethnic clashes throughout the region. The prominence of some political leaders of Jewish descent in postwar revolutions triggered anti-Semitic sentiments. In the case of Hungary, where Béla Kun as well as eighteen of the twenty members of his communist government had been Jewish, a prejudiced discourse developed that entangled communism and Jewish descent.[20] Although they were just "Jews in the technical sense" and identified above all as communists and socialists,[21] the "specter of Jews as Bolshevik agents began to permeate" not only Hungary, but the entire region.[22] The failure of Béla Kun's Bolshevist Republic in August 1919 was "sadly" followed by "new problems" for the Budapest Jewish Community that "joined the existing ones"[23]—a series of riots and violence was committed against Jews associated with the revolution. As Ilse Josepha Lazaroms closely documented, Budapest's Jews were suffering from physical violence and from a "less visible trauma that was unfolding in the years before the war," when their status "abruptly shifted from an insider position of relative comfort to a diminished and persecuted minority in the wake of 1918."[24] A wave of terror against Jews in Hungary, known as the "White Terror," resulted in the torture and execution of several thousand Jews. In addition,

17 "Egy a sok közül," *Egyenlőség*, September 2, 1922, 5.

18 Lajos Szabolcsi, "Gyermekkori emlék," *Egyenlőség*, April 3, 1920, 10.

19 Ibid.

20 Herczl, *Christianity and the Holocaust of Hungarian Jewry*, 25.

21 Mendelsohn, *The Jews of East Central Europe between the World Wars*, 95.

22 Engel, "World War I."

23 Pesti Izraelita Hitközség, *Pesti Izraelita Hitközség Elöljáróságának Jelentése Az 1920 Közigazgatási Évröl* (Budapest: Elek-Várnai-Nyomda, 1921), 6.

24 Lazaroms, "Marked by Violence: Hungarian Jewish Histories in the Wake of the White Terror, 1919–1922," 40.

anti-Jewish legislation such as the *numerus clausus*, limiting, from 1920 onward, the admission of Jewish students to institutions of higher learning to 5,9 percent, gave rise to various forms of anti-Jewish discrimination and a high degree of Jewish unemployment. Yet in postwar Hungary, despite increasing violence against Budapest's Jews, the Jewish community was still driven by the "continuous desire to belong to the newly truncated nation."[25]

Besides suffering from direct violence, members of the local Jewish communities suffered in everyday life from the consequences of unemployment, poverty, and starvation.[26] An information service letter by the JDC in 1920 observed that the "Great War [had] left the Jews of East Europe in rags."[27] Due to the lack of financial resources "[t]housands of men, women and children were forced to wear garments until nothing remained of them but masses of dark, filthy tatters."[28] The "effect of these dirty, decaying garments upon the almost crushed spirits of the poor Jews," the author believed, was their "final degradation."[29] The "rags and filth" had become "part of their everyday lives of suffering and humiliation."[30] Even if many of the Jewish refugees from the former Hungarian territories had been highly educated and had once had well-paying jobs, their move to Budapest often resulted in their unemployment, as the city could not absorb the high number of intellectuals. In 1922, a "family father of six children, handicapped during the war" posted his search for "any kind of job" among the advertisements of a Hungarian Jewish weekly.[31] Here, the threatened well-being of the children was closely linked to the father's physical impairment and resulting unemployment. By appealing to the readers' empathy, the father hoped to find employment that would not only save him, but also his many children. Even years after Trianon, in 1927, a private advertisement appeared in a major Hungarian newspaper from a "Hungarian Jewish refugee from Transylvania," who was "utterly ruined financially due to the Romanian occupa-

25 Ibid., 48.

26 Katzburg, "Louis Marshall and the White Terror in Hungary, 1919–1920." See also Katzburg, *Hungary and the Jews: Policy and Legislation, 1920–1943*; and Hanebrink, *In Defense of Christian Hungary: Religion, Nationalism and Antisemitism*.

27 American Jewish Joint Distribution Committee, *Information Service Letter* no. 10, September 30, 1920, 1. American Jewish Joint Distribution Committee Archive, New York City, New York.

28 Ibid.

29 Ibid.

30 Ibid.

31 "Állást kéreső," *Egyenlőség*, June 24, 1922, 20.

tion" and who called "upon his Jewish brethren to take up the sponsorship of his newborn child."[32]

As the food situation in Hungary and especially in Budapest was highly problematic, parents often struggled with mastering the everyday challenge of providing enough and appropriate food for their children. Contemporary sources report that parents often either failed to secure any food at all or they fed their babies child-inappropriate food. Consequently, the ongoing lack of appropriate, sufficient, and diverse nutrition manifested itself in children's bodily transformation. Dr. Boris Bogen, the head of the JDC, returned in 1919 from a visit to Poland, observing that "[t]he children were emaciated or bloated from starvation."[33] The everyday effects of poverty inscribed themselves first and foremost into the bodies of the weakest—i.e., the youngest—members of the Jewish population. The "catastrophic peril of bodily degeneration" was seen as a serious threat to the "future Jewish generation."[34] Especially bread and milk, the two foods most closely associated with children's healthy growth and development, were at times unknown to Budapest's needy children, as these products were especially scarce at the time: "Thousands of children did not know what bread was, nor had they ever tasted milk."[35] Hunger even distorted children's ability to differentiate between edible and inedible things. In an article from November 1919, Jewish children, reckoned to be the most deprived group of all, were described as being "so hungry that they ate the first soap given to them."[36] Although they received one meal a day at the ARA kitchens, they were still craving food. Hence, when the relief workers "gave out soap, the children ate it. It was plain army issue soap, ordinary laundry soap" that they had bought for them.[37]

While many Jewish children were just suffering from the lack of appropriate housing and food, the war and the geographic displacement had also produced large numbers of orphans. Natan Meir convincingly argued that particularly orphans, but also other categories of social "marginals"—the physically and mentally disabled, widows, servants, and others—were doomed to live a "precarious [...] existence on the periphery of a community

32 *Pesti Hírlap* 49, 17, January 22, 1927, 24.

33 "1,000,000 Children Saved by America," *The New York Times*, November 16, 1919, 20.

34 "Napsugarat, bő táplálékot szegény gyermekeinknek," *Egyenlőség*, May 26, 1928, 2.

35 "1,000,000 Children."

36 Ibid.

37 Ibid.

that was itself already marginal in many ways."[38] The lives of Jewish orphans was especially threatened as orphanages faced serious difficulties in meeting children's most basic needs. "In the length and breadth of Europe there are many war memorials," Evelyn Sharp, a British feminist journalist, wrote in 1923, but there were "few more pathetic than the orphan homes that have sprung up in those countries where famine and pestilence have followed in the track of the armies."[39] She argued that, while the state orphan was usually a national problem, "after war and its accompanying disasters" the war orphan had turned into "an international one, especially in those countries of Eastern Europe where the number is out of all proportion to the nation's resources for coping with them."[40] Yet, the need for extra-familial care for orphaned Jewish children was nothing new in Budapest. Already in 1867 a Jewish Girl's Orphanage (Pesti Izraelita Nőegyesület Leányárvaháza) and two years later, in 1869, a Jewish Boys Orphanage (Pesti Izraelita Hitközség Fiúárvaháza) had been founded that provided care to orphaned, neglected and abandoned children of Jewish descent. Yet, during and after World War I these institutions faced a serious challenge with placing and properly caring for the many Jewish war orphans that flooded Budapest and had nowhere else to go.

Jewish Child Relief

When it came to relieving the suffering of Jewish communities and their youngest generation, local Jewish organizations tried to provide emergency relief. Yet, local Jewish (child) welfare was seriously impaired. Also, when it came to local non-Jewish emergency relief, i.e., war and famine relief, resources were often not distributed equally among Jews and non-Jews.[41] The Hungarian League of Child Protection (Országos Gyermekvédő Liga) and the National Stefánia Association for the Protection of Mothers and Infants (Országos Stefánia Szövetség az anyák és csecsemők védelmére) rather fo-

38 Meir, "From Communal Charity to National Welfare: Jewish Orphanages in Eastern Europe before and after World War I," 19–20.

39 Evelyn Sharp, "The International Orphan: A Foster-Parent Scheme," *Manchester Guardian*, March 14, 1923, 6.

40 Ibid.

41 See Szajkowski: "'Reconstruction' vs. 'Palliative Relief' in American Jewish Overseas Work (1919–1939)."

cused on the general relief of Christian Hungarian children than on the relief of Jewish children. Due to the anti-Semitic tendencies in Horthy's Hungary, there was little awareness of Jewish suffering among the majority society. As Jews were not among the first to be relieved by national nondenominational welfare organizations, the financial means for the emergency relief of Jewish children were very limited. Various Jewish welfare organizations in Hungary found themselves in a situation of financial and social distress.

Yet the "mass politicisation of East European Jewry" affected the local Jewish attitude "towards orphans and other marginal groups" in such a way that their care turned into a "centre piece of national, and nationally minded, Jewish communal life in the interwar period."[42] In Hungary during the White Terror, when large numbers of Jews were imprisoned, the plight of mothers and of children of those fathers who were interned "touched the hearts of many [...] Jewish students."[43] In response, a local Jewish relief organization, Children for Children (Gyermekek a Gyermekekért), was founded in 1921, holding "'tea afternoons' at which school-age girls supplied cakes and ran raffle drawings."[44] This relief organization also raised local funds that would be collected at the Jewish political weekly *Egyenlőség* (Equality) and then further distributed among local Jewish institutions. *Egyenlőség* was a key institution in raising support and money for the relief of Jewish children. Throughout the 1920s this journal reported weekly if not daily about the situation of Hungary's poor Jewish children.

Also, Budapest Neolog Jewry, organized in the Budapest Jewish Community (Pesti Izraelita Hitközség), invested since the mid-nineteenth century much in providing the most basic welfare and health care to its members.[45] It hoped to pursue an "inner mission," closely linking welfare or healthcare to faith and belonging. In 1842 the Budapest Jewish Community opened the doors of its *Hild József* Jewish hospital (Pesti Izraelita Hitközség kórháza). Jewish religious education was a centerpiece of Budapest's private Jewish welfare. From a Jewish doctor, for instance, it was not only expected that he be "a good diagnostician, a good surgeon, an academically trained doctor," but also that he knew "how to serve with his medical knowledge the

42 Meir, "From Communal Charity to National Welfare," 20.

43 Stessel, *Wine and Thorns in Tokay Valley: Jewish Life in Hungary: The History of Abaújszántó*, 167–8.

44 Ibid.

45 Frojimovics and Komoróczy, *Jewish Budapest*, 253.

aims of Judaism" so that the "Jewish patient in the Jewish hospital" could feel "that he belongs to Judaism and that he enjoys such philanthropy that originates from the spirit of Judaism."[46] When it came to schools, in Horthy's "Christian Hungary"[47] most governmental support went to Catholic schools, leaving the Jewish primary schools in Budapest without much public funding. In response, after years of controversy over the need for confessional secondary schools, in 1919 the Budapest Jewish Community, headed by Sándor Léderer, opened both a private gymnasium for Jewish boys as well as one for girls.[48] Yet in 1931, Dr. Arnold Csech, a teacher at the Hungarian Israelite Teachers College (Országos Izraelita Tanitóképző-Intézet), called upon Jewish parents to help "save" "Jewish schools" and to build additional ones, even if they "pull away the state support from our schools."[49] He argued that Jewish schools were the "only place for denominational education" and would thus provide the only "prophylaxis against the deathly illness and the only cure" against the "death" of children's "soul."[50] As families were doubted to be capable of providing their children with the appropriate religious upbringing, schools were seen as the only place to raise children in a "religious atmosphere" that would prevent their souls' "wreckage."[51]

The Budapest Jewish Community played a key role in providing local Jewish relief as it ran schools, orphanages, and centers for religious education. When it came to war orphans, their placement in orphanages and provisioning them with suitable clothing were prime objectives. The National Israelite Patronage Association (Országos Izraelita Patronázs Egyesület) is reported to have provided 400 war orphans with new clothing during a celebration.[52] In 1924, Hanna, a local Jewish child welfare association run by Jewish philanthropic women and headed by Dóra Heiden, not only provided a warm meal to "20 hungry Jewish children," but also gave 250 Jewish children warm winter clothing.[53] Every meal began with a Jewish prayer.[54] The symbolically significant Jewish holiday of Purim, which commemorates the

46 "A zsidó fiuárvaház esete," *Egyenlőség*, July 9, 1927, 2.
47 Hanebrink, *In Defense of Christian Hungary*.
48 Frojimovics and Komoróczy, *Jewish Budapest*, 282.
49 "Kis gyermek halálára," *Egyenlőség*, March 7, 1931, 12.
50 Ibid.
51 Ibid.
52 "Négyszáz hadiárvát 'felruháznak,'" *Egyenlőség*, December 3, 1921, 16.
53 Oszkar Szalai, "A 'Hanna,'" *Egyenlőség*, February 16, 1924, 8.
54 Ibid.

salvation of Jews from extermination at the times of the Persian Empire, provided an opportunity for these and other groups to raise funds for children's rescue from starvation and neglect. In 1922, it was claimed that the "destiny of 500 Jewish war orphans and abandoned children" depended "on the Jewish readiness to donate during the festival of Purim," so that shoes, bread, and clothing could be given to the orphaned and abandoned children.[55]

Transatlantic Jewish Child Relief

Local Jewish relief was to a great extent dependent on help from abroad. In response to eyewitness reports about the often highly problematic local situation of Jews in Central and Eastern Europe, international Jewish philanthropic organizations committed themselves to relieving the suffering of their increasingly impoverished and persecuted Jewish brethren. Since its founding in 1914,[56] the JDC raised relief funds in the United States and thus succeeded in establishing "a common [American] response to the war."[57] It embodied the mixture of "an American identity that expresses benevolence and a religious or ethnic identity that expresses solidarity."[58] But within American society its main purpose was not to "inquire the presumption of difference by the Jewish enclaves within the city," but rather to express the donors' Americanness and thereby strengthen their social standing.[59] In relation to postwar Hungary, Hungarian Jews in the United States were troubled by the news about the White Terror and worried about the destiny of their Jewish brethren at home. Consequently, representatives of the American Jewish Committee, a Jewish advocacy organization, informed the US State Department about the ongoing massive persecution of Jews in Hungary.

Yet, the Western powers' general "considerations of foreign policy," but in particular their "strong anti-Bolshevist position [...] and their consequent attitude of 'understanding' toward Hungary"[60] led them to downplay the

55 "Purim-zsidó gyermeknap," *Egyenlőség*, March 4, 1922, 14.

56 On November 24, 1914, the Joint Distribution Committee was founded by the American Jewish Relief Committee, the Central Relief Committee, and the People's Relief Committee. Albert Lucas, "American Jewish Relief in the World War," *Annals of the American Academy of Political and Social Science* 79 (1918): 223.

57 Wilson, *New York and the First World War*, 93.

58 Ibid., 93–4.

59 Ibid., 93–4.

60 Katzburg, "Louis Marshall and the White Terror," 3.

scope of the terror. In reaction to this, Jewish communities and organizations assumed a watchful eye over the fate and treatment of Jewish communities in Europe. The United States also never ratified the Treaty of Trianon and instead signed an American–Hungarian treaty with Miklós Horthy establishing transatlantic "friendly relations" on August 29, 1921. In December 1919, Ulysses Grant-Smith was sent as the US Commissioner to Hungary and an American legation followed on December 26, 1921.[61] Wishing to maintain good relations with Horthy, who was considered preferable as the Hungarian head of state over Béla Kun, the American and British governments were very careful about criticizing the involvement of Horthy's government in the terror against Jews.[62]

The original move to help the Jews of Central and Eastern Europe came from organizations such as the JDC,[63] which started to lobby in favor of their Jewish brethren in Central and Eastern Europe during the First World War. Having raised funds among American Jews, the JDC shipped large supplies of food, clothing, and medicine to Jewish communities in the target countries that suffered from famine as well as the consequence of pogroms and displacement.[64] In local JDC warehouses in the distressed countries, relief supplies were distributed to Jews. Local relief work was cooperating with local Jewish communities, local charities, and health- and childcare facilities, as they provided the spaces and personnel that were needed for the distribution of relief, be it in schools or other public facilities. The Hungarian government expressed its deepest gratitude towards the American donors, such as the ARA, without ever explicitly mentioning the particular need and relief of Jewish children in Hungary. In a cablegram from Budapest to the ARA's branch office in London on December 17, 1920, Hungary's prime minister promised to provide "every [possible] support" to the further implementation of American relief and promised to devote "all profits [from] transactions Hungary [makes]" to "extending child welfare work [in]

61 Embassy of Hungary, "Key Dates in Hungarian-American Diplomatic Relations," http://washington.kormany.hu/key-dates-in-hungarian-american-diplomatic-relations [last accessed: April 12, 2017].

62 Katzburg, "Louis Marshall and the White Terror," 3.

63 The Alliance Israélite Universelle in Paris also played a central role. For this, see Johnson, "Breaking or Making the Silence?: British Jews and East European Jewish Relief, 1914–1917," 106.

64 On relief to Soviet Jewry, see Beizer, "'I Don't Know Whom to Thank': The American Jewish Joint Distribution Committee's Secret Aid to Soviet Jewry," 112. On relief to Poland, see Tessaris, "The war relief work of the American Jewish Joint Distribution Committee in Poland and Lithuania, 1915–1918."

Hungary."[65] American relief left a long-lasting impact on local charities and welfare institutions, as American relief workers often relied on local institutions and practitioners to distribute the relief to the local population. While the ARA did not focus on relieving Jewish suffering in particular, the JDC was most invested in strengthening the local Jewish communities and to combat anti-Semitism. Throughout the war the JDC established local committees in the relief countries, which regularly "report[ed] to the Joint" so that it could "keep in close, frequent and immediate touch with the various Jewish Committees in the War Zones."[66]

In the case of Hungary, the JDC directly supported the much-impaired Budapest Jewish Community in the postwar years. Via the JDC's Transmission Bureau American Jews of Hungarian descent could send remittances to family members in the former war zones and distressed regions. During the war this system of remittances enabled the direct transfer of money to "wives, parents, brothers, sisters and other relatives" and the direct transmission of "vast quantities of food, clothing, medical supplies and other aid" to the Jews in need.[67] The Hungarian-American "Uncle" Gyula Keszler sent by post thousands of kosher food packages with "three kilos of white flour, a kilo of crystal sugar, a kilo of rice, and two dried figs" as well as "cooking oil instead of fat."[68] The food packages had been financed by "relatives or friends" that had migrated to the United States. Relief in goods was far more effective than money donations, as with the money "hardly anything could be bought at the market," while the "six-kilo packages" with "plaited buns and white bread for the children" and "chocolate for anemic and malnourished toddlers" was greeted with smiling faces.[69] Person-bound relief and remittances were indeed "a mark of ethnic and diasporic ties" between Jewish communities on both sides of the Atlantic.[70] At the same time, the "knowledge and networks of the immigrants" was essential to larger relief organizations like

65 Cablegram, Richardon to Mr. Smith (for action) and Mr. Brown and Captain Quinn (for information. Budapest, December 17, 1920. Hoover Institution Archives, American Relief Administration European Unit, European Children Fund General Files, London Office Cable and Telegram File, Hungary-"Yellow" Budapest to London 1920 Aug.–1922 Feb. F 4 R56.

66 Lucas, "American Jewish Relief in the World War," 221–2. On the British relief, see Johnson, "Breaking or Making the Silence?"

67 Lucas, "American Jewish Relief in the World War," 223.

68 "Szegény pesti gyerekek," *Egyenlőség*, January 1, 1921, 10.

69 Ibid.

70 Granick, "Waging Relief: The Politics and Logistics of American Jewish War Relief in Europe and the Near East, 1914–1918," 58.

the JDC.[71] Once it was conveyed that few goods were available in the target countries, American donors immediately turned the cash they had gathered into goods to be shipped to the distressed region. An article in the Jewish-American newspaper *The Sentinel* acknowledged in 1920 that "even if the Jews in the east are supplied with money, they will still suffer from hunger and cold, and their plight will continue to be what it was in the past." Thus "[i]nstead of money we should send them [the] money's worth in goods," so that "we really would do something great to relieve the situation."[72]

American Humanitarian Collaboration

Since there were problems associated with directly sending supplies to the target communities, the JDC had to rely on the infrastructure and organization of the ARA or the ARC to deliver its relief packages. When it concerned to Jewish child relief items, the JDC relied on the assistance of the ARA's European Children's Fund.[73] However, once the JDC started to transmit supplies in large volume via the ARA, the direct transfer of goods between individuals in the United States and those in Central and Eastern Europe was called off. With Felix Warburg as its chairman, the JDC succeeded in working together with Hoover's ARA. Raised as a Quaker, Hoover believed that no difference should be made on the basis of religious denomination when it came to relieving the suffering of children in Europe.[74] Carleton Bowden, the head of American relief activities in Hungary, strongly argued that American relief organizations "will not look [at] which child is Jewish and which Christian," as there was "no connection between the needy child and religion," which is why the issue of religion did not "interest" them.[75] Yet, as local Jewish communities often suffered not just from poverty and hunger but were also the targets of violent persecution and social marginalization, they were facing additional obstacles when it came to their everyday survival. Furthermore, many Jews followed Jewish dietary laws, which made the consumption of certain nondietary foods delivered and prepared by the

71 Ibid.

72 "The Week," *The Sentinel* 37.6, February 6, 1920, 10.

73 Letter by the Secretary of the Jewish Joint Distribution Committee to Barry Smith, June 25, 1919. Jewish Joint Distribution Committee Archive, New York City, New York.

74 Diner, *The Jews of the United States, 1654 to 2000*, 196.

75 "Valláskülönbség nélkül élelmezik az amerikaiak a magyar gyermekeket," *Egyenlőség*, January 15, 1921, 7.

ARA impossible. Thus, as the ARA did—at least not in Hungary—consider the religious-ethnic dimension of children's poverty and suffering a priority, food relief through the ARA often did not meet the special and often greater needs of Jewish children in Hungary. Therefore the JDC stepped in when it came to the special needs of local Jewish communities.

In Central and Eastern Europe, the ARA and the JDC established child feeding stations "for the children of the very poorest classes, these often being the intellectual classes."[76] Most of the images, such as Figure 6.1, depict children's needs and food relief without explicitely identifying the children's religious denomination.

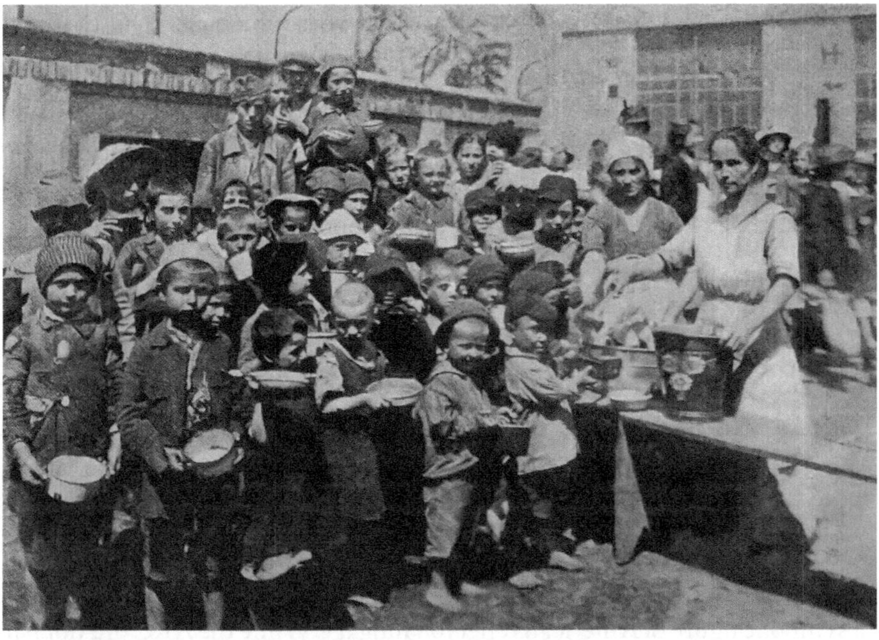

Figure 6.1: ***The Food Line at Újpest.*** **In: American Relief Administration European Children's Fund,** ***Final Report of the Work in Hungary,*** **Budapest, June 1, 1920, 11.**[77]

76 "Hungary," short report in "Salient Extracts from a report made to the Acting Secretary of State by an Official of the Department of State, under date of 15 January 1921, *American Relief Administration Bulletin* 10, March 1, 1921, 3–4, 4.

77 This photograph was taken at one of the largest child feeding stations, a former leather goods factory in Újpest, where 5,000 children received a hearty meal daily through the efforts of the European Children's Fund. As the above image was published before 1923, it is according to the Herbert Hoover presidential library in the public domain. In case I have by any chance and involuntarily infringed any copyright, I hereby declare that the use of the images solely serves educational purposes.

Through the "munificence of the help" afforded by American Jews, soup kitchens could be opened in Central and Eastern Europe, "orphanages reared, hospitals equipped," and even a number of "rabbis and scholars" could be "cared for in special ways."[78] Yet the money that was raised by American Jewry was reported to have gone mostly to bread, "for hunger has been the chief thing to be overcome."[79] In Budapest, the JDC sent money to the Budapest Jewish Community to offer free lunches and distribute urgently needed clothing to impoverished Jewish schoolchildren. The Budapest Jewish Community offered these services in its various schools: "Our schoolchildren, who suffered from ever increasing poverty, received help. Speaking of child relief and its activities we remember with deep gratitude and thankfulness the large-scale generosity with which the JDC Distribution Committee of America [...] supported several hundreds of our pupils with clothing and food."[80] Only through the help of the JDC could the National Jewish Women's Association (Magyar Izraelita Nőegyletek Országos Szövetsége), which since its foundation in 1866 had run a kosher soup kitchen that served a daily warm meal to poor Jews, continue to provide its services.[81] In addition, the JDC's financial help was used to introduce a lunch division in the Jewish schools to provide a "fresh and delicious lunch to our poor."[82] Dr. Nathan Krass, the chief rabbi of the Central Synagogue in New York City and delegate of the JDC, returned from a trip to Eastern Europe, reporting that the JDC's "milk stations" were "wonderful things for the Jewish youngsters."[83] By providing the milk, even if it was only watered condensed milk, within "two weeks a child, who could not stand because malnutrition had softened his bones, could walk and play."[84]

Captain James Pedlow, the representative of the ARC in Hungary, became a symbolic figure of American relief to Hungary. While the ARC did not particularly target Jewish organizations through their relief efforts, Pedlow is remembered for his efforts in relieving the suffering of Jewish children. A Jewish observer wrote in *Egyenlőség* in 1921 that since the "great collapse, since

78 Lucas, "American Jewish Relief in the World War," 227.

79 Ibid., 227.

80 Pesti Izraelita Hitközség, *Pesti Izraelita Hitközség*, 6.

81 "Johanna Bischnitz," *Yivo Encyclopedia of Jews in Eastern Europe*, http://www.yivoencyclopedia.org/article.aspx/Bischitz_Johanna [last accessed: April 12, 2017].

82 Ibid.

83 "With 40,000,000 Aid Jews Still Suffer."

84 Ibid., 17.

[...] despair and poverty" had plagued Hungary, "the name Captain Pedlow" had become "an 'icon' among us." It was considered natural that wherever "poverty rules he appears with his helping hand and his helping heart." Welfare and philanthropic institutions were particularly indebted to him as they found themselves "in such difficult conditions, due to the high inflation rate, that without his help they could have hardly fulfilled any of their tasks." Thus, various Jewish child relief organizations took the celebration of his birthday in 1921 as an opportunity to cherish his great humanitarian deeds, this time jointly with non-Jewish welfare organizations. Yet, a female American social worker at the celebration noted that it had been the first time since her arrival to Budapest that she experienced how "various religious organizations celebrated in such harmony together," and she was "sorry that she experienced this only once."[85] Thus, relief for Jewish and non-Jewish children often took place in distinct areas.

Summer Colonies for Jewish Children

One far-reaching way to relieve the suffering of the Jewish children in Hungary was to send them to the countryside for a month during the summer. The Jewish Child Holiday Association (Izraelita Szünidei Gyermektelep Egyesület) was established in 1909 with the aim of allowing Jewish children between the ages of seven and eighteen to spend their summers in the countryside. Two summer boarding schools, one near Lake Balaton and the other in Diósjenő, were used to accommodate around 500 Jewish children for a period of four weeks during the summer months.[86] In the 1920s, the Jewish Child Holiday Association organized the summer holidays together with the National Hungarian Jewish Educational Association (Országos Magyar Izraelita Közművelődési Egyesület [OMIKE]), which had been established in 1909. While the Jewish Child Holiday Association placed children in holiday colonies, OMIKE arranged for the placement of Jewish children "with better-off Jewish families in Hungary's countryside" so that they would "return in September in a strengthened state."[87]

85 "Pedlow kapitány felekezetközi ünneplése egy zsidó intézményben," *Egyenlőség*, October 15, 1921, 13.

86 Pesti Izraelita Hitközség, *Pesti Izraelita Hitközség*, 6; "Izraelita Szünidei Gyermektelep," *Magyar Zsidó Lexikon*, Budapest 1929, 402, http://mek.oszk.hu/04000/04093/html/0410.html [last accessed: April 12, 2017].

87 Ernő Weller, "Az Omike gyermeknyaraltatása," *Egyenlőség*, June 29, 1929, 17.

Before the children could leave to participate in the summer colonies, they underwent a full physical examination, mostly in school facilities. Throughout the week, in the afternoons, the gym of the Jewish school in Wesselényi Street in Budapest turned into a space for "sad conscriptions"—not those "whose bodies are unharmed and whose health is bursting," but instead those who were "weak, sick, thin, undernourished, and whose stomachs, lungs, and skeletons were functioning poorly."[88] The thinner, sicker, and more destitute a child looked, the more likely it was to become part of the "army, which is year after year dragged to the holiday colonies at Lake Balaton or in the mountains."[89] While the peak of these colonies was the immediate postwar period, they continued throughout the 1930s and found their historical continuation in the socialist children's holidays at Lake Balaton.

When it came to finding temporary foster parents in the countryside, appeals were published in the Jewish weekly *Egyenlőség* calling upon "Jewish mothers and fathers" to relieve the suffering of the poor Jewish children from the capital. An article from 1920 starts with an image of "destitute urban childhoods in Budapest," where in "tiny flats of the large tenement houses thousands and thousands of anemic, pale Jewish children with broken hearts" were "awaiting the burgeoning spring and were longing for the hot summer."[90] Employing the idea of a philanthropic community in faith, the organizers of the summer colonies appealed to the emotions of their "[d]ear brethren in the countryside!"[91] They went on with employing gendered forms of address to separately gain male and female supporters: "We turn to your fatherly humanitarian heart. And to you: beloved sisters, who with both your Jewish heart and your motherly goodness feel the great and life-threatening poverty of the poor children from Budapest."[92] Ensnaring mothers and fathers separately, they pleaded with them to "give—at least for four weeks—one or two Jewish children from Budapest [...] a corner in your house and a place at your family table."[93] While throughout the history of childhood, children's life in rural areas had mostly meant a life of pov-

88 "Ahol a szegénység hadseregét sorozzák," *Egyenlőség*, June 13, 1931, 11.
89 Ibid.
90 "Zsidó gyerekek nyaralása," *Egyenlőség*, March 20, 1920, 4.
91 Ibid.
92 Ibid.
93 Ibid.

erty and deprivation, industrialization, war, and postwar population movements transformed the notion of rural life. Life in the countryside was considered an ideal setting for children's healthy and prosperous upbringing, promising Jewish children "air, sun, and health" as well as "plenty of food,"[94] which were seen as a means to "save the only hope for the future: the Jewish youth."[95]

In response, many Jewish families in the countryside invited poor urban children to their homes. While before the war OMIKE could accommodate "around 5,000 impoverished middle-class children," the war and its aftermath reduced its ability to host such numbers at the holiday colonies. In an article in *Egyenlőség* from 1929, Ernő Weller complained that "[u]nfortunately, due to the—from year to year—worsening economic situation [...] we are able to bring fewer and fewer children to the countryside."[96] Thus, in 1921 only 500 out of 4,000 needy children could participate in the OMIKE summer holiday, and only 600 out of 2,000 children in the programs of the Jewish Child Holiday Association, because "not enough friends and supporters of this humane project could be found."[97] Thus, the Jewish child colonies also relied on financial support from abroad. Krass reported that the JDC had sent "7,000 Jewish children to the country," about which he wrote that he had "never known anything more wonderful than those happy colonies of little ones, who, a week or two before, were starving."[98] Krass reported that "[o]ne little boy wrote about his first night in the colony" that he had "turned over on one side and could not go to sleep, and then turned over on the other side and could not go to sleep."[99] He then "looked up at the ceiling and could not sleep." He could not fall asleep not because of fear, but "because he was so glad that he had had his dinner."[100] Employing the language of the child's overtly positive emotions[101] was instrumental in gaining the support of families for this rather far-reaching relief activity.

94 Original title of an article in *Egyenlőség*: "Napsugarat, bő táplálékot szegény gyermekeinknek," *Egyenlőség*, May 26, 1928, 2.

95 "Zsidó gyerekek nyaralása," 4.

96 Weller, "Az Omike gyermeknyaraltatása."

97 "A zsidó gyermekek nyaraltatása," *Egyenlőség*, July 9, 1921, 7.

98 "With 40,000,000 Aid Jews Still Suffer."

99 Ibid.

100 Ibid.

101 For a recent study on the history of emotions, see Plamper, *The History of Emotions: An Introduction*.

Financial (and Real) Adoption

Beyond providing material support, the JDC also arranged for the financial adoption of Jewish orphans by American Jews by developing a foster-parent scheme for war orphans. It was perceived as "both impracticable and unwise" to attempt to solve the problem of Central and Eastern Europe's war orphans "through the emigration of any large number of orphans, either to America or the South."[102] Instead, a foster-parent scheme was to be developed "in which individuals" were to be found to "adopt a particular child and provide for his maintenance."[103] By keeping up a regular correspondence, the child could "feel he is of importance to somebody who cares for him."[104] In order to realize this plan, the JDC enlisted a "great number of American Jews who will agree to give $100 a year a piece for the support of the orphans in Europe."[105] This "system of financial adoption" was based on the premise that future "financial foster-parents in this country" would "not contribute impersonally to a fund."[106] Instead, they were asked to provide "care" for a "given child."[107] In order to establish human contact between foster parent and foster child, the financial foster parent was to be "supplied with photographs and a history of the child and kept informed of the child and [...] of his or her progress."[108] Personal "correspondence between the foster-parent and the child" was also arranged.[109]

Evelyn Sharp was convinced that the "foster-parent scheme" would incidentally "sow many seeds of future friendships in Europe."[110] While she considered the real adoption of foreign children, where the children would be brought up in the country of their adoption, a good option, she was convinced that it would be better to "still adopt them" but "allow them to grow up in their own country."[111] In this way, the orphans would "remain citizens of their own country"[112] but possess foster parents in another country. This

102 "Plan to Aid to 300,000 Jewish Orphans: Distribution Committee's Program Includes System of Financial Adoptions," *The New York Times*, November 15, 1920, 26.
103 Sharp, "The International Orphan."
104 Ibid.
105 "Plan to Aid to 300,000 Jewish Orphans."
106 Ibid.
107 Ibid.
108 Ibid.
109 Ibid.
110 Sharp, "The International Orphan."
111 Ibid.
112 Ibid.

would create a "new relationship that should tend to break down those racial barriers that help to make racial antagonisms."[113] In her report she referred to the foster-parent scheme that had been created in Switzerland, which had enlisted the "sympathy of its children who send both money and parcels to the orphans they adopt as brothers and sisters."[114]

The JDC sometimes allowed for the "real" adoption of war orphans and arranged for their transportation to the United States. An article in *The New York Times* from 1921 reported that "[f]ifty orphaned Jewish children arrived here yesterday in the care of the Joint Distribution Committee on the steamship *Polonia* of the Baltic American Line."[115] This, however, was the exception. Financial adoption was far more widespread and easier to arrange. Felix Warburg, too, was convinced that it would be best to raise the orphans in each country into the "most useful and patriotic citizens of the country of which they are natives."[116] Warburg appealed to American Jewry to raise funds to secure the "future of the children of Europe," as he was sure that their well-being affected "not alone the future of the Jewish people through the world, but the well-being of all the countries of Europe."[117] The yearbook of the Budapest Jewish Community reports in 1920 on the financial support of the Jewish Boys' Orphanage in Budapest through the JDC. The "long-lasting war, but especially the following general turmoil and economic depression brought our orphanage into a very critical situation. [...] [Last year] it was uncomfortable for the orphanage to halve the number of its orphans and [...] expose them to an uncertain fate. In the following year we did everything [...] to again increase the number."[118] As the orphanage's ability to further maintain its services had been the result of the JDC's financial support, the article explicitly addressed the American donors: "At this point we would like to express our deep gratitude for their noble-hearted support."[119] In addition to the institutional support through the JDC, individual American "brothers in faith" were also reported to have donated great sums to the Jewish orphanage.[120]

113 Ibid.
114 Ibid.
115 "Ship Brings 50 Jewish Orphans," *The New York Times*, December 2, 1921, 14.
116 "Plan to Aid to 300,000 Jewish Orphans."
117 Ibid.
118 Pesti Izraelita Hitközség, *Pesti Izraelita Hitközség*, 15.
119 Ibid., 15.
120 Ibid., 16.

Transatlantic Fund-Raising Campaigns

In order to initiate and implement the financial support of Jewish communities in Central and Eastern Europe, broad fundraising campaigns were conducted in the United States for the suffering Jews in the distressed parts of Europe. New York City, with its large Hungarian Jewish minority, served as a bridge between the Hungarian and American Jewish communities. In 1922, three representatives of the Budapest Jewish Community[121] were sent to New York City to set up the cooperation with the Hungarian and American Jews in New York, helping them organize the relief to Hungary. While local relief inside Hungary was very limited, in New York these three important figures experienced the "really noble mission of great importance," without which the maintenance of Jewish relief was thought to be impossible.[122] Leading "Jewish orators" went on fundraising mission in every part of the United States "to tell the story of the sufferings and privations of the Jews in the War zones."[123] The fundraising campaign targeted particularly Jewish émigrés from Eastern Europe and their descendants in the United States, who had ancestral connections to the region and thus cared about the destiny of their Jewish brethren. An article in *Egyenlőség* on May 15, 1920, noted that the "Hungarians living in America" had already started "fighting poverty in Hungary" by collecting a huge "amount of dollars" by means of which "more bread to the poor, baby equipment for the infants, and nutritious food for the sick" could be provided.[124] In this way, Hungarian-Americans joined into this "great humanitarian work."[125]

The American Relief Committee for Hungarian Sufferers in New York, established in September 1919, played a central role in coordinating the efforts of Hungarians in the United States to relieve the suffering in their home country.[126] A number of Jewish delegates were sent to this committee, yet with no particular religious objective, because, as the above-mentioned article from 1920 stated, "the Hungarian-Americans do not know any de-

121 The three representatives were Ferenc Székely, Illés Adler, and Emil Zahler.

122 "Bizottság alakult Amerikában a magyar zsidók megsegitésére," *Egyenlőség*, January 7, 1922, 14.

123 Lucas, "American Jewish Relief in the World War," 226.

124 "Az Amerikában élő magyar zsidók akciót inditottak az itthoni nyomor leküzdésére," *Egyenlőség*, May 15, 1920, 2.

125 Ibid.

126 "A Nemzeti Ujság, America és a magyar zsidók," *Egyenlőség*, May 29, 1920, 3.

nominational difference among each other."[127] Although not focused in particular on relieving the suffering of Jewish children, this committee contributed much to the general relief of Hungarian children. In its "Notice to Hungarian-Americans" (1920), the author called upon the entire Hungarian population of the United States to provide "sufficient aid" for the "children of Hungary, and to prevent their destruction."[128] Uncomfortable with the fact that national "strangers"—the ARA and the JDC—were taking "care of this very important [Hungarian] matter," the author demanded that the "entire Hungarian population [...] stand together, and become a mother, who lovingly embraces her starving children," thereby saving "the future of our homeland."[129]

Even child victims of hunger and recent recipients of American relief turned into relief mediators. In early May 1920, the fourteen-year-old Jewish Hungarian boy Lajos Turteltaub, who had fled from Hungary because of hunger, caused a huge sensation among Hungarian-Americans in New York City, where he filled "theater and concert halls" for his fundraising speeches.[130] Turteltaub allowed New York donors to hear the personal story of one of those starving Hungarian children who had been saved through American money. But Turteltaub did not stop here, because he had promised to his suffering comrades in Hungary to raise further funds for those children whose parents were unable to earn enough money to dress and feed their children. In his printed speech, he not only described how "hunger, inflation, and epidemics" ruled in Hungary, but also aroused fears about the planned dismemberment of the "fervently loved mother country."[131] As the Treaty of Trianon was signed only a few weeks later, on June 4, he trusted that with his speech he could not only save the life of starving comrades at home, but also alter the country's geopolitical destiny through Hungarian-American help. The call for explicit Hungarian patriotic relief to save the Hungarian nation and state fundamentally questioned the internationalization of relief in the postwar period, disqualifying international or American donations as highly problematic to the proud Hungarian nation. Yet,

127 "Az Amerikában élő magyar zsidók."

128 "A Notice to Hungarian-Americans," *Magyar Tribune*, February 13, 1920, http://flps.newberry.org/article/5422061_2_1067/ [last accessed: April 12, 2017].

129 Ibid.

130 "Turteltaub agitál Magyarországon," *Egyenlőség*, May 8, 1920, 7.

131 Ibid.

without relying on the transnational infrastructure of the large relief organizations, Hungarian-American support would have lacked much of its efficiency. Both the JDC and the ARA allowed for the massive collection, transmission, and distribution of relief goods in Europe.[132]

In 1920, American Jews as well as non-Jewish Americans were reported to have raised over $40 million for the "suffering Jews of Eastern Europe" since 1916, yet this amount was still considered "inadequate to do constructive relief work."[133] The JDC stated that they had "kept millions of children and adults alive in the hopes that the coming peace would so alter living conditions [so] as to enable the Jews to care for themselves."[134] By 1920, however, they realized that their "hopes were in vain," as the conditions of the Jewish communities had worsened practically everywhere since 1914.[135] Therefore, further funds were necessary. Public appeals addressed the "American generosity" for "saving the lives of the children, among whom tuberculosis has reached calamitous proportions."[136] In 1921, Louis Marshall, president of the American Jewish Relief Committee, wished to find "words powerful enough to bring this terrible tragedy home to all the Jews of America."[137] Images such as "the cry of 300,000 orphans, robbed by the European war of their natural protectors and now suffering from both hunger and cold" were used by the American Jewish Relief Committee to attract the solidarity and compassion of donors, in order to collect another $14 million in 1920.[138]

Beyond the "propaganda in person," Jewish relief organizations also employed modern written and visual propaganda means. They sent out several hundred thousand copies of newsletters in which the situation of starving and sick Jewish children in hospitals in Budapest was visually documented.[139] One newsletter was illustrated with a picture of "three emaciated infants in one bed looking up with their open mouths," carrying the caption "Children in Budapest Are Suffering from Starvation."[140] They also arranged for a great number of lantern lectures, accompanied by such visual slides about

132 "Bizottság alakult Amerikában a magyar zsidók megsegitésére."
133 "With 40,000,000 Aid Jews Still Suffer."
134 Ibid.
135 Ibid.
136 "Found Mid-European Jews in Great Need," *The New York Times*, September 12, 1921, 2.
137 "Cry of 300,000 Orphans in Europe," *The New York Times*, November 27, 1921, 6.
138 Ibid.
139 "Az Amerikában élő magyar zsidók."
140 Ibid.

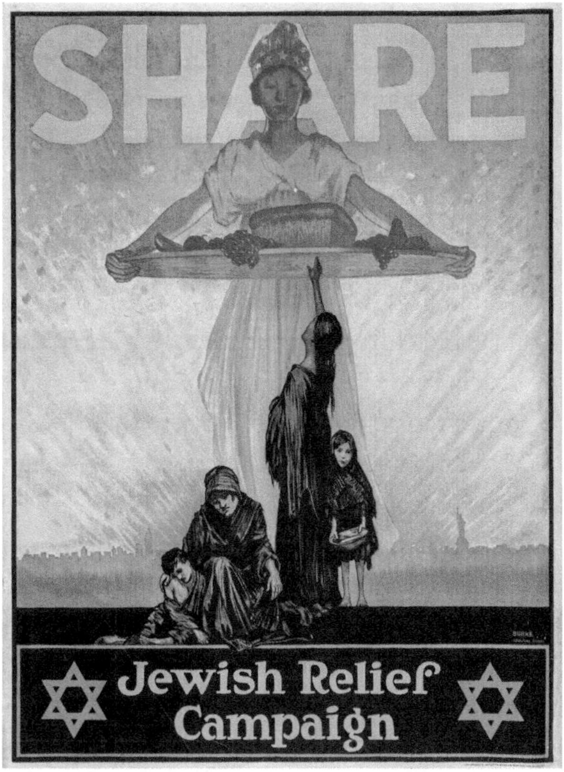

Figure 6.2: *Share-Jewish Relief Campaign*. Burke, Johnstone Studios, lithographed by Sackett & Wilhelms Corporation, Brooklyn, N.Y. 1917. Washington, Library of Congress, Prints & Photographs Division, WWI Posters, Courtesy of the Library of Congress, LC-DIG-ppmsca-05663. [141]

"poverty in Budapest" which left the audience crying. After such lectures "thousands of dollars could be collected."[142] Posters and visuals were also used to raise funds among Jewish and non-Jewish donors. The poster "Share" by the JDC used Columbia, the female personification of the United States, to call upon New York's Jewish and non-Jewish citizens to share their food with Central Europe's starving Jews.

This image, however, exists in various versions of which some carry even a non-denominational slogan which calls upon New York's wealthy for do-

141 Accordingly to the Library of Congress no restrictions on publication are known. In case I have by any chance and involuntarily infringed any copyright, I hereby declare that the use of the images solely serves educational purposes.

142 Ibid.

nations to the "European Relief Council" and thus for non-Jewish relief.[143] But here, this unequivocal image of suffering and relief is combined with the slogan "Jewish Relief Campaign" and two stars of David, which is meant specifically to address New York Jewish émigrés from Eastern Europe to relieve the suffering of their European Jewish brethren. Such Jewish relief visuals linked two messages. First, by identifying the Jewish donor with the female personification of America suggests the successful assimilation and Americanization of Jewish émigrés in the United States. Secondly, offering food to poor Jewish women and children in their home country, these integrated Jews were able to reach out to fellow Jews in Central Europe and thereby strengthen or re-create transnational social ties to their Jewish home communities in Europe. Such advertisements perfectly visualized the "fundamental tension in East European immigrant Jewish life" between, on the one hand, the "drive to integrate more fully into American society," and, on the other, the high "inclination to maintain active ties to people in the immigrants places of origin," as Daniel Soyer observed.[144] This ambivalent tendency of émigrés toward "'Americanization,' on the one hand, and 'transnationalism,' on the other" found perfect expression in their fundraising and lobbying activities for the poor in their home countries. At the same time, such humanitarian commitments contributed to the social recognition and integration of Hungarian émigrés into American life.

In this way, émigrés could confirm and consolidate their new status both in America as well as in world Jewish affairs. Thus, despite their inner ambivalence, "Americanization and transnationalism" were to some degree "compatible."[145] It is quite telling that the same visual was used three years later, as a poster for "The Invisible Guest" dinner of the European Relief Council that took place on December 29, 1920. While it is mentioned that the poster had been contributed by the JDC, its caption no longer identifies its purpose as a "Jewish Relief Campaign" but calls upon relief in general. Here we can see how Jewish relief, and its visual language, became incorporated into the making of non-denominational transatlantic humanitarian relief.[146]

143 For a discussion on the non-Jewish "Share"-poster, see my article "Compassion for the Distant Other: Children's Hunger and Humanitarian Relief in Budapest in the Aftermath of WWI," 145–6.

144 Soyer, "Transnationalism and Americanization in East European Jewish Immigrant Public Life," 47.

145 Ibid.

146 On the invisible guest dinner, see my article "Compassion for the Distant Other."

Yet, in terms of transatlantic relations, relief also turned into an arena of paternalistic intervention of the West in the life of the starving Eastern European child. Material relief helped to deepen the inequality between receiving and donating societies, proving Central and Eastern European societies to be backward. Social unrest and conflicts could also be triggered between Hungarian social workers and Hungarian recipients of relief. Aladár Kaszab, a social worker of the JDC in Budapest, remembered, in article from 1927, how once, after he had finished the distribution of relief donation, a "crying woman who had received shoes and clothing came back angrily and shouted at me: What made me think that she could wear a black dress and high heels?" He recalled that she made such a fuss that they had to call the police to remove her. He concludes that this inappropriate reaction expressed the ungratefulness of some relief "profiteers" that not only harmed the real poor, but equally disappointed and disillusioned the donors.[147] As relief was supposed to be gratefully received, allowing the donor societies to appear generous and humanitarian, any reaction that did not fit this expectation was considered inappropriate. If this pattern of humanitarian aid did not work, transatlantic aid could trigger misunderstandings and social unrest between donors and recipients. The Jewish woman's emotional reaction to the dress and the high heels might as well reflect the cultural and religious misunderstandings. This was especially the case when relief donations, be it in the form of clothing or food, did either not consider or conform to certain denominational conventions.

Conclusion

Beyond the general problems involved in transatlantic relief, Jewish relief did face a number of particular obstacles, both locally and transnationally. Relief for Jewish children in Central and Eastern Europe was often just a part of general, i.e., non-denominational, relief, diminishing the particular neediness of Jewish communities and their children in the aftermath of the First World War. Although the news of Horthy's White Terror against Jews in Hungary had quickly spread across the Atlantic, it did not manage to substantially alter official Hungarian-American (relief) politics. Transatlantic

147 Kaszab, "A zsidó jótékonyság hibái és tévedései," 9.

economic and political concerns were of such value that the scope of anti-Semitic persecution in Hungary was slightly downplayed. In response, only Hungarian-American Jewish initiatives and above all the JDC could help to meet needs of Hungarian Jewish communities. The successful provision of transatlantic Jewish child relief was dependent on the personal ties between Hungarian-American Jewish émigrés and local Jewish communities in Hungary. The immense influx of transatlantic goods, in the form of food and clothing, guaranteed the saving of the masses of impoverished Hungarian Jewish children. In this way, the Great War and its troublesome aftermath created new needs as well as an "enabling space" for transatlantic health and food intervention. Yet complementary humanitarianism was not immune to furthering transatlantic political and economic dependencies.

CHAPTER VII

The Bodily Disabled as a Poster Boy-Veteran: War Invalids in the Soviet Union after the Second World War[1]

Alexander Friedman

Western and post-Soviet researchers have demonstrated that numerous war veterans and, foremost, war invalids led pitiful lives in the Stalinist Soviet Union after the Second World War. These "destitute war victors," in the words of historian Beate Fieseler, had to deal with significant problems in their work and private lives. With poor medical provisions and insufficient support from the socialist state, many came to depend on help provided by their families, friends, and acquaintances. In their despair, some disaffected war invalids who felt marginalized and abandoned, succumbed to alcoholism. Although the conditions for war invalids gradually improved under Nikita Khrushchev (1953–1964) and, especially, after the increasingly pronounced valorization of the victory over the "Third Reich" in the Soviet Union under Leonid Brezhnev (1964–1982), they nevertheless remained poor.[2]

As such, the Soviet press rarely reported on the drab daily lives of disabled Red Army veterans and their problems, neither under Stalin nor his succes-

1 This chapter was translated by Tudor Georgescu.

2 On this see, for example, Beate Fizeler [Beate Fieseler], "'Nishchie pobediteli': invalidy Velikoy Otechestvennoy voyny v Sovetskom Soyuze," *Neprikosnovennyy zapas: debaty o politike i kul'ture* 2/3 (2005): 290–7; Fieseler, "The Bitter Legacy of the 'Great Patriotic War': Red Army Disabled Soldiers under Late Stalinism"; Fieseler, "De la 'génération perdue' aux bénéficiaires de la politique sociale? Les invalides de guerre en URSS, 1945–1964"; Fieseler, "Soviet-Style Welfare: The Disabled Soldiers of the 'Great Patriotic War.'" On the living conditions of war veterans in the USSR, see Edele, *Soviet Veterans of the Second World War: A Popular Movement in an Authoritarian Society, 1941–1991.*

sors. The most important Soviet newspaper, *Pravda* (Truth), and other Soviet media such as literature and cinematography conveyed the exaggerated propagandistic image of the "happy, brave war invalids"—the "real Soviet men" widely revered by the people—who had defeated National Socialism and freed Europe from fascism, who had not let themselves be disheartened by their disability, who were comprehensively cared for in the USSR, and who were making a considerable contribution to the socialist reconstruction of their fatherland.[3] The Soviet state, which had neglected its war invalids for decades, was anxious to present itself as the "most humane and philanthropic country in the world" and instrumentalized disabled soldiers and officers for propaganda purposes.

This thesis is examined through the following discourse-analytical case study of the individual fates of disabled veterans and the ways in which they were perceived in the Soviet Union (Moscow as well as the periphery). Such an approach has not been commonly used in post-Soviet and international historiography. This study deals with two characteristic examples: the fighter pilot Aleksey P. Mares'ev (1916–2001) and the sharpshooter Gurban Durdy (1917–1976). As people with "perfect socialist profiles" who suffered from serious injuries and showed outstanding heroism in the fight against fascism, Durdy and Mares'ev entered the Soviet propaganda spotlight. While Mares'ev was famous throughout the Soviet Union and the socialist domain and was even seen in the West as the Soviet "poster boy-veteran,"[4] Durdy was a rather more local hero, predominantly celebrated in his Turkmen homeland during and after the war. Scholars have barely noticed these and other individual biographies, although they allow for a more thorough investigation and more differentiated perspectives of the propagandistic instrumentalization of war invalids in the USSR. First, I illuminate Mares'ev and Durdy's lives before the German attack on the Soviet Union. Then I examine their lives in the Soviet Union after the Second World War, and conclude with the ambivalent reception of these socialist heroes in the post-Soviet space after the collapse of the USSR.

---

3 See Fieseler, "Soviet-Style Welfare," 19–20. On this, see also Iarskaia-Smirnova and Romanov, "Heroes and Spongers: The Iconography of Disability in Soviet Posters and Film," 76–8.

4 Manfred Quiring, "Russischer Kampfflieger ohne Beine. Generationen wuchsen auf mit der Heldengeschichte Alexei Maresjews," *Die Welt*, May 26, 2001, http://www.welt.de/print-welt/article453279/Russischer-Kampfflieger-ohne-Beine.html?config=print [last accessed: October 1, 2016].

Aleksey Mares'ev and Gurban Durdy: "Heroes of the Soviet Union"

In 1967, the Soviet Ministry of Defense's military publisher released a tract addressed to Soviet youth to familiarize future soldiers and officers with the Soviet armed forces, its battle traditions, and its history. The print run was an impressive 100,000 copies. Among others, this booklet also mentioned Gurban Durdy and Aleksey Mares'ev. The authors presented the sharpshooter Durdy as a heroically brave Turkmen Red Armist who was badly wounded at the front; with regards to Mares'ev, it was just succinctly emphasized that the legendary "fighter pilot without legs" was famous worldwide.[5]

Aleksey Mares'ev and Gurban Durdy were born in Tsarist Russia during the First World War (1916 and 1917, respectively), experienced the establishment of Soviet rule as children, and were socialized in the Stalinist Soviet Union. The fatherless Mares'ev—his father died in 1919—grew up in the city of Kamyshin on the Volga. His mother worked as a cleaning lady in a wood-processing factory. After leaving school, Mares'ev completed his vocational training as a lathe operator and left his hometown in 1934. He was part of the group of youths the local committee of the All-Union Leninist Young Communist League (Komsomol) sent to help build the new Siberian city of Komsomol'sk-on-Amur. In 1937, Mares'ev was conscripted into the Red Army and realized his life's dream: as an adolescent Mares'ev had wanted to become a pilot and study at flight school. Due to his poor health and constitution—Mares'ev suffered from rheumatism—he was initially turned down. He did not give up, and in 1940 graduated from the Serov Flight School in Bataysk (Rostov region) as a junior lieutenant and, after the German invasion of the USSR, was deployed first to the southwestern (August 1941) and then to the northwestern (March 1942) front.[6]

In March 1942, the war had already been long over for the Komsomol member Durdy. He recovered at a military hospital and later returned to Turkmenistan. Durdy came from the village of Kongur-Yab in the Mary re-

5 Beshkarev et al., *V pomoshch' doprizyvniku*, 43, 70, 72.

6 On Mares'ev, see *Konets povesti: Mares'ev* [The end of the story: Mares'ev], documentary film directed by Aleksandr Slavin (Russia 2001), 25:51 minutes; *Aleksey Mares'ev. Sud'ba nastoyashchego cheloveka* [Aleksey Mares'ev: The destiny of the real man], documentary film directed by Aleksandr Slavin (Russia 2005), 44:08 minutes; *Aleksey Mares'ev. Rozhdennyy letat'* [Aleksey Mares'ev: Born to fly], documentary film directed by Andrey Vladimirov (Russia 2016), 44:45 minutes.

gion and worked on a Voroshilov collective farm (*kolkhoz*) during the latter half of the 1930s. Conscripted into the Red Army in 1938, Durdy participated in the Soviet campaign in Eastern Poland (September 1939). He experienced the German attack as a junior sergeant of the 4th Company of the 389th Regiment of the 176th Rifle Division in Moldova, where the Red Army tried to repel a German–Romanian offensive. At the end of June 1941, Durdy led a troop of scouts that killed eleven "German–Romanian" soldiers, wounding another three and taking several others prisoner. This successful campaign and the story of his dramatic injury can be reconstructed through a certificate of commendation issued on August 8, 1941. In this document, in the military archive of the Russian Federation in Podol'sk near Moscow, the regiment's leader, Major Kramskoy, and War Commissary Zekin emphasized that the Turkmen lost his arm during a battle on July 27, but had remained on the battlefield and continued fighting with his torn "arm in his armpits." With this act of heroism, he thoroughly deserved to be honored as a "Hero of the Soviet Union."[7] Durdy received this most important of Soviet decorations on November 9, 1941, when the Presidium of the Supreme Soviet of the USSR awarded the daring sharpshooter the Order of Lenin and the Medal of the Red Star.[8]

Aleksey Mares'ev was honored as a "Hero of the Soviet Union" on August 24, 1943. The impetus for the decoration was a dogfight during the battle for Kursk on July 20, 1943. On that day, the fighter pilot shot down two German fighters and saved two comrades. An important tributary to the commendation was surely also the fact that the Soviet flying ace accomplished this heroic feat while wearing prosthetic legs. On July 4, 1942, the German Luftwaffe in the Novgorod region shot down Mares'ev's fighter plane. The wounded Soviet pilot spent eighteen days in a forest, before being found by local farmers. Moscow doctors managed to save his life, but his legs had to be amputated below the knee. Officers of the People's Commissariat for Internal Affairs ruled out that the pilot, who had lost his documents in the forest, was a German spy.[9] Owing to an extraordinary strong will, Mares'ev re-

7 Certificate of commendation issued on August 8, 1941, http://www.podvignaroda.mil.ru/?#id=150009516&tab=navDetailDocument [last accessed: October 1, 2016].

8 Decree of the Presidium of the Supreme Soviet from 9 November 1941, http://www.podvignaroda.mil.ru/?#id=2020224&tab=navDetailDocument [last accessed: October 1, 2016].

9 Kolesnichenko, *Aleksey Mares'ev. Ya—ne legenda! Ya—prosto chelovek!* 12:10–12:50; *Aleksey Mares'ev*, Television program *Legendy armii s Aleksandrom Marshalom* [Legends of the army with Aleksandr Marshal] (May 17, 2016, Channel *Zvezda*), 37:50 minutes, esp. 00:10–14:00.

turned to the Red Army, continued his career as a pilot, and shot down a total of seven German planes.[10]

Despite his remarkable life story, Mares'ev was hardly known in the Soviet Union during the war. The first Soviet publication about him appeared in 1945 in the newspaper *Pravda*.[11] *Pravda* war correspondent and author Boris N. Polevoy (1908–1981),[12] thought to have discovered the pilot, met Mares'ev in 1943 and subsequently wrote a piece on him. The story caught Stalin's attention, but its publication was delayed—probably due to the significant educational and propagandistic potential of Mares'ev's case—until the immediate postwar period.[13] In contrast to Mares'ev, Durdy appeared in several of *Pravda*'s wartime publications. Brigade Commissar I. Bidyukov praised the Red Armist's heroic deeds on February 4, 1942, and referred to Durdy's "tremendous heroic bravery."[14] On February 27, 1942, an anonymous *Pravda* lead article honored the Komsomol soldiers who heroically fought the "German fascist bands" at the front. Gurban Durdy from Turkmenistan, among others, served as an example of these young heroes.[15] At the end of March 1942, another anonymous article in the newspaper discussed "junior commanders" (*mladshie komandiry*) as constituting a "basic element of the military organization." Durdy was characterized as an "example of selfless bravery and heroism."[16]

Bidyuskov's article, in which Durdy's injury was highlighted, and the anonymous articles, in which his injury was not discussed, were reprinted by Soviet provincial presses[17] and made the Turkmen known throughout the

10 See Slavin, *Konets povesti*; Slavin, *Aleksey Mares'ev; Aleksey Mares'ev. Ya—ne legenda! Ya—prosto chelovek!* [Aleksey Mares'ev: I am not a legend! I am a man!], documentary film directed by Irina Kolesnichenko (Russia 2016), 41:45 minutes, esp. 00:30–25:00.

11 See Pravdisty, "Pamyat' o nem ne umret," *Pravda*, May 22 and 23, 2001, 1.

12 In the Second World War's immediate aftermath, Boris Polevoy was among the leading *Pravda* correspondents. In 1945 and 1946, he reported for the Moscow newspaper from Nuremberg on the war crimes trials conducted there. See G. Kaurova, "Nevydumannye geroi i zhizn'," introduction to *Povest' o nastoyashchem cheloveke. Doktor Vera*, by Boris Polevoy (Leningrad: Lenizdat, 1980), 548–54, esp. 548; Irmtraud Gutschke, "Wie sich der Traum vom wahren Menschen im Leben erfüllt hat," *Neues Deutschland*, January 26, 1982, 4; Gutschke, "Die Größe unserer Zeit zeigte er im Menschen. Heute wäre Boris Polewoi 75 Jahre alt geworden," *Neues Deutschland*, March 17, 1983, 4.

13 See Slavin, *Aleksey Mares'ev*, 29:00–31:40; Kolesnichenko, *Aleksey Mares'ev. Ya—ne legenda! Ya—prosto chelovek!* 26:05–28:00. Also see Kirill Aleksandrov, "Umer nastoyashchiy chelovek," *Kommersant*, May 19, 2001, 1.

14 I. Bidyukov, "Boevoe stalinskoe plemya," *Pravda*, February 4, 1942, 2.

15 See "Vpered k pobede, boevoe stalinskoe plemya!" *Pravda*, February 27, 1942, 1. See also *Tekhnika—molodezhi*, May 6, 1942, 8.

16 "Mladshiy komandir—osnova voennoy organizatsii," *Pravda*, March 26, 1942, 1.

17 See, among others, "Vpered k pobede, boevoe stalinskoe plemya!" *Sovetskaya Sibir'*, March 1, 1942, 1.

Soviet Union. In 1943, the Moscow Komsomol press Young Guard (Molodaya gvardiya) published a brochure titled *About the Komsomol's Work in Rural Areas.* The brochure contained the sketch "Oath of a Young Turkmen," in which the "brave son of the Turkmen nation" Gurban Durdy was celebrated for having distinguished himself in battle against the "German fascists," having fulfilled his patriotic duty and suffered serious injuries.[18] On April 13, 1943, *Pravda* published a "Letter from the Turkmen Nation to the Turkmen Red Armists," in which Red Army soldiers were called upon to fight at the front as bravely as their famous compatriot Durdy. Among the signatories were Durdy himself, the author Berdy Kerbabayev, and several other prominent Turkmen.[19]

Probably the most famous Turkmen author of the Soviet epoch, Kerbabayev, who led the Union of Writers of the Central Asian Turkmen Soviet Socialist Republic between 1942 and 1950,[20] made a crucial contribution to the creation of the myth of the "Turkmen Warrior"[21] Gurban Durdy in Turkmenistan and beyond. In 1942, he wrote the play *Gurban Durdy,* which was performed in Turkmenistan after the war.[22] The personage of Turkmen

18 See M. Mitrokhin et al., *O rabote komsomola na sele* (Moscow: Molodaya gvardiya, 1943), 54.

19 See "Pis'mo turkmenskogo naroda frontovikam-turkmenam," *Pravda,* April 13, 1943, 3.

20 Kerbabayev was also well-known within the wider socialist domain (such as, for example, in the GDR). On this, see D. Schunski, "Blühende Wüste Kara-Kum. Wasser in den schwarzen Wüstensand Turkmeniens," *Berliner Zeitung,* September 18, 1960, 5; I. G., "Das Buch ist geschrieben, jetzt hat der Leser das Wort. 'Literaturnaja gazeta' schreibt über 'Leser und Schriftsteller,'" *Neues Deutschland,* November 6, 1972, 4; Helga Radmann, "Dem Leben auf der Spur. Beiträge der sowjetischen Schriftsteller zum Fünfjahresplan," *Neue Zeit,* March 20, 1973, 4; Christoph Trilse, "Zeitgenössische Autoren dominieren im Spielplan. Eindrücke von einer Theaterreise in den Sowjet-Orient," *Berliner Zeitung,* September 21, 1985, 7. The author visited the GDR; see "Gäste...," *Berliner Zeitung,* May 15, 1965, 6. His works were translated into German and published in the GDR; see "Bücher im Überblick," *Berliner Zeitung,* January 9, 1952, 3; "Freiheit für Artyk und das ganze Volk. Aus dem Roman 'Der entscheidende Schritt' von Berdy Kerbabajew," *Neues Deutschland,* November 7, 1953, 5; "Neu im Buchladen," *Berliner Zeitung,* August 5, 1978, 10. As with Mares'ev, Durdy, and other famous personalities, Kerbabayev also participated in various Soviet propaganda campaigns. At the end of February 1971, for example, he signed a public appeal by Soviet intellectuals addressed to Belgian scientists and artists and to the wider Belgian public to protest against the anti-Soviet World Conference on Soviet Jewry that convened in Brussels. ADN, "Sowjetische Persönlichkeiten: Zionisten säen Völkerzwist," *Neues Deutschland,* February 26, 1971, 7. On Kerbabayev, see Aylar Kerbabaeva, "'Zhizn'—kak dom: fundament ee nado zakladyvat' gluboko i prochno!,'" *Velikoross* 6 (2012): 120–36.

21 "Ot uchastnikov respublikanskogo sleta peredovikov sel'skogo chozyaystva Turkmenskoy SSR, Moskva, Kreml', tovarishchu Stalinu," *Pravda,* March 31, 1944, 3.

22 Regarding this work, see N. Klado, *Turkmenskaya sovetskaya dramaturgiya* [The Turkmen Soviet dramaturgy] (Moscow: Iskusstvo, 1956), 5; O. Saparov, *Rasskazy i povesti Berdy Kerbabaeva (1928–1958 gg.)* [Tales and stories by Berdy Kerbabayev (1928–1958)] (Ashgabat 1966), 14, 22; Dzhuma Seyitniyazov, *Bibliograficheskiy ukazatel' po tvorchestvu Berdy Kerbabaeva* [The biographical register of Berdy Kerbabayev's works] (Ashgabat: Turkmenistan, 1974), 11, 13.

Durdy—the first of a total of seventy-eight Turkmenistan-born Red Armists who were honored as "Heroes of the Soviet Union" during the Second World War[23]—also served as inspiration for other artists: Turkmen sculptors and painters featured Durdy in their works.[24] The Turkmen composer Ashir Kuliyew wrote the cantata *Gurban Durdy* (1942)[25]; and the Kirgiz poet Kubanychbek Malikov compared the "Hero of the Soviet Union" to a fierce lion in his poem "Gurban Durdy" (1943).[26] In 1944, the leadership of the Soviet military forces in Central Asia counted Durdy among the heroic and courageous "Sons of the Central Asian Nations."[27]

"Real Soviet Men"

Upon his return to Turkmenistan in 1942, Durdy assisted in the military training of young Turkmen.[28] In 1947, he completed his history degree at the Turkmen State Pedagogical Institute in the capital, Ashgabat, and later became the director of the History Museum of the Academy of Sciences of Soviet Turkmenistan.[29] During the Second World War, Soviet authors spread the image of the "selfless Turkmen warrior" Durdy, who came to embody the heroic deeds of the Komsomol members, the great importance of petty officers, and, above all, the battle of the Soviet people against Nazi Germany—and did so with the aim of fortifying the patriotism and willingness of the people to make sacrifices in Soviet Central Asia and Turkmenistan in particular. Durdy was perfectly suited to the Turkmen "Hero of the Soviet Union" role Moscow assigned him: as a kolkhoz farmer, a member of Kom-

23 See Vladimir Pavlov, "Podvig vash bessmerten! Vklad turkmenistantsev v bor'bu za svobodu Otechestva," *Turkmeninstan* 2 (2005): 16–31, 20.

24 See, for example, "Turkmenskoe iskusstvo vtoroy poloviny 40-kh–50-kh gg.," http://artdepot.ru/article/izobrazitelnoe-iskusstvo/turkmenskaja-ssr/kartiny-40–kh-50–kh-gg.htm [last accessed: October 1, 2016].

25 See V. A. Gurevich, "Turkmenskaya muzyka" [Turkmen music], in *Muzykal'naya entsiklopediya* [The encyclopedia of music], ed. Yuriy V. Keldysh (Moscow: Soviet Encyclopedia, Soviet Composer, 1981), vol. 5, 645–50, 648.

26 Published in Sergey S. Narovchatov and Yakov A. Chelemskiy, *Svyashchennaya voyna... Stikhi o Velikoy Otechestvennoy voyne* [The holy war: Poems on the Great Patriotic War] (Moscow: Chudozhestvennaya literatura, 1966), 402–4.

27 TASS, "Torzhestvennye zasedaniya, posvyashchennye godovshchine Krasnoy Armii," *Pravda*, February 24, 1944, 2.

28 See Pavlov, "Podvig vash bessmerten!" 20.

29 See Nurgozel' Bayramova, "Pavshie i zhivye," *Gündogar: For Democracy and Human Rights in Turkmenistan*, 11 May 2004, http://gundog.newhost.ru/?0221041031000000000000011000000 [last accessed: October 1, 2016].

somol and later of the Communist Party, and a Red Armist, he presented an "immaculate biography" from a Soviet perspective; his wartime heroism and merits were undisputed.

After the war, Durdy was no longer suitable for the role of an All-Union identification figure in the Russian-dominated USSR because of his non-Russian (non-Slavic) origin, and he gradually disappeared from the view of the main Soviet press and was featured only rarely in Moscow's publications. For example, *Pravda* published a short piece by Durdy on July 7, 1971, in which he showed himself to be affected by the Soyuz 11 Soviet space mission accident and compared the deceased Cosmonauts Georgiy Dobrovolskiy, Vladislav Volkov, and Viktor Patsaev to the heroic Soviet Red Armists who had fought in the war against Germany.[30] On April 16, 1974, and again ten years later, Durdy was mentioned in *Pravda* publications with the accolade "Hero of the Soviet Union."[31]

In Turkmenistan, though, Durdy continued to be exalted and considered a worthy Turkmen veteran, one of the "distinguished" people of Soviet Turkmenistan and a symbol of the Turkmen contribution to victory over the "Third Reich."[32] The characteristic tendency, as seen in the Komsomol brochure from 1943, to portray Durdy's wartime opponents in Moldova exclusively as "fascists"—that is, "German fascists"—can be observed in several postwar Turkmen publications. Among such examples are Turkmen history textbooks from the 1960s, as well as the 1967 documentary *V sem'e edinoy... (In the United Family...)*.[33] Romanian regiments were not discussed explicitly so as to not dampen the heroic deeds of the Turkmen in the battle against a—compared to Nazi Germany—reputedly weaker enemy, and to not damage the image of the postwar Romanian socialist state in the USSR. The injury that ended the Turkmen's military career was mentioned only peripherally, if at all. This was, presumably, to avoid having to confront

30 See Kurban Durdy [Gurban Durdy], "Vstanut novye boytsy," *Pravda*, July 2, 1971, 2.

31 V. Filatov, "Zolotoe sozvezdie. Sorok let nazad bylo uchrezhdeno zvanie—Geroy Sovetskogo Soyuza," *Pravda*, April 16, 1974, 6; I. Shkadov, "Simvol vysshey doblesti," *Pravda*, April 16, 1984, 3.

32 G. Nepesov, "Vozniknovenie i razvitie Turkmenskoy Sovetskoy Sotsialisticheskoy respubiki" [Formation and development of the Turkmen Soviet Socialist Republic], *Voprosy istorii* 2 (1950): 3–24, 19.

33 See Aga K. Karryev, *Istoriya Turmenistana (uchebnoe posobie dlya vuzov)* [History of Turkmenistan (A textbook for students)] (Ashgabat: Turkmenistan, 1966), 407; Ovlya K. Kuliev et al., *Istoriya Turkmenskoy SSR dlya VII-VIII klassov* [History of Turkmenistan: For 7th and 8th Grades], 5th ed. (Ashgabat: Turkmenistan, 1967), 65; *V sem'e edinoy* [In the united family], documentary film directed by Aleksandr Pavlov (USSR 1967), 28:31 minutes.

the war invalids' circumstances, most of whom fared far worse than the museum director Durdy. Durdy died on December 2, 1976 at the age of fifty-nine and was buried in the village of Keshi near Ashgabat.[34] In contrast, fate gave the fighter pilot Mares'ev a long life. He died on May 18, 2001, two days before his eighty-fifth birthday.

Soviet propaganda seized on Mares'ev shortly after the Second World War. At the end of 1946, the literary journal *Oktyabr'* (October) published Boris Polevoy's largely factually accurate novel *Povest' o nastoyashchem cheloveke* (*A Story About a Real Man*).[35] In 1948, a film version was released, directed by Aleksandr Stolper and featuring Pavel Kadochnikov in the lead role.[36] That same year, the composer Sergey Prokof'ev penned his opera *A Story About a Real Man*, which, while criticized heavily in contrast to the widely acclaimed novel and the widely seen movie, was not performed until 1960, when it was first staged.[37] The novel, which had become mandatory reading in Soviet middle school, and the feature film tell the story of a conscientious, willful pilot who would not allow himself to be captured, overcame fate's calamity, and was ready to die for his fatherland. These works were honored with the Stalin Prize, captured the hearts of Soviet citizens, and made Aleksey Mares'ev the very symbol of the Red Army's heroics during the war against Nazi Germany.

In his novel, Boris Polevoy changed the protagonist's name and turned Aleksey Mares'ev into Aleksey Meres'ev, with an "e." In Stopler's film, the pilot is also called Aleksey Meres'ev. Asked about this in the 1990s, Mares'ev joked that in 1946, Polevoy could not have known whether the disabled pilot would become an alcoholic after the war, and he probably wanted to change the protagonist's name in order to be able to avoid a possible ban of the work if that happened.[38] Given the multitude of tragedies that befell war invalids,

34 See Bayramova, "Pavshie i zhivye."

35 See Boris Polevoy, *Povest' o nastoyashchem cheloveke* [A Story About a Real Man] (Moscow: Chudozhestvennaya literatura, 1947).

36 See *Povest' o nastoyashchem cheloveke* [A story about a real man], feature film directed by Aleksandr Stolper (USSR, 1947). About this movie, see Fieseler, "The Wounds of War: Experiences of War Related Disablement in Soviet Feature Films," 280–2; Fieseler, "Keine Leidensbilder. Die Invaliden des 'Großen Vaterländischen Krieges' im sowjetischen Spielfilm," 83–4.

37 See Slavin, *Aleksey Mares'ev*, 35:30–40:00.

38 See Vladimir Shunevich, "Posle voyny Mares'evu, letavshemu bez obeikh nog, ne khoteli davat' prava na vozhdenie avtomobilya," *Fakty i kommentarii*, May 5, 2011, http://fakty.ua/133189-posle-vojny-mediki-i-gaishniki-ne-hoteli-davat-letchiku-alekseyu-maresevu-letavshemu-bez-obeih-nog-prava-na-vozhdenie-avtomobilya [last accessed: October 1, 2016].

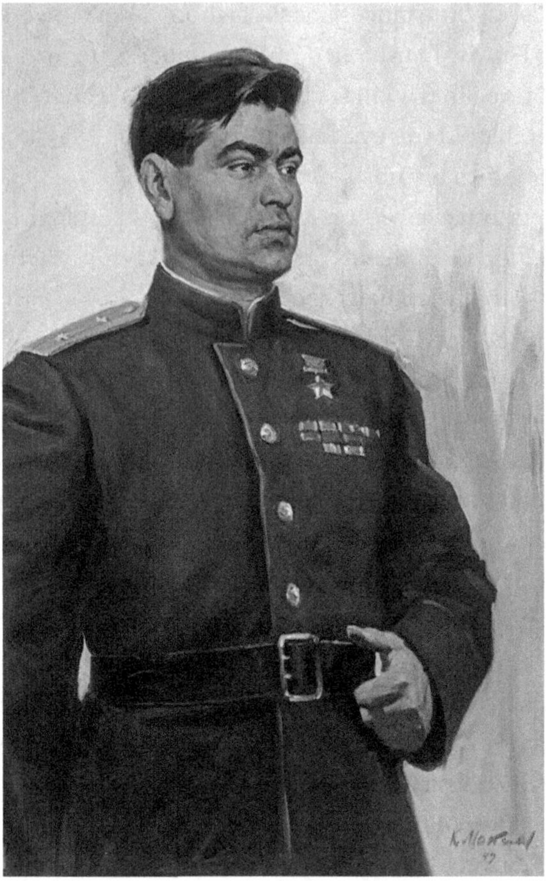

Figure 7.1: *Aleksey P. Mares'ev (1949),*
Artist: Konstantin M. Maksimov (1913–1994).

Mares'ev's comment is clearly more than just an anecdote; it reflects the circumstances of disabled Red Armists in the USSR in the immediate aftermath of the Second World War.[39]

The decision to exploit Mares'ev's biography was most probably made by Stalin himself. Stalin, who in the late 1940s decided to "clean" big Soviet cities of the impoverished former Red Armists (such as blind persons or amputees)—many of whom had been honored with orders and medals for their exploits—and to move them into special homes for disabled veterans in the neglected monasteries throughout the USSR, including one on Va-

39 See, for example, Fizeler, "'Nishchie pobediteli.'"

laam Island in Karelia,[40] was touched by the pilot's personality and openly expressed great respect for him.[41] Indeed, the Russian Aleksey Mares'ev—his Russian origin having been emphasized in both the novel and the film—was a perfect fit for the profile of the heroes of the late Stalinist period, in which Russian nationalism and Soviet patriotism assumed central roles. Also, the pilot came from a humble background, had the "right proletariat origins," owed his career to Soviet might, was a Komsomol and Communist Party member, had proven his ideological resolve,[42] and had performed superhuman feats. The dictator, as well as his son, Vasiliy Stalin (a general in the Soviet Air Force), who himself had become disabled during the war,[43] supported Mares'ev.

After the war, Mares'ev had settled in Moscow and lived with his family—his wife, Galina, and their sons, Viktor and Aleksey—in a three-bedroom apartment in a building on the prestigious Gorkiy Street and was allocated a dacha, two cars, and even a driver. Mares'ev had access to supplies that were out of the reach of "mere mortals"—high-quality foodstuffs, consumables, and medical provisions.[44] Soviet painters and sculptors dedicated their works to the "Hero of the Soviet Union,"[45] and in several schools so-called Mares'ev corners were created.[46]

By the late 1940s, and especially from the second half the 1950s onwards, Mares'ev, having been promoted to major (and, in 1978, to colonel), played a remarkable role in Soviet public life. Taking Boris Polevoy's advice, he ended his military career and began his studies at the Communist Party's Higher Party School. He graduated from this Soviet elite cadre factory in 1952 and subsequently completed a doctoral degree in 1956 at the Commu-

40 See *Predany i zabyty* [Betrayed and forgotten], documentary film directed by Maksim Katushkin (Russia, 2010), https://www.youtube.com/watch?v=d5_6FkYe-yw [last accessed: October 1, 2016]; Aleksandr Dobrovol'skiy, "'Samovary' tovarishcha Stalina," *Moskovskiy komsomolets*, September 2, 2011, 16.

41 See Aleksandr Khokhlov, "Nastoyashchiy chelovek posle voyny. Personal'nuyu mashinu Mares'evu vruchil Stalin, i ee ne smog otobrat' dazhe El'tsin," *Novye izvestiya*, May 18, 2004, 7.

42 On this, see for example B. Polevoy, "Nash molodoy sovremennik," *Pravda*, October 29, 1948, 3; B. Polevoy, "Pobediteli," *Pravda*, May 9, 1949, 3.

43 See *Vasiliy Stalin. Syn za ottsa* [Vasiliy Stalin: The son is responsible for his father], documentary film directed by Sergey Kozhevnikov and Galina Ogurnaya (Russia, 2011), 48 minutes, 22:40–23:55.

44 See Slavin, *Aleksey Mares'ev*, 34:00–35:30. Also see Kolesnichenko, *Aleksey Mares'ev. Ya—ne legenda! Ya—prosto chelovek!* 29:55–30:10; Vladimirov, *Aleksey Mares'ev. Rozhdennyy letat'*, 13:25–13:35, 31:40–32.10; Khokhlov, "Nastoyashchiy chelovek posle voyny."

45 See, for example, A. Navozov, "Eto—Palekh! K 50-letiyu sozdaniya khudozhestvennykh masterskikh," *Pravda*, December 4, 1974, 3.

46 See Heinz Stern, "Eine Heldin und ihre Paten," *Neues Deutschland*, August 25, 1973, 11.

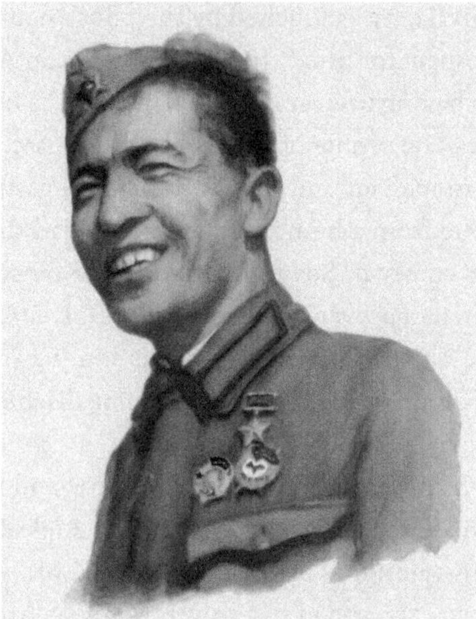

Figure 7.2: ***Gurban Durdy.*** **Collection Legendarnye geroi-komsomol'tsy (Moscow: Izobrazitel'noe iskusstvo, 1973). Edited by I. Sobol', Artist: S. Yakovlev.**

nist Party's Academy of Social Sciences, writing a military history dissertation on the Battle of Kursk.[47] The fact that Mares'ev and Durdy combined their lives after the Second World War with the study of history is not astonishing in the context of the USSR, as in this country history and propaganda were very closely connected.[48]

Stalin's death in 1953 and his son Vasily's rapid downfall, having been persecuted and repeatedly arrested under Khrushchev,[49] had no nega-

47 See Yuriy Makhnenko, "Svet muzhestva," *Pravda*, July 7, 1985, 3. Also see Khokhlov, "Nastoyashchiy chelovek posle voyny."

48 On the role of history and historians in the USSR, see Geyer, *Klio in Moskau und die sowjetische Geschichte*; Hösler, *Die sowjetische Geschichtswissenschaft 1953 bis 1991. Studien zur Methodologie- und Organisationsgeschichte*.

49 Vasiliy Stalin died on March 19, 1962. News of his death first reached the Western world a few weeks later. The Hamburg-based journal *Der Spiegel* printed a curt obituary: "VASILIY STALIN, 41, the airforce general demoted to major and son of a dictator—first marriage to a daughter of Marshall of the Soviet Union Timoshenko, second marriage to the Soviet record-breaking swimmer Kapitolina Vasil'eva, third marriage to Molotov's daughter Svetlana—and who, under the influence of alcohol, fatally ran over a women and was committed to an alcohol-dependency clinic for a prolonged time, [died] of a heart attack in Kazan." *Der Spiegel* 18 (1962), 97.

tive consequences for Mares'ev, who maintained excellent relationships with both Khrushchev as well as his successor, Brezhnev. Mares'ev was highly rated by the Soviet leadership as a loyal Communist Party member and honest patriot who devoted his life to serving his social homeland. In 1956, Mares'ev was entrusted with the post of secretary of the newly founded Soviet War Veterans Committee. Several of his contemporaries, in their personal recollections, describe Mares'ev as a modest and righteous person who did not draw attention to his heroic past. He was aware of the reality that he, as a privileged veteran, led a far better life than most other war invalids, and used his position on the committee as well as his contacts in the Ministry of Health and other institutions to make life more bearable for disabled veterans. In particular, he fought for the improvement of the economic situation and medical care of disabled veterans, as well as for qualitative improvement in a medical service that was notorious for its poor quality.[50]

Despite his efforts, Mares'ev's successes were modest, and ultimately he was unable to substantially improve the situation of disabled veterans and other disabled people. The numerous complaints by disabled veterans and in data collected by Soviet dissidents paint a gloomy picture. On paper, veterans enjoyed a range of privileges such as special consideration in terms of housing allotments, free cars, holiday vouchers, access to food in special shops, and the free use of public transportation. In reality, though, they received small pensions, were isolated from the outside world, spent their lives in poverty, had poor medical treatment, and were treated without dignity by social authorities, doctors, and officials. They could only dream of apartments equipped for the disabled, motorized wheel chairs, suitably adapted small cars, good quality medical equipment, or visits to health resorts. Dissatisfied disabled veterans and disabled persons who fought for their rights, particularly those who insistently or openly criticized

50 On this, see also Anatoliy Dokuchaev, "Nastoyashchiy Chelovek ostaetsya s nami. Mirovaya istoriya ne znaet primera muzhestva, podobnogo tomu, chto proyavil Aleksey Mares'ev," *Krasnaya zvezda*, May 22, 2001, 1; Vladimir Shunevich, "'Prezhde chem poznakomi'sya s budushchey zhenoy, Aleksey Mares'ev poprosil priyatelya—nachal'nika otdela kadrov—vyzvat' devushku k sebe na besedu'," *Fakty i kommentarii*, May 17, 2002, http://fakty.ua/91691-quot-prezhde-chem-poznakomitsya-s-buducshej-zhenoj-aleksej-maresev-poprosil-priyatelya----nachalnika-otdela-kadrov----vyzvat-devushku-k-sebe-na-besedu-quot [last accessed: October 1, 2016]. See also Kolesnichenko, *Aleksey Mares'ev. Ya—ne legenda! Ya—prosto chelovek!* 31:45–35:30; Vladimirov, *Aleksey Mares'ev. Rozhdennyy letat'*, 17:30–20:00.

the Soviet system, were branded mentally ill and sent to psychiatric institutions, harassed, frightened, arrested, or exiled from the USSR.[51]

The KGB persecuted the activists of the Committee for the Defense of the Rights of Disabled People in the USSR, which was founded in May 1978 by Yuriy I. Kiselev, Valeriy A. Fefelov, and Fayzulla Khusainov. As a result, the wheelchair-bound Fefelov was forced to leave the Soviet Union in 1982. In 1986, he published an internationally acclaimed book in London about the situation of disabled people in the USSR. Describing the provisions for disabled war veterans, he emphasized their privileged status compared to other disabled people: disabled veterans stood a far better chance of defending their rights. Overall, however, the socialist state did nothing for other disabled people. In his book, Fefelov blamed official Soviet propaganda and indicated a serious discrepancy between this propaganda and reality, but he did not deal directly with the "poster boy-veteran" Mares'ev (probably due to his respect for the imposing figure of the fighter pilot).[52]

With regards to Mares'ev's propagandistic instrumentalization in the Soviet Union, it is possible to differentiate between three aspects. First, Mares'ev's personal history helped sustain the memory of the war and the Red Armists' heroic achievements in Soviet society. The charismatic veteran was deployed pedagogically and assumed the function of a role model in the "patriotic education" in the USSR and socialist realm. He wrote books, published articles, and engaged with children and adolescents.[53] Mares'ev discussed his own experiences of war as well as his trips abroad and appealed

51 See "Gräber für Lebende," *Der Spiegel* 33 (1979), 112, 113; Lyudmila Alekseva, *Istoriya inakomysliya v SSSR. Noveyshiy period* [Soviet dissent: Contemporary movements for national, religious, and human rights], 3rd ed. (Moscow: Moscow Helsinki Group, 2012), 347–8; Vyacheslav Dolinin, "Invalidy protiv TSK KPSS" [Invalids against the Central Committee of the Communist Party of the Soviet Union], *Pchela* 18 (1999), http://www.pchela.ru/podshiv/18/ck.htm [last accessed: October 1, 2016]; Nikita Pivovarov, "'Zabota' ob invalidakh voyny" ['Care' for the war invalids], http://www.world-war.ru/zabota-ob-invalidax-vojny/ [last accessed: October 1, 2016].

52 See Valeriy Fefelov, *V SSSR invalidov net!...* [There are no invalids in the USSR...!] (London, 1986). Fefelov (1949–2008) settled down in the Federal Republic of Germany, worked there for the Russian-speaking section of the US broadcasting service Radio Free Europe/Radio Liberty in Munich, and got a job at the International Society for Human Rights in Frankfurt am Main. In his book he responded positively to the Western policy toward disabled people (105–21). After the breakdown of Communism, Fefelov reversed his pro-Western attitude, rejected the transformation in Russia under Boris Yeltsin, openly supported revanchist, nationalist, and communist political forces in Russia, and in his Russian publications portrayed himself as a disabled person being harassed in Germany due to his Russian origin. Valeriy Fefelov, "'Brys', bydlo!'" *Pravda*, June 22, 1994, 6; Valeriy Fefelov, "Vot tak 'prava cheloveka'! Pis'mo russkogo emigranta," *Zavtra*, April 10, 2000, 6.

53 See Makhnenko, "Svet muzhestva."

to the youth to be courageous, dogged, and fight for the truth.[54] Second, as a respected Soviet war veteran, Mares'ev was responsible for contacts with foreign veterans and tried to win them over to the Soviet Union.[55] He also profiled himself as a peace activist—greeted with great respect abroad.[56] He celebrated his first big success on the international stage at the end of April 1949 in Paris, where the—communist-dominated—World Peace Conference met. As a member of the Soviet delegation, Mares'ev delivered a speech in which he reviewed his own destiny, glorified the Stalinist Soviet Union, and aggressively attacked the recently founded NATO.[57] Third, Mares'ev published several pieces in the Soviet press in which he responded to current internal and international affairs. In May 1967, following the military coup in Greece, he protested the arrest of the prominent antifascist resistance fighter Manolis Glezos, who was highly respected in the Eastern Bloc and whom he knew personally.[58] Mares'ev condemned the "imperialist" foreign policy of the United States and raged against critics of the Soviet regime.[59] On January 24, 1974, for example, he scolded the vilified and then banned author Aleksandr Solzhenitsyn in *Pravda* as a "liar," "lunatic," "renegade," and "traitor to the fatherland."[60] It can be assumed that Mares'ev was aware of the Committee for the Defense of the Rights of Disabled People in the USSR. However, he did not mention the movement in his publications: the protest movement by the disabled was a phenomenon that was embarrassing to the "philanthropic country" of the USSR, and this is why the Soviet press preferred to keep quiet about this development.[61]

As early as 1949, in a speech in Paris, Mares'ev noted that after his injury and leg amputation he could have stayed in the Soviet hinterland, but his goal had been to drive the enemy out of the Soviet Union as quickly as pos-

54 See N. Shasherina, *Vospityvay kharakter. Sbornik* [Bring up your character: A collection] (Moscow: Young Guard, 1957), 14–20, 20.

55 See, for example, TASS, "Sovetskie veterany pribyli v Vashington," *Pravda*, April 23, 1958, 5; A. Lerua, "Tovarishchi po oruzhiyu—za mir bez voyn!" *Pravda*, April 29, 1960, 6; Makhnenko, "Svet muzhestva."

56 See, for example, Viktor Gorlenko, "Simvol voli," *Krasnaya zvezda*, March 31, 2009, 1, 4.

57 See TASS, "Vystuplenie Geroya Sovetskogo Soyuza Alekseya Mares'eva," *Pravda*, April 24, 1949, 4.

58 See A. Mares'ev, "'Net' razgulu reaktsii," *Pravda*, May 3, 1967, 5.

59 Klaus Haupt, "Ein Buch und sein Held. Gespräch mit dem ehemaligen Flieger Alexej Petrowitsch Maresjew," *Neues Deutschland*, May 3, 1980, 11.

60 Aleksey Mares'ev, "Zhalkiy udel otshchepentsa," *Pravda*, January 24, 1974, 3.

61 The fact that many activists lived in the provinces rather than in Moscow might also be essential. The activists were attacked by the provincial press. See Fefelov, *V SSSR invalidov net!...*, 142–4.

sible and free the Soviet people from misery and suffering.[62] In his recollections, Mares'ev's son Viktor emphasizes that his father was offensive in dealing with his disability, did not want to feel disabled, and even refused to use a walking cane, against medical advice.[63] This attitude correlated with the requirements of communist propaganda that wanted to make the disabled "useful" to society, extolled the allegedly disabled-friendly communist social policy, and stylized Mares'ev into a role model for disabled citizens. In the Soviet Union and other socialist states, the press reported on Latif M. from the Sudan,[64] Georgi B. from Bulgaria,[65] Fausto D. from Cuba,[66] Hanna L. from the GDR,[67] and other people with disabilities that let themselves be inspired by Mares'ev. In 1976, the Soviet author Nikolay A. Meysak proudly emphasized that the USSR had numerous Mares'ev's at its disposal.[68]

In the late 1970s, the name Captain Yuriy V. Kozlovskiy, whom the Moscow journalists were quick to label "the next Mares'ev," created a stir throughout the Soviet Union. Midway through the night of March 27, 1973, the 30-year-old was piloting his MiG-17 fighter plane in the Transbaikal region. While flying over the city of Chita, the plane engine failed; Kozlovskiy managed to direct the plane away from the city, where it crashed in the taiga, or boreal forest. Kozlovskiy survived, but he was severely injured. He spent three days in the taiga, where the temperature was about 30 degrees below zero, before being rescued. The captain survived, but his legs had to be amputated.[69]

Yuriy Kozlovskiy became the "Alexey Mares'ev of the Brezhnev era." The official images of Mares'ev and Kozlovskiy were constructed in the USSR in the same way: both Mares'ev and Kozlovskiy became the highlight of Soviet propaganda several years after the tragic events that led to the amputation of their legs. In Kozlovskiy's case, the role of Boris Polevoy (the journal-

62 See TASS, "Vystuplenie Geroya Sovetskogo Soyuza Alekseya Mares'eva."

63 See Chochlov, "Nastoyashchiy chelovek posle voyny."

64 See "Pomoshch' sovetskikh vrachey," *Pravda*, January 9, 1958, 4.

65 See L. Zhmyrev, "Podnyatyy na krylo," *Pravda*, June 8, 1987, 3.

66 See Gisela Wenck, "Held der Schlacht von Playa Giron," *Neues Deutschland*, February 21, 1981, 6.

67 See Inge Kania, "Ein wahrer Mensch," *Neues Deutschland*, October 30, 1966, 3. For the perception of Aleksey Mares'ev in the GDR, see Friedman, "'Der wahre sozialistische Mensch'. Der sowjetische Kampfflieger Aleksej P. Mares'ev (1916–2001) und seine Rezeption in der DDR."

68 See Nikolay Meysak, *Skol'ko u nas Mares'evykh?* [How many Mares'evs do we have?] (Moscow: Young Guard, 1976), 246–54.

69 See *Vtoroy Mares'ev* [The Second Mares'ev], TV program *Istorii spaseniya* [Stories of rescue] (January 21, 2014, Channel *TV Center*), 25:37 minutes.

ist who "discovered" Mares'ev) was played by Gennadiy Bocharov (born in 1935), a journalist from *Komsomol'skaya Pravda* (Komsomol Truth). Much like Polevoy, who had written an article for *Pravda* and then a novel about Mares'ev, Bocharov published an article in *Komsomol'skaya Pravda* and then a sketch about Kozlovskiy.[70] In the last period of the war and its aftermath, Mares'ev received support from General Vasiliy Stalin; Kozlovskiy received the patronage of the influential Evgeniy M. Tyazhel'nikov (born in 1928), first secretary of the Central Committee of the All-Union Leninist Young Communist League (1968–1977) and head of the propaganda department of the Central Committee of the Communist Party of the Soviet Union (1977–1982). Tyazhel'nikov appreciated the propaganda potential of "the second Mares'ev." Publications and TV documentaries about Kozlovskiy as well as meetings of Mares'ev and Kozlovskiy with children aimed to show a generational continuity of "the real Soviet people" in the USSR. Kozlovskiy admitted that his role model was Mares'ev.[71]

There are notable differences in the biographies and constructed images of Mares'ev and Kozlovskiy. The Soviet authorities emphasized that Mares'ev resumed his career as a pilot during the war, after having his legs amputated. Kozlovsky's career came to the end in 1973 after he lost his legs, but he continued working in the aviation world by becoming an aircraft engineer.[72] Mares'ev's aircraft crashed during the fight against the Nazis; the MiG-17 piloted by Kozlovskiy crashed due to a technical problem. The reasons for the technical failure and the fact that Kozlovskiy had prevented his plane from plunging into a city were kept secret so as not to cast a shadow on the Soviet Air Force. This method of dealing with tragedies involving military aircraft was quite typical in the USSR under Brezhnev. For example, a military aircraft crash in Svetlogorsk, a small resort town in the Kaliningrad region, on May 16, 1972, which had multiple casualties (thirty-four victims, twenty-three of them children), was completely ignored by the Soviet press.

70 Gennadiy Bocharov, "Nepobezhdennyy," *Komsomol'skaya Pravda*, February 4, 1977, 4; Gennadiy Bocharov, *Nepobezhdennyy* [An invincible man] (Moscow: Young Guard), 7–21. Also see Valeriy Ganichev, "Pravo byt' pervym," *Pravda*, March 21, 1979, 3.

71 See *Sud'ba cheloveka. Yuriy Kozlovskiy—letchik, povtorivshiy v mirnoe vremya podvig Alekseya Mares'eva* [The destiny of the man: Yuriy Kozlovskiy—A Pilot, who followed Aleksey Mares'ev's deed in peace time], Radio program *Osobyy sluchay* [A special case] (November 9, 2013, Radio *Komsomol'skaya Pravda*), 29:28 minutes, http://www.kp.ru/radio/26511/3471881/ [last accessed: October 1, 2016].

72 *Sud'ba cheloveka.*

In order not to cause damage to the reputation of the Soviet Air Force and the Baltic navy, the Soviet government decided to cover up the disaster.[73]

While the heroism of Durdy, Mares'ev, and Kozlovskiy were highlighted in Soviet propaganda, the fortunes of "simple" veterans and disabled people were of very little interest to the Soviet press and filmmakers. The experience of the renowned Soviet writer, singer, and actor Vladimir S. Vysotskiy (1938–1980) exemplifies the nervousness of the authorities about dealing with disabled war veterans. During the Brezhnev era, numerous movies about the Second World War were released in the USSR. In the 1970s, Vysotskiy was invited to act in a new Soviet film about the war to play a cameo role as a disabled soldier telling a boy about his war experiences.[74] Vysotskiy grew up in Moscow in the second half of the 1940s; he had met disabled veterans and listened to their stories, later describing their fates in his poetry.[75] He had a deep-seated respect for disabled veterans and understood that the Soviet government had not treated them adequately.[76] The scene in which Vysotskiy brilliantly played the disabled soldier was cut from the film, as such images were unwelcome on the Soviet big screen.[77]

Reception After the Collapse of Communism

Coming to power in 1985, the last Communist Party leader of Turkmenistan, Saparmurat "Türkmenbaşy" Niyazov, managed to assert his power and remained head of the Turkmen state until his death in 2006. Niyazov sealed his country off from the outside world, pursued a "Turkmen special path," and established a brutal dictatorship with an absurd cult surrounding himself and his family. The "Hero of the Soviet Union" Gurban Durdy became a victim of these politics and this personality cult. After his death in 1967, Durdy initially remained a respected personality in Turkmenistan;

73 See Elena Ruzhinskaya and Alexander Friedman, "'Menschen und Städten ändern sich. Nur die Ostsee bleibt…' Zelenogradsk (Cranz) und Svetlogorsk (Rauschen)—ostpreußische Seebäder und sowjetische Kurorte," *Virus. Beiträge zur Sozialgeschichte der Medizin* 12 (2013): 135–46, 142.

74 See *Vospominanie* [Memorials], documentary film directed by Vladimir Savel'ev (USSR, 1986), 65:38 minutes, 11:35–13:40; Natal'ya A. Krymova, *Imena. Kniga chetvertaya. Vysotskiy. Nenapisannaya kniga* [Names: Volume 4: Vysotskiy: An unwritten book] (Moscow: GKCM "Vysotskiy," 2008), 73.

75 See Vladimir Vysotskiy, *Sobranie sochineniy* [Selected works], ed. Ol'ga Novikova and Vladimir Novikov (Moscow: Vremya, 2008), vol. 1, 6; vol. 3, 40, 41.

76 See Nikolay Andreev, "'Ya ne lyublyu kholodnogo tsinizma…,'" *Rodina* 7 (2015), http://www.rg.ru/2015/07/24/rodina-vysotsky.html [last accessed: October 1, 2016].

77 See Krymova, *Imena*, 73.

several enterprises and a street in the capital, Ashgabat, were named after him.[78] Under Niyazov's rule, though, there was a rapid depreciation of Soviet history and an expulsion of Russian influences from the country's cultural and public life. Under these circumstances, Durdy, who was firmly rooted in Russian culture and language[79] and remained a great hero of the Soviet era, faded into the background. Although Niyazov acclaimed Durdy and other Turkmen "Heroes of the Soviet Union" posthumously as "Heroes of Turkmenistan" for their participation in the fight against National Socialism, Durdy nonetheless was no longer seen as the symbol of the Turkmen contribution to the victory over fascism. This role was taken over by the soldier Atamyrat Niyazov, the president's father, who lost his life in 1943.[80]

The collapse of the Soviet Union also meant the collapse of Aleksey Mares'ev's world. The country he had served his entire life no longer existed. As a convinced communist, Mares'ev categorically rejected the economic and political transformation Russia experienced under Boris Yeltsin (1991–1999), and was indignant about the neoliberal reform policies and the reputed cultural and moral decline in the postcommunist Russian Federation. According to the recollections of his son Viktor, Mares'ev had bitterly insisted in the 1990s that Yeltsin's Russia, with its "predatory capitalism," was not the country for which he had fought and risked his life.[81]

The veteran's economic situation worsened at the end of the 1980s and the beginning of the 1990s. He lost his savings to rampant inflation and had to make due with a modest pension, while also providing for his ill wife and disabled son Aleksey. But as deputy leader of the Russian veterans association, he must have been particularly stricken by the reality that the memory of the Second World War increasingly faded in Russia. Polevoy's

78 See Bayramova, "Pavshie i zhivye."

79 See, for example, a letter from Gurban Durdy to the journalist Nikolay A. Nikiforov, May 21, 1966, http://forums-su.com/viewtopic.php?f=194&t=553179 [last accessed: October 1, 2016].

80 See "2004 god ob'yavlen v Turkmenii godom otsa Saparmurata Niyazova," *lenta.ru*, March 6, 2004, http://lenta.ru/world/2004/03/06/bashi/ [last accessed: October 1, 2016]. See also Alan Peskov, "Novye vremena—novye geroi," *Khroniki Turkmenistana*, May 25, 2011, http://archive.chrono-tm.org/?id=3123 [last accessed: October 1, 2016].

81 See Ol'ga Khodaeva, "Alekseyu Mares'evu ne khvatalo deneg dazhe na lekarstva," *sobesednik.ru*, April 21, 2011, http://sobesednik.ru/print/incident/alekseyu-maresevu-ne-khvatalo-deneg-dazhe-na-lekarstva [last accessed: October 1, 2016]; Anatoliy Sul'yanov, "Moi vstrechi s Alekseem Mares'evym," *Belorusskaya voennaya gazeta. Vo slavu Rodiny*, April 21, 2014, 7. See also Kolesnichenko, *Aleksey Mares'ev. Ya—ne legenda! Ya—prosto chelovek!* 37:10–39:20; *Aleksey Mares'ev*, Television program *Legendy armii s Aleksandrom Marshalom*, 31:30–34:10.

novel *A Story About a Real Man* was no longer considered mandatory reading; Stolper's film of the same title was rarely screened. The legendary hero was gradually forgotten.[82] In this context, the last significant decoration Mares'ev was awarded is indicative. In 1996, for his 80th birthday, President Yeltsin awarded him the Order for Merit to the Fatherland, 3rd class.[83] His service to Russia was valued less than, say, the service of the French president Jacques Chirac, who received the same Order, 1st class, in 1997.[84]

Subsequent to the regime change in the Kremlin, Mares'ev witnessed a growth in the estimation for Soviet history and especially the Second World War at the hands of Vladimir Putin, who paid tribute to Mares'ev's "years of work supporting the patriotic education of youth, the social protection of veterans, and the solidification of friendship among the nations."[85] Over the following years interest in the Second World War and the "Heroes of the Soviet Union" increased, and was further amplified in the context of the 70th anniversary of the victory over Nazi Germany (2015), and particularly within the context of the dramatic conflict in Ukraine (since 2014). This conflict is being stylized by the Russian side and pro-Russian separatists in Ukraine as principally a conflict of values between the "good antifascist Russian world"—with its glorious history and heroes Mares'ev, Durdy, as well as other Red Armists from the different parts of the former USSR—and the "Ukrainian fascists" (successors of the Ukrainian collaborators in the Second World War) supported by the West.[86] Considering this context, the activities of the Mares'ev Foundation, which Aleksey Mares'ev created shortly before his death, are worth noting in that it supports the separatist "People's Republics" in Eastern Ukraine through the collection of donations, among other activities.[87] In 2016, Russia car-

82 See Khodaeva, "Alekseyu Mares'evu ne khvatalo deneg dazhe na lekarstva"; Sul'yanov, "Moi vstrechi s Alekseem Mares'evym."

83 See "Decree No. 731 of the President of the Russian Federation, May 16, 1996," http://kremlin.ru/acts/bank/9364 [last accessed: October 1, 2016].

84 See "Decree No. 1056 of the President of the Russian Federation, September 23, 1997," http://kremlin.ru/acts/bank/11519 [last accessed: October 1, 2016].

85 "Arrangement No. 245-rp of the President of the Russian Federation, April 27, 2001," http://www.kremlin.ru/acts/bank/16883 [last accessed: October 1, 2016. See also Quiring, "Russischer Kampfflieger."

86 On this, see for example Dar'ya Andreeva, "Misha Matvienko: Mir nastupit, kogda lyudi poymut, chto idet voyna," *novorossiapress.ru*, February 8, 2015, http://novorossiapress.ru/blog/misha-matvienko-mir-nastupit-kogda-lyudi-pojmut-chto-idet-vojna [last accessed: October 1, 2016]. On Durdy, see the blog of Oleg G. Artyushenko, http://artyushenkooleg.ru/index.php/velikaya-otechestvennaya-vojna-1941-1945-g/geroj_sssr_kurban-durdi/ [last accessed: October 1, 2016].

87 See "Pomoshch" Novorossii," http://маресьевцы.рф/?page_id=157 [last accessed: October 1, 2016].

ried out a big celebration of the Mares'ev's centenary: leading national TV channels (Channel One and Russia 1) broadcasted new documentary films about the famous pilot[88]; articles appeared in Russian newspapers[89]; several monuments were erected[90]; and the Russian post released a special postage stamp into circulation.[91]

Conclusion

On June 7, 1947, *Pravda* published a piece in which the author Vsevolod Vishnevskiy discussed the literary works that had been awarded the Stalin Prize. With regard to the novel *A Story About a Real Man*, the author highlighted that the protagonist's situation would have been hopeless in both the Russian Tsarist Empire prior to the October Revolution and in a capitalist state. In the Soviet Union, though, he had been saved and provided for.[92] Vishnevsky suggested to *Pravda* readers that the conditions for war invalids were far worse abroad than in the Soviet Union. The article ignored the reality that most Soviet war invalids had to wage a constant fight for survival after the war and that those who were instrumentalized by propaganda and celebrated in the press, literature, and film—like the heroes Aleksey Mares'ev and Gurban Durdy—constituted an exception among disabled Red Armists.

88 *Aleksey Mares'ev. Rozhdennyy letat'* [Aleksey Mares'ev. Born to fly]; *Aleksey Mares'ev. Ya—ne legenda! Ya—prosto chelovek* [Aleksey Mares'ev. I am not a legend! I am a man!]. See also *Aleksey Mares'ev*, Television program *Legendy armii s Aleksandrom Marshalom* [Legends of the army with Aleksandr Marshal] (May 17, 2016, Channel *Zvezda*), 37:50 minutes.

89 See for example Ivan Zubkov, "100 let letchiku Mares'evu—geroyu "Povesti o nastoyashchem cheloveke," *Izvestiya*, May 19, 2016, http://izvestia.ru/news/614382 [last accessed: October 1, 2016]; Valeriy Korneev, "100 let legende: zhizn' i podvig Alekseya Mares'eva," *TASS*, May 20, 2016, http://tass.ru/info/3295714 [last accessed: October 1, 2016]; Naum Aranovich, "Russkiy kharacter Alekseya Mares'eva," *Vechernyaya Moskva*, May 20, 2016, http://vm.ru/news/2016/05/20/russkij-harakter-alekseya-mareseva-320833.html [last accessed: October 1, 2016]; Andrey Sidorchik, "*Zhizn' nastoyashchego cheloveka. Chem Aleksey Mares'ev otlichalsya ot geroya knigi*," Argumenty i Fakty, May 20, 2016, http://www.aif.ru/society/history/zhizn_nastoyashchego_cheloveka_chem_aleksey_maresev_otlichalsya_ot_geroya_knigi [last accessed: October 1, 2016].

90 Inga Bugulova, "Na Valdae otkryli pamyatnik letchiku Mares'evu," *Rossiyskaya gazeta*, May 14, 2016, https://rg.ru/2016/05/14/reg-szfo/na-valdae-otkryli-pamiatnik-letchiku-maresevu.html [last accessed: October 1, 2016]; Igor' Klenevich, "Pamyatnik-samolet Yak-1 v chest' Alekseya Mares'eva otkroyut 22 iyunya na maloy rodine letchika," *TASS*, June 21, 2016, http://tass.ru/obschestvo/3386045 [last accessed: October 1, 2016].

91 TASS, "'Pochta Rossii'" vypustila marku k 100-letiyu legendarnogo letchika Mares'eva," *TASS*, May 20, 2016, http://tass.ru/obschestvo/3299208 [last accessed: October 1, 2016].

92 See Vsevolod Vishnevskiy, "Lautreaty Stalinskich premiy po literature," *Pravda*, June 7, 1947, 5.

The ambivalent reception of these figures in the Soviet Union and the post-Soviet space reflects the historic developments of these countries as they were shaped by internal and foreign political developments. Durdy was briefly feted in the Soviet press during the war and after 1945, first of all in Turkmenistan. He was presented in the role of the "Turkmen Warrior," a symbol of the fight of the Soviet peoples against fascism and the strong connection between Soviet Turkmenistan and the USSR. Durdy was also supposed to promote pro-Soviet sentiments among the people of Central Asia. In post-Soviet Turkmenistan, the dictator Niyazov preferred to remove this "undesirable" hero of the Soviet epoch from the consciousness of the Turkmen people. The ableist tyrant Stalin and his successors in the Kremlin appreciated the value of using the figure of the "Russian fighter pilot without legs" Aleksey Mares'ev in Soviet propaganda. Mares'ev, who was conscious of his role as a poster boy and a role model, used his status in society to help war invalids and other veterans, and embodied the idealized image of the "real" socialist man and also that of the widespread Eastern Bloc ideal image of disabled persons who did not want to be a burden on society and did everything to make themselves "useful." In Boris Yeltsin's Russia, he sank into oblivion, but under Putin, who praises the "glorious Soviet past" and "Russian battle traditions," Mares'ev has once again become a great hero.

CHAPTER VIII

Afflicted Heroes: The Rise and Fall of Yugoslav War Neurosis after the Second World War

Heike Karge

Today, scholarship conceives of psychiatry as the medical discipline that is most closely and obviously bound to culture, society, and politics. What was perceived as a normal mental state in one society could easily be diagnosed as abnormal and pathologic in another. This especially holds true for the issue of the mental breakdown of soldiers as a result of wartime combat, which first appeared en masse during the First World War. From that experience, a psychiatric diagnosis was established—war neurosis—which made it possible, at least for a short while, for people to embrace the diverse symptoms of suffering men and to trace them back to the devastating effects of war. There is a body of literature relating to the complex Western and Central European experience of 1914–1918 as an event that produced mentally broken soldiers classified with diagnoses of shell shock or war neurosis. This scholarship has documented the varying practices and discourses of excluding and enclosing soldiers' mental conditions not only in psychiatric discourse, but also in public, actuarial, and military-medical discourses.

One of the most intriguing questions of military psychiatry, therefore, was whether the mentally broken state of a soldier in combat was caused by the war itself. Different societies gave different answers to this question at various times, and in their answers they revealed their changing—and sometimes unchanging—perceptions of the male—and sometimes female—psyche and body, the hero-soldier, and bravery and cowardice in war and peace.[1] In recent decades, scholars have approached this question by focusing on the experience of the Second World War. Most remarkably, these studies—which mainly deal with Western contexts—make it clear that there was no unique tradition, no linear "Western" way of learning from the experience of the First World War for the next world war to come.[2] While the issue of mental breakdown in wartime was a major topic in most countries after 1914 and in the early postwar period, the image of the mentally broken soldier and the issue of their social and medical needs mostly disappeared from the headlines of European newspapers in the interwar period. The reappearance of the issue of mental breakdown in wartime during the Second World War was, as a rule, short-lived, and it did not have an impact on the wider public before the end of the Vietnam War. Only then, after the new diagnosis of posttraumatic stress disorder (PTSD) was introduced in 1980 (replacing the older diagnoses of war neurosis, shell shock, and the like), was it finally accepted that, without doubt, war was an event that could produce a mentally broken state.

The Yugoslav case does not differ from this finding. In Yugoslavia in 1945, there were hundreds or even thousands of Partisan fighters who, having successfully fought for the liberation of the country and the socialist revolution, returned as broken men. The new socialist state had to deal with these men; the way it did so confirms the findings of historians Allan Young and Ben Shephard, namely that medical diagnoses relating to a mentally broken state likely caused by war—such as PTSD, war neurosis, anxiety neurosis, or shell shock—are culturally and sociopolitically embedded concepts of the twentieth century, which do not exist outside of their historical contexts.[3] Diagnosing is not merely medicine, but culture and poli-

1 See, for instance, Bourke, *Dismembering the Male: Men's Bodies, Britain, and the Great War,* 107–23; for Russia, see Phillips, "Gendered Dis/ability: Perspectives from the Treatment of Psychiatric Casualties in Russia's Early Twentieth Century Wars." See also Lerner, "Psychiatry and Casualties of War in Germany, 1914–18"; and Brunner, "Will, Desire and Experience: Etiology and Ideology in the German and Austrian Medical Discourse on War Neuroses, 1914–1922." For a comparative perspective, see the introduction to a special journal issue on shell shock: Winter, "Shell-Shock and the Cultural History of the Great War."

2 In fact, there is lively discussion with regard to this question. While Bourke and Leese argue that Britain did not truly learn its psychiatric lessons from the First to the Second World War, Shapira argues the converse. See Bourke, "Der Heilberuf und das Leiden. Die Erfahrungen der Militärmedizin in den beiden Weltkriegen"; Leese, *Shell Shock: Traumatic Neurosis and the British Soldiers of the First World War;* and Shapira, "The Psychological Study of Anxiety in the Era of the Second World War."

3 See Young, *The Harmony of Illusions: Inventing Post-Traumatic Stress Disorder;* and Shephard, *A War of Nerves: Soldiers and Psychiatrists, 1914–1994.*

tics, and therefore each warring society in the twentieth century produced its own way of dealing with and conceptualizing the mental breakdowns of soldiers during war. Therefore, the process of diagnosing and understanding soldiers' mental breakdown in and after the Second World War in Yugoslavia bears its own cultural and ideological specifics.

In order to understand how Yugoslav society dealt with the issue of the mentally broken fighter for freedom and communism, or, in the words of historian Peter Leese, "to understand how a mental condition is culturally shaped,"[4] in what follows I will try to historically and culturally contextualize this condition. As Yugoslavia was after 1944 to transform into a socialist state, one might rightfully expect that this profound political, ideological, and social rupture would have repercussions on psychiatric discourse. As historian Marius Turda has highlighted, healthcare systems were conceived by the new communist regimes in Eastern and Southeastern Europe after 1945 "as part of the general transformation of society according to the principles of socialism and communism."[5] Psychiatry and military psychiatry in Yugoslavia formed part of this new healthcare system and therefore of the aim to transform Yugoslav society according to the ideological principles formulated by the communist elite. However, as Mat Savelli and Sarah Marks have recently argued, this should not be equated with a totalitarian perception of a sole instrumentalization of healthcare—in this case psychiatry—by the new socialist states.[6] Instead, scholarship has to address the uncertainties and shifts in this instrumental relationship in state-socialist societies, as well as in any other society, through a close examination of the diverse interactions between the state, the healthcare system, and society.

Looking at how mentally broken Yugoslav Partisan fighters were dealt with in the first two decades after 1944, one is struck by the ambiguities evident in this instrumental relationship. In my reading, military psychiatry was a complicated tool, used by the new socialist state in order to engineer its population to create the "new man." I call the relationship between psychiatry and the state in Yugoslavia "ambiguous," because there was only one concrete—albeit short-lived—attempt by the political elite of the new

4 Leese, *Shell Shock*, 3.

5 Turda, "Private and Public Traditions of Healthcare in Central and South-Eastern Europe, from the Nineteenth to the (Mid-)Twentieth Centuries," 103.

6 Marks and Savelli, "Communist Europe and Transnational Psychiatry."

country to incorporate the mentally broken Partisan fighter into the heroic image of the officially propagated war narrative. Emblematic of this attempt is the diagnosis of "Yugoslav war neurosis" developed by psychoanalyst Hugo Klajn, who was entrusted at the war's end by the political elite of the new country with the task of treating mentally suffering Partisan soldiers. At the core of Klajn's diagnosis was an interpretation of war neurosis as being caused by war. This was neither new nor unique, but it did constitute a break with the views held by military psychiatrists in interwar Yugoslavia. At the end of the 1920s, they had established a position toward mentally broken former soldiers that did not acknowledge the soldiers' suffering as being caused by war. Instead, malingering, unspoken desire for a military pension, and personal predisposition were established as the main causes of the soldiers' "misbehavior." In contrast, Hugo Klajn believed the mentally broken Yugoslav Partisan soldiers were suffering from a type of war neurosis unique to the Yugoslav experience, a diagnosis neither related nor comparable to mental breakdown in any other war or during the Second World War by any other military forces.

In addition, Klajn made it quite clear that in his interpretation, war was the central factor that brought the neurosis to light—but he did not infuse his interpretation with pacifist undertones. Instead, Klajn attempted to incorporate the mentally broken Partisan fighter into the officially communicated image of the hero who fought in the War of Liberation. Here, we find the close link between a fully developed and unique medical psychiatric diagnosis and the new ideology, norms, and values of the young socialist Yugoslav state. However, we will see that Klajn's attempt to therapeutically treat the mentally broken Partisan soldiers failed after a couple of months. What took place in Yugoslavia was a return to earlier military and mainstream psychiatric interpretations of wartime mental breakdown based on older ideological and discursive notions; in other words, a renewal of the interwar discourse that corresponded with the psychiatric discourse of the new socialist Yugoslavia.

In what follows, I will argue that the cultural shaping of mental breakdown in war in post-1944 Yugoslavia had its origins not only—and not primarily—in socialist ideology, but rather in the interwar period. In the long run, the (Yugoslav) socialist ideology would prove unable to absorb the Partisan fighter who collapsed when faced with the horrors of war. In order to develop my argument, I will examine the psychiatric and military psychiatric discourse of the first two decades of postwar Yugoslavia. Here, the professional psychiatric experts and their reasoning about the mentally broken soldiers interest me. Therefore, the source material consists mainly of Yugoslav psychiatric and military-psychiatric articles and monographs from the interwar period up to the 1960s.

The Rise of A Debate

The psychiatric debate about mentally broken Yugoslav Partisan fighters started in 1944. At this time, the Serbian physician and neurologist Isak Alfandary published an article about his experiences working with mentally broken Yugoslav soldiers in a British Army hospital in Grumo close to Bari.[7] From January to September 1944, he treated 141 Yugoslav Partisan fighters suffering from nervous symptoms. Among others, he described the hysterical attacks experienced by Partisan soldiers, at that point the most widespread form of psychoneurotic reaction to war by Yugoslav soldiers.[8] When these hysterical attacks started to occur after the Kozara Offensive from spring 1943 onward, they were called "Kozara psychosis" by contemporary physicians, "battle attack" by the soldiers, and "Partisan disease" by citizens.[9]

In contrast to the interpretation of Hugo Klajn, Alfandary did not yet frame the symptom of the hysterical attack as something unique to the Yugoslav war experience. Rather, his interpretation was that these reactions were comparable to those experienced by the combatants of other warring nations. It was Hugo Klajn, a year later, who was to identify the hysterical attacks of Yugoslav Partisan fighters as a uniquely Yugoslav psychiatric phenomenon. From November 1944 to August 1945, Klajn had been working in the neuropsychiatric ward of the Main Military Hospital in Belgrade. In the latter half of 1945, he became one of two neuropsychiatrists at the newly established Military Psycho-Hygienic Institute in Kovin. In addition to Klajn, Stjepan Betlhajm, also a psychoanalytically trained neuropsychi-

7 Isak Alfandari, "Ratne psihoneuroze," *Vojnosanitetski pregled* 1.1 (1944): 24–8.
8 Ibid., 26.
9 Ibid., 27, and Hugo Klajn, *Ratna Neuroza Jugoslovena* (Beograd: Tersit, 1995; rpt. 1955), 59.

atrist, was employed at the institute.[10] The institute was opened in August 1945 in the building of the former Kovin Hospital for Mental Diseases. According to Klajn, the institute was founded because "[a]t the beginning of 1945 the neuropsychiatric ward of the Main Military Hospital in Belgrade had to face the problem of war neuroses due to an ever increasing influx of the sick."[11] Accordingly, the directorate of the hospital's neuropsychiatric ward suggested the founding of a special institute for war neurosis, and in July 1945, the Medical Department of the Yugoslav Ministry of Defense consulted neuropsychiatrists about this question. During August and September 1945, there were 150 patients being treated at the institute. According to another source, all the patients were Partisan soldiers from the Third Yugoslav Army unit. This source also mentions that until the dissolution of the institute in December 1945, a total of 219 patients were treated there.[12]

Klajn developed his diagnosis of the Yugoslav war neurosis primarily in Kovin. It was rooted in his psychoanalytical understanding of soldiers' mental breakdown being caused by war, or, more precisely, by an inner conflict between the desire to survive and the will to fight.[13] Yet this did not make the Yugoslav soldier unique. What was unique about the Yugoslav case—according to Klajn—was the fact that Yugoslav Partisan fighters as a rule became soldiers voluntarily; they deliberately joined the communist Partisan forces in order to take part in the liberation of the country and to build a new and better (communist) future. This was the source of the neurosis, which manifested itself in the form of "battle attacks." The deliberate decision to fight for the liberation of the country unleashed an attribute intrinsic to the Yugoslav fighter, namely, a particular "fighting spirit" (*borbenost*). Klajn emphasized that whereas anxiety and the inner wish to escape dan-

10 Stjepan Betlhajm was also of Jewish origin. He was a doctor specializing in neurosciences with great interest in psychoanalysis. Betlhajm worked with neurotic soldiers before the war's end. From late 1944 onward, he was the director of the then newly founded hospital for war neurosis of the Fifth Krajina Corps of the National Liberation Army of Yugoslavia in the former village of Čipuljić close to Bugojno, in Bosnia and Herzegovina. See Jovo Kovačević, "Pregled teritorijalnih bolnica narodnooslobodilačke vojske i partizanskih odreda Jugoslavije 1941–1945," in *Sanitetska služba u narodnooslobodilačkom ratu Jugoslavije: 1941–1945*, ed. Ivan Pantelić (Beograd: Vojnoizdavački i novinski centar, 1989), vol. 4, 425–520.

11 Klajn, *Ratna Neuroza Jugoslovena*, 57. For the following, see ibid.

12 Mihajlo Funtek, "Nastanak i razvoj sanitetske službe u oružanim snagama u NOR-u Vojvodine 1941–1945," in *Sanitetska služba u narodnooslobodilačkom ratu Jugoslavije: 1941–1945*, ed. Ivan Pantelić (Beograd: Vojnoizdavački i novinski centar, 1989), vol. 3, 377.

13 For the following, see Klajn, *Ratna Neuroza Jugoslovena*, 72–112.

ger were characteristic of war neuroses among soldiers in other armies, the Yugoslav soldier, with his high morale, his voluntary entry into the military forces, and his "fighting spirit," did not want to flee, but was instead drawn to the front line. In order to feel healthy, he had to continue fighting, or at least to imagine continue fighting, even when peacetime arrived in Yugoslavia. Those who were unable to reintegrate these combative, military values into peacetime behavior would start to display the kind of neurotic reaction that Klajn described.

Klajn had been looking at—and understanding—his soldier patient as one who could not stop being attracted by battle, fighting, and the very event of war. Thus, Klajn attributed war and warlike values a prominent role in the psychiatric understanding of the mental neurotic state, and he even adapted this role to the specifics of Yugoslav communist Partisan warfare. He did not interpret the value of the "fighting spirit" as an ethno-psychological peculiarity of the Yugoslavs, but as evolving out of certain military and social characteristics of the experience of time and place.[14] For Klajn, these combative values evolved (1) because until 1943 there had been a strong imbalance between enemy and Partisan forces; (2) because in 1943 the Partisan units started to be transformed into regular Yugoslav army forces; and (3) because the Partisan forces included very many underage volunteers, both male and female. It was, according to Klajn, foremost this young group of Partisans who suffered from the Yugoslav war neurosis because, due to their youth, they were emotionally and socially less developed than the average soldier and thus more vulnerable to neurotic breakdown.

The qualities highlighted by Klajn as unique to the Yugoslav soldier and as evolving out of the conditions surrounding the Yugoslav War of Liberation were long part of the epic South Slavic tradition, and had also been analyzed by interwar authors such as the human geographer Jovan Cvijić and others.[15] These stalwart values also ranked prominently in the new, socialist state ideology, since it interpreted the National War of Liberation as a glorious event fought by fearless Partisan heroes. The war was also understood

14 Psychiatrist Žarko Trebješanin wrote a preface to the 1995 edition of Klajn's monograph. Here, he emphasized that Klajn deliberately abstained from ethno-psychological interpretations because of Yugoslav communist postwar ideology. See Žarko Trebješanin, "Klajnova analiza ratne neuroze," in Klajn, *Ratna Neuroza Jugoslovena*, 22.

15 Ibid.

to be a conflict that had produced specific kinds of victims—in Yugoslavia called "victims of fascist terror"—but during the 1950s, the Partisan fighter was seen not as a victim, but always as a hero. Thus, the communist ideological interpretation of Partisan warfare as a heroic struggle, and Klajn's interpretation of the adolescent Partisan fighter as suffering from "battle attacks" (in the words of the soldiers), the "Kozara psychosis" (in the words of wartime physicians), or Yugoslav war neurosis, formed an ideal pairing. Klajn's interpretation bolstered—at least in part—the heroic principle communicated to the public by the new Yugoslav state under the leadership of the Communist Party during the 1950s. Interpreting underaged, mentally suffering Partisan fighters as men who could not stop fighting or attacking the enemy and who perceived war as a stimulus, enabled them to be understood as "afflicted heroes."

Klajn's interpretation only partly bolstered the heroic principle; he emphasized that many of the afflicted Partisans were in fact infantile, uneducated, and even mentally challenged. This, as psychiatrist Žarko Trebješanin rightfully argued, did not sit well with the officially communicated image of the deliberately fighting brave communist hero.[16] Historian Ana Antić convincingly argued that Klajn's interpretation of the Partisan neurosis was in fact a way for "middle-class or upper-middle-class psychiatric professionals to express their anxiety over, and even open disapproval of, the increasing upward social mobility and related sociopolitical transformations following the socialist revolution of 1945."[17] There is much to support these theses, but it terms of analyzing the psychiatric discourse on mental breakdown in war other aspects seem to be more important. Klajn's aim was to establish a radically new diagnosis that brought war back into the arena of psychiatric reasoning. This was indeed groundbreaking, because interwar psychiatry, as I argue below, had been moving in the opposite direction. It was not an abstract war, or just any war, which Klajn tried to bring back into focus, but the Yugoslav Communist National War of Liberation. Klajn attempted to link the Yugoslav Partisan war to the positively connoted warlike values of his suffering patients, and thus to make them visible as part of the heroically fought battle.

16 Ibid., 20.

17 Antić, "Heroes and Hysterics: 'Partisan Hysteria' and Communist State-building in Yugoslavia after 1945," 351.

The establishment of the Military Psycho-Hygienic Institute in Kovin can be interpreted as an early sign that the emergence of the diagnosis of Yugoslav war neurosis was strongly welcomed by the political leadership of the country. I have no documents clarifying the position of the leadership toward Klajn's interpretation of the mentally wounded Partisans as afflicted heroes, but the very founding of such an institute, at the war's end, in a socialist country, is more than unexpected. Scholars have much to do to understand how society and the state dealt with mental breakdown in war in Yugoslavia (as well as in other socialist countries) after 1945, but the founding of such an institute, led by two psychoanalytically trained neuropsychiatrists, was a rather exceptional—and telling—case.[18]

Klajn's interpretation of the mentally broken Partisan fighter as suffering from peace and longing for the "just war" was supported by the Yugoslav political elite—if at all—for less than six months. The institute in Kovin no longer existed at the end of 1945. We do not have much information about what happened in Kovin. There are a few pages in Klajn's writings, as well as a letter from Betlhajm to his wife indicating that the psychiatric experiment of dealing with the Yugoslav war neurosis failed after a few weeks. As opposed to official sources, which claimed that the institute was dissolved in December 1945 because the mental epidemic had ended,[19] Klajn blamed the failure of the institute primarily on the failings of the staff. In an article published at the end of 1945, he complained that the therapy failed because the staff did not carry out their responsibilities. In response to being treated, the patients "established a compact fighting unit" and adopted a general rebellious stance.[20] In a letter to his wife, Betlhajm wrote in October 1945: "I very much hope that the hospital will be dissolved soon. It is impossible to work here. The staff is running away, nobody dares to do anything against them [the patients]. They smash windows, go wild in the town, and terrorize everybody."[21]

18 Historian Mat Savelli, without dealing with military psychiatry, has carefully analyzed the openness of Yugoslav psychiatry toward psychoanalytical approaches. See Savelli, "The Peculiar Prosperity of Psychoanalysis in Socialist Yugoslavia."

19 Funtek, "Nastanak i razvoj sanitetske službe u oružanim snagama u NOR-u Vojvodine 1941–1945," 377.

20 Hugo Klajn, "Ratna neuroza Jugoslovena," *Vojno-Sanitetski Pregled* 10–11.2 (1945): 57; and Klajn, *Ratna Neuroza Jugoslovena*, 142–3. After the experiment in Kovin ended, Klajn changed careers and became a well-known theater director.

21 Stjepan Betlheim, *Radovi, Pisma, Dokumenti. 1898–1970* (Zagreb: Antibarbarus, 2006), 348.

The Fall of a Debate

At the end of 1945, with the closing of the Kovin institute, the phenomenon of the Yugoslav war neurosis—and, in fact, any other form of soldiers' mental breakdown caused by war—suddenly and completely disappeared in Yugoslavia, at least for a decade. The participants of the first postwar Yugoslav conference of neurologists and doctors stated quite optimistically in 1946 that "[w]ar neuroses in the form of 'mental attacks,' which, in any case, occur rarely among civilians, have almost entirely disappeared in the army and among the demobilized."[22] In 1949, Klajn's close colleague Betlhajm closed this chapter completely at the second postwar gathering of Yugoslav neuropsychiatrists, which was held in Opatija, when he insisted that "[t]he problem of the war neurosis has been solved thanks to our uniform position toward those who suffered from it."[23]

From a medical-psychiatric point of view, it is unlikely that the sudden disappearance of war neurosis happened all at once and so quickly. As argued above, the issue of soldiers' mental breakdown has never been a subject solely bound to narrow psychiatric knowledge and practice. In fact, actuarial science, social politics, economy, gender images, and images of the national collective always figure as influential factors, and thus the solution to the problem of war neurosis after 1945 could not have been a spontaneous collective recovery of the afflicted soldiers. Rather, the solution consisted of a radical psychiatric reinterpretation of the established diagnosis of Yugoslav war neurosis. In fact, from then on the majority of early postwar psychiatrists held a position that not only negated the very existence of the diagnosis of Yugoslav war neurosis, but that neglected any other psychiatric diagnosis that linked the mental suffering of Partisan soldiers to the cause of war.

Following the closing of the Kovin institute, Klajn, who attempted to completely change the direction of how wartime neurosis was diagnosed, faded from view. In his place, his former wartime fellow psychiatrists took the lead in developing the discourse on mental breakdown in war. Amongst them was Betlhajm, who adopted a severe and strict position regarding the

22 Boško Niketić, "O organizaciji psihijatrijske službe u FNRJ," *Narodno zdravlje* 2.3 (1946): 18.

23 Stjepan Betlhajm, "O radnoj sposobnosti neurotika," in *Zbornik II. naučnog sastanka neuro-psihijatara FNRJ u Opatiji 1949g.*, ed. Savez Lekarskih Društava FNRJ (Beograd, 1951), 106.

suffering soldiers. In a conference lecture in 1949, he equated the "alleged" war neurotic with a phrase that was well established in Croatian and Middle European psychiatry from 1916 onward, namely the "pension neurotic." Claiming that the pension neurotic was not suffering from a mental disease, but that his symptoms occurred out of "unspoken desires" (*Begehrensvorstellungen*), he insisted: "In general they are able to work. They do not belong in the hospital. [...] Before the war, our social insurance system did not accept this kind of pension. This is how the example of other countries has demonstrated the most effective way to bring this pension neurotic back to work."[24] Thus, Betlhajm linked the postwar professional psychiatric perception of the neurotic soldier with regulations stemming from the evolving social welfare system of interwar Yugoslavia. In this view, the neurotic soldier was not sick at all. Instead, while displaying his symptoms to the public, the soldier unmasked himself as a social welfare scrounger.

The most forceful spokesman for the exclusion of Yugoslav war neurosis from the catalog of medical diagnoses was military psychiatrist Josip Dojč from Zagreb.[25] Dojč published regular contributions on simulation, psychopathic personalities, and the nonexistence of psychoneuroses as a real disease in general and as a war psychoneurosis in particular. In his articles, he expressed the opinion that Yugoslav war neurosis never existed, and that most of the documented nervous attacks it was based on were in fact faked by the patients.[26] In autumn 1945, he delivered two lectures to military doctors and the political and military elite of the Yugoslav Army, discussing two cases of "nervous attacks" in which the patients deliberately imitated and simulated their condition. As he spoke, no one in the audience realized that the cases were based on fabricated evidence. The simulation that took place in these two cases indicated for Dojč that all cases of mental attack among Yugoslav Partisan fighters—including those studied by Klajn—consisted of imitation and simulation.[27]

24 Betlhajm, "O radnoj sposobnosti neurotika," 106.

25 At the end of 1943, Dojč became director of the hospital of the 6th Lika Division of the National Liberation Army of Yugoslavia. See Ivan Kralj, "Nastanak i razvoj sanitetske službe u narodnooslobodilačkom ratu u Hrvatskoj," in *Sanitetska služba u narodnooslobodilačkom ratu Jugoslavije: 1941–1945*, ed. Ivan Pantelić (Beograd: Vojnoizdavački i novinski centar, 1989), vol. 2, 277.

26 Josip Dojč, "O biti živčanih napadaja u ratu (ratna neuroza)," *Vojnosanitetski pregled* 3.3 (1946): 117–19; also Dojč, "Psihička trauma i njezino lečenje," *Vojnosanitetski pregled* 3.1 (1946): 24–7; and Dojč, "Simulacija i simulanti sa psihijatrijskog gledišta," *Srpski Arhiv za Celokupno Lekarstvo* 78.12 (1950): 848–66.

27 Dojč, "O biti živčanih napadaja u ratu (ratna neuroza)," 117–18.

Dojč's position toward the mental attacks experienced by the former Partisan fighters was instead that these constituted a kind of infantile reaction of defiance, which could be successfully cured by strict education and consequence.[28] He divided the 2,000 military-psychiatric cases he had been working on in Zagreb at the end of the war into three categories: psychopaths and hysterics (a small group), infantile and underaged persons (the biggest group), and persons simulating war neurosis. Regardless to which group an alleged war neurotic was classified, "[i]n all three groups it is not about diseases, but about a phenomenon which can be mastered, if the respective person is really trying to behave in a disciplined way and if he is willing to devote his mental energy to fighting these phenomena."[29] For Dojč, the problem of war neurosis was not a psychiatric one, but merely an educational one. Therefore, he criticized the wartime practice of evacuating mental patients by airplane to Grumo and elsewhere as a "misguided action,"[30] since this simply fortified the spreading of the attacks among military staff. He concluded in a quasi-ironic style: "But now our rich experience has directed us to the right assessment of the very nature of this phenomenon, so that it is high time now that with respect to therapy all responsible factors take on an appropriate [and] proper 'therapeutic' position."[31] The essence of this "proper therapeutic position" was nicely summarized in 1952 by Dojč himself in an article discussing the issue of psychoneuroses from the viewpoint of modern military psychiatry. Dojč argued that, hypothetically, war could produce serious psychoneurotic reactions among military staff, but that war neurosis diagnosed in wartime Yugoslavia was a different phenomenon, which could by no means be labeled a disease. Instead, the "sick," as he would claim, were reacting with nothing else than a public self-display, which in turn would infect its spectators and thus, finally, lead to the kind of epidemic which befell the mostly underaged and premature Yugoslav Partisan fighters.[32]

In this view, Yugoslav war neurosis as diagnosed by Klajn as a very special type of mental breakdown in wartime never ever truly existed. Instead, Dojč and his colleagues interpreted the mental attacks of the Partisan sol-

28 Ibid., 118.
29 Ibid.
30 Ibid., 119.
31 Ibid.
32 Josip Dojč, "Ratne psihoneuroze sa gledista savremene vojne psihijatrije," *Vojno-Sanitetski Pregled* 7–8.9 (1952): 233.

diers as a variety of common psychoneurosis, which was by no means bound to war, but could occur in peacetime as well.[33] Dojč emphasized that even though anyone could react slightly neurotically under the prolonged strains of modern warfare, it was only "the constitutionally labile, the psychopath, and the moronic" who displayed serious neurotic reactions.[34] Dojč's psychiatric views had become judgmental and unforgiving as compared to his own early postwar position. While in 1946, Dojč was still suggesting (socialist) education as a proper means to "master the phenomenon" and to raise the "new man," his later classification of the afflicted soldiers as "psychopaths" and "morons" moved the discourse of interpretation into the sphere of antisocial and inherited personal predisposition.

As mentioned earlier, this interpretation was surprisingly close to military-psychiatric interpretations developed in the interwar period. Starting in the 1930s, psychiatric understanding of soldiers' mental breakdown in wartime was characterized by the view that sufferers were somehow mentally weak or inferior, as well by the assertion that it was not the war that triggered the sickness. For example, a 1930 article in the *Vojnosanitetski glasnik* (*Military-Medical Herald*) about mentally broken Yugoslavian veterans of the First World War stated that "[m]ental disorders among the injured that are in shock are manifested particularly among individuals with abnormal psychological constitutions (alcoholics and syphilitics)."[35] Additionally, in the late 1930s the psychiatric files of diseased soldiers would typically contain a doctor's note asserting that "the sickness was already there before military service."[36] Thus, in interwar Yugoslavia, war was preemptively excluded from the catalog of potential catalysts of a soldier's mentally broken state.[37] This view returned after the closing of the Kovin institute, as seen by the move to eliminate the war from the list of possible causes of soldiers' mental illness, according to socialist Yugoslav psychiatric diagnostics.

33 Ibid., 226–7. Interpreted in the very same way in Gojko Nikoliš and Zdenko Kraus, "Nacionalna organizacija zdravstvene službe u ratu. Koordinacija gradjanskog i vojnog saniteta. Priprema za vreme mira," *Srpski Arhiv za Celokupno Lekarstvo* 83.4 (1955): 429–43.

34 Dojč, "Ratne psihoneuroze sa gledista savremene vojne psihijatrije," 229.

35 Gavrilo Petrović and Ivo Jovanović, "O traumatičnom šoku. Mehanizam, simptomatologija i lečenje," *Vojnosanitetski glasnik* 1.3–4 (1930): 198.

36 Vojni Arhiv Srbije (VA) [Military archive of Serbia], Fond Vojske Kraljevine Srbije (FVKS) [Portfolio Army of the Kingdom of Serbia], P-17, k-911, f-2, d-7.

37 For more details, see Karge, "Making Sense of War Neurosis in Yugoslavia."

By the beginning of the 1950s, a situation was in place that more or less would be the dominant military psychiatric position for years to come. From then on, the main military-medical and medical journals kept quiet about Yugoslav war neurosis and any other possible war neurosis associated with the Yugoslav Partisan fighter. Even though the *Vojnosanitetski pregled* (*Military-Medical and Pharmaceutical Review*) published regular contributions on military psychiatry, these mainly dealt with the potential of a future (nuclear) war to affect the mental health of military personnel and the civilian population, issues of recruitment, and psychological testing. Experiences resulting from the work in Kovin, or references to Klajn and his Yugoslav war neurosis in regards to other forms of mental breakdown caused by the Yugoslav War of Liberation, rarely appeared. There were some exceptions, but the few studies presented to the public after the mid-1950s did so admitting their limited scope.[38] In all, the retreating position of mainstream military psychiatrists, such as Josip Dojč, regarding the existence of Yugoslav war neurosis (it did not exist) and, more importantly, toward war as a significant variable affecting soldiers' mental problems (it was not) meant that the subject was not addressed in any significant way. This silence characterized not only Yugoslavian military-psychiatric and medical journals, but also the views of the general public throughout the 1950s.

The Reemergence of the War Neurotic

Tracing the mentally broken Partisan soldier in postwar Yugoslavia proves difficult. During the first decade after the war, silencing the existence of soldiers' mental breakdowns seems to have been the dominant strategy not only for psychiatrists, but also for patients. At the beginning of the 1960s, neuropsychiatrist Slavka Morić-Petrović stated: "It is interesting to observe that wartime neurotics are today reluctant to confess to the physician that they have attacks."[39] This reluctance of patients to admit to mental symp-

38 One of these studies was led by Betlhajm, who obviously changed sides again. In 1957, he reported on a pilot study with 34 former Partisan fighters from the territory of Croatia suffering from neurotic symptoms. See Stjepan Betlhajm, "Adaptacija ratnih neurotika. Analiza rezultata probne ankete," *Vojnosanitetski pregled* 14.9 (1957): 506–10.

39 Slavka Morić-Petrović, "Neuropsychiatric After-effects on a Group of Participants in the People's Liberation War of Yugoslavia," *International Conference on the Later Effects of Imprisonment and Deportation, The Hague, November 20–25, 1961* (The Hague: World Veterans Federation, 1961), 96.

toms is telling, and it suggests the nature of the psychiatric and general discursive climate, which aimed at hushing up the disease and the suffering people experienced.

However, it is clear that public and professional views were changing by the end of the 1950s. This had to do most of all with the increasing public visibility of mentally damaged Partisan fighters, who wandered around Yugoslavia's city streets without being cared for. There is also some plausibility to the argument that the increased visibility was a Yugoslavian response to a changing international discourse, which started to broach the issue of medical support for victims of war, including antifascist resistance fighters and the former inmates of concentration camps. At the end of the 1950s, former deportees and internees in many European countries started to raise their voices in public to demand acknowledgement of their mental and physical suffering, which had outlasted the war.

After the war, many of the former Partisan fighters in Yugoslavia formed the League of Associations of Fighters of the National War of Liberation (Savez Udruženja Boraca Narodnooslobodilačkog Rata [SUBNOR]), and it seems logical that this would be the place where the issue would eventually reappear. It was not until the end of the 1950s that the mental health problems of former fighters found their way onto the agenda of SUBNOR's leadership, however. Neda Božinović, herself a former Partisan fighter and until the early 1970s a high-ranking member of the Yugoslav political leadership, stated in 1957:

> It is a problem that there are people who wander around in Belgrade with a badge and a certificate [identifying them as war veterans]. Another problem is that there are people admitted to neuropathic clinics who, upon release, do not have a home to go to. [...] Slovenia has carried out a survey and it reveals that the relative majority of inmates in the clinics for mental patients and in the neuropathic clinics is made up of former fighters.[40]

Božinović also mentioned that a commission was founded in Slovenia to take care of former fighters suffering from mental problems. In Bosnia and Herzegovina, however, where the problem was even more pressing, no sim-

40 Arhiv Srbije i Crne Gore (ASCG), f. 297, 15, document dated May 29, 1957.

ilar commission existed; nor were there any neuropathic clinics for veterans who needed help. The position of SUBNOR as well as of the general political leadership of the country was problematic regarding this issue—indeed, their concern was to conceal the problem. When asked about which medical specialist should be consulted regarding this issue, Božinović warns: "The main thing is that this is done as silently as possible!"[41]

The politically mandated silence did not last forever. The 1960s saw new developments, which finally resulted in the foundation of new care centers for mentally wounded war veterans and former deportees and internees. What factors triggered this new development? Morić-Petrović, a neuropsychiatrist from Belgrade, argued in an article from 1961 that SUBNOR "was keenly interested, on the one hand, in helping these men and, on the other, in examining and establishing whether there was any link between the symptomatology of these patients and the trauma they were exposed to during the war."[42] In contrast to Morić-Petrović, it seems to me that much more important than SUBNOR's activities were the actions of former deportees and internees in bringing the subject of the consequences of the war to the table. Internees and deportees had been part of SUBNOR since its foundation in 1947, but their status in the war veterans' organization remained marginal for the entire period of its existence. The emphasis within SUBNOR—and within the overall official Yugoslav war narrative and state ideology—was instead always focused on the heroic, active fighter, the one who fought at the front lines, and not on the needs of those who had been deported elsewhere during the war.

Nonetheless, May 1960 saw the organization of the first federal conference of former internees and deportees in Yugoslavia. Not surprisingly, one participant warned that, although more and more former internees and deportees had become "mentally ill," nothing had been done to address the problem: "That is why we have a lot of mentally ill people and often we meet people on the street who suffer from this. For a long time these people did not get any attention."[43] Views like this showed that from the early 1960s, even though it was slow and silent, there was a shift of attention toward ad-

41 Ibid.

42 Morić-Petrović, "Neuropsychiatric After-effects on a Group of Participants in the People's Liberation War of Yugoslavia," 97.

43 ASCG, f. 297, 19, document dated May 8, 1960.

dressing mental problems that had (possibly) been caused by the war in Yugoslavia. This change would not lead to major revisions of military psychiatric understandings of mental breakdown caused by war—at least not until the beginning of the 1980s. But one important result of the gradual rise of public awareness in Yugoslavia toward the problem was the founding of institutions that could and did provide medical and psychiatric care for the mentally broken former Partisan fighters.

In Sarajevo, the capital city of the republic of Bosnia and Herzegovina, a building with a fifty-bed capacity was constructed next to the neuropsychiatric institution on the initiative and with the support of the Bosnian branch of SUBNOR.[44] In the 1964 schedule of the Croatian branch of SUBNOR, the foundation of a center for psychoneurotic patients was envisioned in cooperation with the secretaries of social policy and national health: "The necessity of this establishment's foundation is due to the diffusion of alcoholism and psychoneuroses in the combatants' union, which is a result of the long-term effects of the war and of the abuse of the people in the prisons and camps."[45] Slovenian and Croatian sources suggest that in addition to the creation of specialized institutions, public hospitals also regularly treated former Partisans. In the Ljubljana Psychiatric Hospital, for instance, former Partisans made up at least three percent of all patients treated from the mid-1950s to the mid-1970s, and most of these suffered from either neuroses or alcoholism.[46]

In Belgrade, a special medical center was founded in 1960 for the purpose of conducting research into the etiology and the symptomatology of the later effects of war.[47] Thanks to the above-mentioned Morić-Petrović, who published an article about the work of this center in an edited volume of the World Veterans Federation, we know that in the first eighteen months of its existence, 110 patients went through this medical center. The tone of the article is very cautious, stating that even in the group of patients who were of more or less sound health prior to the war, "war stresses played

44 Ibid.

45 Hrvatski Državni Arhiv (HDA), f. 1241/2, 291, document dated October 1, 1963.

46 See J. Kostnapfel, "Katamnestički nalaz bivših boraca sa duševnim smetnjama poslije 5 godina," in *Psihijatrija. Zbornik radova 6. kongresa neurologa i psihijatara Jugoslavije.* (Sarajevo: Udruženje neurologa i psihijatara Jugoslavije, 1980), 124–5.

47 Morić-Petrović does not mention the exact name of the center in her article.

their part in forming an apparent vulnerability in the later years of life."[48] Although Morić-Petrović admitted that only systematic research with larger numbers of veterans could confirm the results, this was a revolutionary statement indeed, as—except for the interpretation of Klajn—personal predisposition and immaturity were the main frames for the interpretation of soldiers' mental breakdown within Yugoslav military psychiatry. Morić-Petrović's article, except for the writings of Klajn, was one of the very few official statements from a Yugoslav psychiatrist regarding the correlation between mental breakdown and war that addressed the issue without pejorative undertones.[49]

But what kind of knowledge about the effects of the World War on the mental health of Yugoslav Partisan fighters had all these hospitals and mental care centers produced? There are strong indicators that the actions of these newly founded institutions did not really result in an increase in public knowledge about the issue, despite an increase in public awareness. Psychiatric textbooks, for instance, do not give the impression that there was a major change before the 1980s. As Christiane Wildgrube et al. show, psychiatric textbooks published in Serbia display a very mild change of perception of the war neurosis over time. Real change started only in the 1980s, with the introduction of the concept of PTSD. Before, textbooks dealt with the issues of war neurosis, pension hysteria, and also Klajn's concept of Yugoslav war neurosis, but always with the underlying assumption "that war neurosis only affected predisposed persons."[50] This statement went far beyond the preliminary results mentioned by Morić-Petrović. Also, take the example of the 1982 monograph on military psychiatry by Yugoslav military psychiatrist Gojko Kapor. It is clear that Kapor's review of the field did not use any knowledge produced during the 1960s or 1970s. Kapor's view is that:

> The analysis and interpretation (even from the side of [...] outstanding neuropsychiatrists) of the dynamics of mental dysfunction among the fighters

48 Morić-Petrović, "Neuropsychiatric After-effects on a Group of Participants in the People's Liberation War of Yugoslavia," 98.

49 Antić mentions in this regard yet another Belgrade-based wartime psychiatrist, Stojan Kulić. See Antić, "Psychiatry at War: Psychiatric Culture and Political Ideology in Yugoslavia under the Nazi Occupation."

50 Wildgrube et al., "Psychological Trauma in German, Serbian and British Psychiatry since 1945: A Comparison of Textbooks," 253.

> of the National War of Liberation, on the basis of material stemming from [the period] of the National War of Liberation, that is, based on statements of participants of the [...] war, after the end of the [...] war, above all, many years after its end, bears the danger of arbitrary interpretations and conclusions, first of all because of the fact that many biological, psychological, and sociocultural factors which influenced the emergence of the mental dysfunction are unknown.[51]

His 400-page-long monograph contains only three pages referring to the Yugoslav case. He mentions Klajn and his interpretation of Yugoslav war neurosis, but there is no discussion of the results of later postwar psychiatric treatment of former Partisan fighters. As the quotation above makes clear, Kapor even warns professionals about (or, at least, he saw no use in) analyzing and interpreting these phenomena almost four decades after the end of the war, because misinterpretation—from the side of the patient as well as the doctor—would be almost inevitable.

One could also take as a further example the war memoirs of Gojko Nikoliš, the medical consultant to the Supreme Military Staff (Vrhovni Štab) of the Yugoslav Partisan Army during the war. Nikoliš had taken part in the military-psychiatric debate of the 1950s, which had excluded the war as an etiological factor of a soldier's mentally broken state. He was obviously familiar with the military-psychiatric discourse of the time. His memoirs were published in 1980, that is, two decades after the founding of the special medical center in Belgrade for the treatment of war neurotics. However, the more than 600 pages of the memoir do not contain any discussion of mental breakdown among Yugoslav Partisans, let alone of its (therapeutic) treatment during or after the war.[52] Finally, the silencing of the subject matter in the Yugoslav public and in psychiatric discourse becomes evident when one considers the topics discussed at the Seventh Congress of Yugoslav Psychiatrists held in 1984, which dealt exclusively with neuroses and psychoses. The publication of the conference papers, which included contributions from military psychiatrists, does not contain a single contribution regarding the question of war neuroses or mental breakdown caused

51 Gojko Kapor, *Ratna psihijatrija* (Beograd: Vojnoizdavački zavod, 1982), 66.
52 Gojko Nikoliš, *Korijen, stablo, pavetina. Memoari*, 3rd ed. (Zagreb: Liber, 1981).

by war.[53] One paper, ironically, did observe that there were no long-term studies about the issue of neuroses among war veterans since there had been always too many different conceptions of what the neurosis actually was.[54] Whatever knowledge the few special institutions for the treatment of war veterans' mental problems did produce, it seems that it did not really find its way into the practice of Yugoslav psychiatry, nor into the understanding of the issue by the wider public.

Conclusion

It is difficult to arrive at a reliable estimate of the total number of Yugoslav Partisan fighters who suffered from mental breakdown in the war. Contemporaries admit that Yugoslav war neurosis—which was just one among many other possible mental diagnoses—had been spreading since 1943 in quasi-epidemic form. Alfandary described the neurosis as a collective neurosis, which easily spread among soldiers of military units. Paul Parin, a Swiss doctor and psychoanalyst who joined the Yugoslav Partisans as a physician during the war, described the neurosis as a kind of infectious disease.[55] There are some estimates by contemporary observers, but these vary tremendously between 3,000 (Klajn) and 100,000 (Parin).[56] At the start of the 1980s, Yugoslav military psychiatrist Kapor interpreted Klajn's estimate of 3,000 to refer to the number of cases in a single month (October 1945) rather than an overall total. Accordingly, Kapor concluded that the number of mental casualties among Yugoslav Partisan fighters for the whole war period must have been much larger.[57]

Finally, one should not forget that Klajn, Parin, and (partly) Alfandary, in fact, only spoke about one group among mentally affected Yugoslav soldiers—namely, those who, according to Alfandary, suffered from hysterical

53 *Psihijatrija: Zbornik Radova VII kongresa psihijatara Jugoslavije, Budva, 3–6. oktobar, 1984 g.* (Titograd: Udruženje psihijatara Jugoslavije, 1984).

54 A. Marković, "Invalidogenost neurotskih bolesti u Dalmaciji," in *Psihijatrija: Zbornik Radova VII kongresa psihijatara Jugoslavije*, 479–85. Similarly, see also D. Milovanović et al., "Klinička fenomenologija psihičkih obolenja," in *Psihijatrija. Zbornik radova 6. kongresa neurologa i psihijatara Jugoslavije* (Sarajevo: Udruženje neurologa i psihijatara Jugoslavije, 1980), 207–12.

55 Paul Parin, "Die Kriegsneurose der Jugoslawen," *Schweizer Archiv für Neurologie und Psychiatrie* 61 (1948): 3–24. See also his later account recalling his experience among the Yugoslav Partisans; Parin, *Es ist Krieg und wir gehen hin. Bei den jugoslawischen Partisanen.*

56 See Klajn, *Ratna Neuroza Jugoslovena*, 59; and Parin, *Es ist Krieg und wir gehen hin*, 188.

57 Kapor, *Ratna psihijatrija*, 317.

attacks and, according to Klajn, suffered from Yugoslav war neurosis. However, as we know today, Yugoslav Partisans did also suffer from other kinds of mental breakdown. Kapor eventually admitted in 1982 that besides Yugoslav war neurosis, there had also been anxiety, panic, and depressive reactions, as well as reactions of split personality.[58]

In their discussion about the politics of war trauma after 1945 in a European comparative perspective, Jolande Withuis et al. rightfully emphasize that there was no single, unique way of coming to terms with the mental effects of war in the long postwar period. The way nations dealt with the mental aftereffects of war varied and were deeply rooted in the way these nations dealt with concepts such as trauma, along with how their social insurance system worked, their experiences with soldiers' mental breakdown during the First World War, etc.[59] This holds true, of course, for Yugoslavia as well, with its distinct history of the sudden rise and fall of the psychiatric diagnosis of "Yugoslav war neurosis."

Except for a brief initial period, throughout the postwar years the issue of mental breakdown in war remained a marginal one in Yugoslavia. The reasons for silencing any discussion of Yugoslav soldiers' mental breakdown in war are to be found, in part, in the politics of the postwar period, which would not allow the brave Partisan hero to be a mentally suffering victim of a war that had been fought to achieve the new socialist state. More significant reasons are to be found in the continuation of a psychiatric and sociopolitical discourse that stemmed from the period 1914–1918 and the interwar period, when issues of simulation, pension neurosis, and personal predisposition held great discursive importance. There is, however, nothing special about this. It was only after the Vietnam War that mental breakdown caused by the very event of war received the public and psychiatric attention it deserved. All of a sudden, wartime mental breakdown became a valid psychiatric diagnosis all over the world through its standardization in terms of PTSD. This acknowledgement of the issue in the 1990s had a significant impact on Yugoslav psychiatry as well.[60]

58 Ibid., 65.

59 Jolande Withuis, "Introduction: The Politics of War Trauma," in *The Politics of War Trauma: The Aftermath of World War Two in Eleven European Countries*, 1–11.

60 Wildgrube et al., "Psychological Trauma in German, Serbian and British Psychiatry since 1945," 265.

What was special about the Yugoslav case was that for a brief period in 1945, Partisan soldiers suffering from mental breakdown were offered the chance to be seen as afflicted heroes. In Klajn's interpretation, these soldiers, although acting strangely under the mental attacks they were suffering from, were still heroes. Klajn was, in fact, the only psychiatric professional who attempted—in a positive way—to make sense out of the war neurotic within the new state ideology and the war narrative of the heroically fought National War of Liberation. If Klajn's efforts had lasted for more than just six months, one could claim that his interpretation was a successful example of adopting psychiatric knowledge to socialist state ideology. As we have seen, it was not, but other psychiatrists and other interpretations were to succeed in this. After Klajn, mainstream postwar Yugoslav psychiatry was to neglect any heroism to the mentally distressed soldiers of the National War of Liberation by successfully adopting to the new circumstances the knowledge and practices that dated back to the European interwar period. Thus, there was indeed an instrumental relationship between psychiatry and the socialist state in the period following 1945. However, in my reading, this relationship was less inspired by controversies about the by-products of the socialist transformation than by the resurgence of sociopolitical and psychiatric arguments that, though originating from a nonsocialist past, finally and successfully amalgamated with Yugoslav socialist realities.

PART III

Regulating Societies After 1945: State-Socialist Policies and Legacies

CHAPTER IX

Politics and Family Conflicts through the Psychiatric Lens: East Berlin's Charité in the early GDR[1]

Fanny Le Bonhomme

> Overall, their marriage is pretty good. Their financial situation is more than satisfactory. But she often gets into ideological quarrels with her husband over how to raise their children. The husband is a Marxist and wishes to raise their children accordingly, whereas the patient wants to raise them in a religious setting. This is obviously why fights are frequent.[2]

This is an extract from the medical record of patient Gisela R., who in the summer of 1962 spent a month in the psychotherapy unit of the psychiatry and neurology clinic of the Charité hospital in East Berlin. This young woman, aged thirty, had had difficulty walking for about three years. According to her medical record, she was believed to suffer from a "hysterical symptom." The director of the clinic, psychiatrist Karl Leonhard, explained that this symptom had its roots in "a conflict between what the

---

1 This chapter was translated by Delphine Silberbauer. It is part of my PhD project *Psychiatry and Society in the German Democratic Republic: Stories of Patients from the Charité Psychiatry and Neurology Clinic (East-Berlin, 1960–1968)* (University of Rennes 2/University of Potsdam, 2016).

2 "Die Ehe sei im allgemeinen gesehen relativ gut. Auch die wirtschaftlichen Verhältnisse seien durchaus ausreichend. Nur habe sie öfter weltanschauliche Auseinandersetzungen mit ihrem Ehegatten hinsichtlich der Erziehung der Kinder. Der Mann, welcher Marxist sei möchte seine Kinder in diesem Sinne erziehen und die Pat im Gegenteil, religiös erziehen, dadurch gäbe es selbstverständlich oft Streik." HPAC [Historisches Psychiatriearchiv der Charité] F 373a/62, Krankengeschichte, Anamnese, Eheverhältnisse.

person desires, and, in contrast, the external demands made upon her,"[3] which led to a "flight into illness." But the only conflict that Gisela R. mentioned during her stay in the clinic concerned her relationship with her husband, who wanted to raise their children in line with the official state ideology and in accordance with Marxist doctrine. About two weeks after his wife was admitted to the clinic, he was invited to have a discussion with the doctor. This is what the record states concerning the conflict between his wife and himself:

> Regarding the upbringing of the children, he is of the opinion that they should be raised according to state guidelines. He believes religious education is a sentimental issue [Gefühlssache]. When he was told that he needed to show more tolerance in this regard, he indicated that he was prepared to do so in future.[4]

This passage shows that the doctor clearly advised the husband to be more flexible with regard to the religious education of his children. In doing so, the doctor took a position that went against the educational norms defined by the socialist state. According to the "Ten Commandments of Socialist Morality," promulgated in 1958, it was indeed "in the spirit of peace and socialism" that "the socialist man" must raise his children.[5] The 1965 Family Code, in which socialist law and morality were intertwined,[6] stipulated that one of the main tasks of parents was to instill socialist ideology in their children[7] within the "smallest unit of society,"[8] namely the family. In this perspective,

3 Karl Leonhard, *Differenzierte Diagnostik der endogenen Psychosen, abnormen Persönlichkeitsstrukturen und neurotischen Entwicklungen* (Berlin: Verlag Volk und Gesundheit, 1964), 82.

4 "Wegen der Erziehung der Kinder wäre er der Ansicht, dass man die Kinder im Sinne des Staates erziehen soll. Die religiöse Erziehung sei seiner Meinung nach eine Gefühlssache. Als er darauf hingewiesen wird, dass es notwendig sei, in dieser Frage toleranter zu sein, war er bereit, in Zukunft, dies zu respektieren." HPAC, F 373a/72, Krankengeschichte, Rücksprache mit dem Ehemann am 6 Juli 1962.

5 See *Zehn Geboten für den neuen sozialistischen Menschen*, 1958 (commandement no. 8: "Du sollst deine Kinder im Geiste des Friedens und des Sozialismus zu allseitig gebildeten, charakterfesten und körperlich gestählten Menschen erziehen.").

6 In the words used by Justice Minister Hilde Benjamin in her speech to the Volkskammer (People's Chamber) on December 20, 1965, "Das Grundgesetz der Familie im Sozialismus," in *Ein glückliches Familienleben—Anliegen des Familiengesetzbuches der DDR* (Aus der Tätigkeit der Volkskammer und ihrer Ausschüsse), Staatsverlag der DDR, 1965. On the subject, see also Friedrich W. Busch, *Familienerziehung in der sozialistischen Pädagogik der DDR* (Düsseldorf: Schwann, 1972), 106–8.

7 FGB, § 42 Abs. 2.

8 Familiengesetzbuch [FGB], Preambule.

parents were discouraged from providing religious instruction to their children. Nevertheless, when dealing with the conflict between Gisela R. and her husband, which obviously played a part in the patient's medical condition, the doctor did not seem to relay the orders of the communist authorities. On the contrary, as evidenced by this issue in the context of the GDR of the 1960s and in the context of therapeutic interviews, the medical response issued within the psychiatric clinic did not follow systematically the behavioral standards promulgated by the official discourse.

This situation, documented by the clinic's archives, calls for a fresh look at the relations between psychiatry and politics in the GDR.[9] This initiative fits in with the renewed historiographic interest in the history of psychiatry under Communism. As evidenced by the book published in 2015 by historians Sarah Marks and Mat Savelli, psychiatric systems east of the Iron Curtain have become the object of historical research concerning Czechoslovakia, Yugoslavia, Romania, Hungary, and the USSR.[10] Filling a gap in the historiography, these studies have challenged the monolithic image of a "communist psychiatry," thought to have been used for political purposes and as a tool for brainwashing political opponents. The case of the USSR, where psychiatry placed itself at the service of the regime to silence opponents between the 1960s and the late 1980s, continues to generate suspicion concerning the practice of psychiatry in the entire Eastern Bloc. In the absence of systematic research on the topic, however, it is impossible to assess the exact extent of this phenomenon throughout the Communist Bloc.[11]

Beyond the issue of instrumentalization, an analysis of sources provides a complex and nuanced picture of psychiatric care systems in the Eastern Bloc, systems whose stories are embedded in contexts that extend be-

9 Eghighian, "Was There a Communist Psychiatry? Politics and East German Psychiatric Care, 1945–1989."

10 Savelli and Marks (eds.), *Psychiatry in Communist Europe.*

11 In the USSR, and from the mid-1960s onward, political dissidents were indeed unduly confined in "special" psychiatric hospitals under the control of the Ministry of Interior, in order to silence their voices. This practice was intensified in the 1970s. This instrumentalization of psychiatry, which aroused criticism and indignation among the international community as well as several Soviet psychiatrists, only came to an end in the late 1980s. For more on the abusive use of psychiatry for political purposes in the USSR, see, in particular, Bloch and Reddaway, *Russia's Political Hospitals: The Abuse of Psychiatry in the Soviet Union*; idem, *Soviet Psychiatric Abuse: The Shadow over World Psychiatry*; Smith and Oleszczuk, *No Asylum: State Psychiatric Repression in the Former USSR*; Spencer, *An Investigation of the Relationship of Soviet Psychiatry to the State.* For a brief overview on the subject, see Süß, *Politisch missbraucht? Psychiatrie und Staatssicherheit in der DDR*, 18–27.

yond the communist era. Psychiatry appears as "an excellent prism through which to explore the different facets of the social, political, and intellectual history of Eastern Europe under communism."[12] In line with the objectives of these studies, my research seeks to place the history of psychiatry under Communism in a broader context, paying attention to the sources it has produced. In the context of this study, which examines the situation in the GDR in the 1960s, my aim is not to focus on the possible instrumentalization of psychiatry for political purposes (which has been denied by several scientific investigations and studies[13]), but to shift the perspective from which the interaction between the psychiatric institution and the socialist state can be approached, by ceasing to regard the former as an instrument serving the latter.

It was the discovery of patient files that made this shift possible. Contrary to the image of psychiatry as being instrumentalized by the regime, these sources reveal a very different situation: the psychiatric arena could become the place that allowed both patients and healthcare professionals to distance themselves from the official political line. The three axes around which this volume revolves—the state, the healthcare system, and society—interact here in an original dynamic process. In the context of the GDR, the healthcare system—characterized by free access to care—played a key role in the political system of the country. Healthcare policy—as part of social policy—can be considered an "instrument of domination" in that one of its objectives was to "softly" mobilize support from citizens. In this perspective, the concept of "welfare dictatorship" (*Fürsorgediktatur*) points to a specificity of the GDR and differentiates it from other modern dictatorships of the twentieth century.[14] Though it constituted a component of the official legitimization discourse and contributed to the acceptance of socialism in society, the healthcare system could also be a place for interactions in which individuals enjoyed relatively unheard of leeway in the socialist society. The sources show that during therapeutic interviews, a relative freedom of tone was acceptable and could be indicative of reservations toward state injunctions. This type of situation is observed in cases when the patient refers to family tensions of a

12 Marks and Savelli, "Communist Europe and Transnational Psychiatry," in *Psychiatry in Communist Europe*, 20.

13 Süß, *Politisch mißbraucht?*

14 Jarausch, "Realer Sozialismus als Fürsorgediktatur. Zur begrifflichen Einordnung der DDR."

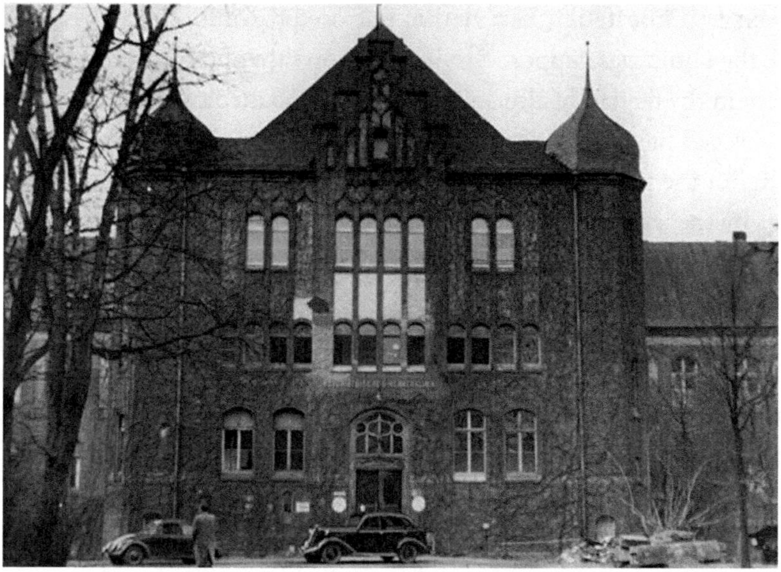

Figure 9.1: *The psychiatry and neurology clinic of the Charité (East Berlin, 1950).* Heinz Funk, January 11, 1950, Bundesarchiv, Bild 183-S91935/CC-BY-SA 3.0.

political nature. Although those conflicts—because they have a political or even an ideological dimension—were generally not openly talked about in the socialist society, they could be discussed by the patient in his or her interactions with the therapist. Through hints left in the patients' record, one can find a complex and nuanced version of the individuals' relation to the political regime in its most intimate dimensions. As for the response of therapists, it did not necessarily follow the dictates of the official discourse. It is around this twofold discovery in the sources that I have structured this study, which focuses not only on the family tensions experienced by the patients, but also on the physician's or psychologist's perspective on those conflicts.

I have based my study on a corpus of records on patients who were treated in the psychiatry and neurology clinic of the Charité in East Berlin during the 1960s.[15] This clinic occupied a prominent place in the psychiatric landscape of the GDR. Indeed, it was part of the Charité university hospital, the largest hospital complex in the GDR, which was associated with Humboldt

15 I would like to thank the Institute for the History of Medicine and Ethics in Medicine of Berlin, and especially its director, Volker Hess, for having given me access to the clinic's archives.

University.[16] Located in East Berlin, in close proximity to its West German rival, the clinic was supposed to be the showcase of the socialist healthcare system in the field of healthcare, education, and medical research. Thus, the framework I have used for my study is not just any mental institution in the GDR, but the top clinic in the country. This institution was marked in the 1960s by the leadership of the new director, Karl Leonhard, who took office in 1957, two years after emigrating from West to East Germany for professional reasons.

The highly hierarchical structure of university clinics explains the influence wielded by the person at their head. Against all expectations, the head of the first psychiatric clinic in the GDR was a professor who came from the West. The authority of this character, whose attitude toward the communist regime was, if not reserved, at least pragmatic, had a strong impact on the running of the clinic throughout the 1960s.[17] In the course of this decade, the establishment underwent many transformations, both in terms of spatial organization (creation of open-door psychiatric services, more flexibility in the partitioning practices, etc.) and of the therapies practiced in the institution (opening of a psychotherapy unit). Thus, although the observatory I have chosen was, indeed, located to the east of the Iron Curtain, the changes it experienced are situated within trends in the European and world history of psychiatry.

I have based this study on a corpus composed of psychiatric and psychotherapeutic records, in which the patient indicates experiencing family conflicts with a political dimension. These records consist of various types of documents—administrative and medical documents, personal letters, etc.—all relating to the patient. One of the key documents in the file is the *Krankengeschichte* (history of the patient), which is divided into two stages. The first is related to the anamnesis: transcription of the information provided by the patients themselves (or by one of their relatives) about the patient's past and the history of their illness. The *Krankengeschichte* is followed by the *Verlauf*, which pertains to the treatment process and pathway and provides an account of the patient's stay in the facility.

16 For a history of the clinic of the Charité, see Bleker and Hess (eds.), *Die Charité. Geschichte eines Krankenhauses*; Herrn and Hottenrott (eds.), *Die Charité zwischen Ost und West 1945–1992*.

17 In this regard, he does not distinguish himself from most other professors of medicine. On the subject, see Jessen, *Akademische Elite und kommunistische Diktatur*.

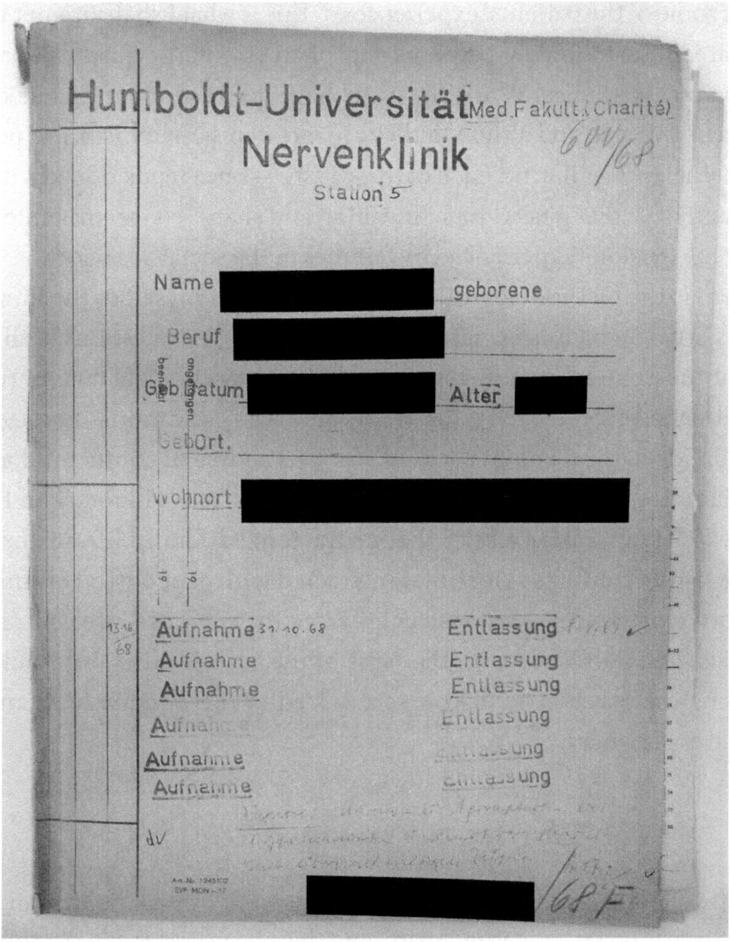
Humboldt-Universität Med.Fakult.(Charité)
Nervenklinik
Station 5
600/68

Name [redacted] geborene
Beruf [redacted]
Geb.Datum [redacted] Alter [redacted]
Geb.Ort.
Wohnort [redacted]

Aufnahme 31.10.68 Entlassung
Aufnahme Entlassung
Aufnahme Entlassung
Aufnahme Entlassung
Aufnahme Entlassung
Aufnahme Entlassung

[redacted] 68 F

Figure 9.2: *A cover of a patient record* (HPAC F 600/68) with the friendly authorization from the HPAC, Institute for the History of Medicine and Ethics in Medicine, Charité Berlin.

The documents were written by physicians or psychologists, who chose to mention certain events or some of the statements made by the patient, which could provide clues toward making a diagnosis. Central to the production of this document were, therefore, processes of translating, rewording, and excluding some of the statements or information provided by the patient, processes conducted by the writer for demonstrative purposes. Though the patients' voices were filtered through the expertise of medical practitioners, they are far from inaudible to the historian who, from this source, can reconstruct some of the patients' experiences.[18] This is what I shall attempt to demonstrate in the following pages, as part of an essentially qualitative analysis based on case studies. While the files I have used represent unique cases in the archived data, and although they are rare items, their historical potential is nonetheless significant. Each of these cases—once repositioned within the "context[s] ... that give[s] them meaning and shape"[19]—seems quite revealing of the tensions experienced by families in the socialist society.

Such is the methodological challenge I have set myself in the framework of this study, which is structured around three key questions. I shall first look at the political tensions that could affect the conjugal lives of the clinic's patients. Secondly, the issue of the children's education—because it implied an ideological choice—could also be a source of conflict in East German families. Finally, the third stage of the analysis will focus on the "*jeu d'échelles*" (game of scales)[20] that characterized family life in the GDR, where family conflicts sometimes interacted with geopolitical events. If the patients' experiences—reconstructed from the sources—are central to my analysis, I will also need, on the basis of the cases studies, to examine the meaning the psychiatric discourse ascribed to these individuals and their unique experiences.

Politics and Conjugal Tensions

> SI [sexual intercourse] occurs once or twice a week, because the husband wishes it. She has no sexual desire. Apart from this, the marriage appears to be functional, from an outsider's perspective. There are no political disagreements.[21]

18 Regarding the field of French-speaking historiography, several recent studies are based on this source and were performed using a micro-historical approach, by focusing on reconstructing the trajectories and experiences of patients: Majerus, *Parmi les fous*; Hervé and Tison, *Du front à l'asile. 1914–1918*. For the field of German historiography, see the works of Viola Balz (patient records used as a source for a history of the use of psychotropic drugs): Balz, *Zwischen Wirkung und Erfahrung*; idem, "Terra Incognita: An Historiographic Approach to the First Chlorpromazine Trials Using Patient Records of the Psychiatric University Clinic in Heidelberg." See also her fascinating case study on the consumption of psychotropic drugs in the GDR, with consumption examined from the consumer/patient's perspective: idem, "'Für einen Aktivisten wie mich muß es in einem sozialistischen Staat doch effektive Medikamente geben.'"

19 Revel, "Présentation," in *Jeux d'échelles*, 12.

20 Revel, "Présentation."

21 "GV findet 1 bis 2 mal in der Woche statt, weil der Ehemann es wünscht. Sie selbst hat kein Verlangen. Die Ehe wäre sonst in äusserer Beziehung in Ordnung. Politische Missverständnisse gebe es nicht." HPAC, F 604/61, Krankengeschichte, Nachexploration.

In this excerpt taken from the file of a patient who was hospitalized at the clinic in the fall of 1961, the absence of any "political disagreements" between the spouses is mentioned immediately after notes concerning the couple's sex life. This mention suggests that the therapists did ask the question to the patient during an exchange concerning the state of her marital relationship with her husband. Thus, just like sexuality, politics appears to the therapist as a potential source of conflict; the same assumption can be found in the other files.

In June 1963, Hannelore E. was admitted into the psychotherapy unit.[22] This unit was created in 1959 under the leadership of the new director of the clinic, Karl Leonhard. It practiced a particular type of psychotherapeutic treatment, referred to as "individualized therapy" (*Individualtherapie*), which was intended primarily for patients with neuroses.[23] In this unit, the diagnosis needed to be determined very precisely, and the *Individualtherapie* had to be adapted to each individual form of neurosis. It was structured around four key concepts: deflection (*Ablenkung*), incrimination (*Belastung*), addiction (*Gewöhnung*), and rehabilitation (*Umerziehung*). While the theoretical framework could differ—especially with regard to the conception of neurosis—the therapeutic practices involved in *Individualtherapie* were comparable in some respects to those of the first behavioral therapies, initiated on the other side of the Iron Curtain.[24] It is this therapy that Hannelore E. underwent during her stay in the clinic in 1963. This woman, aged twenty-six, suffered from multiple fears accompanied by sleeping problems and headaches. The diagnosis indicated in the end-of-stay report (*Epicrisis*) indicated the occurrence of an "ideohypochondriac evolution"[25] in the form of multiple phobias in an anankastic personality suffering from anxiety and growing "vegetative irritability."[26] The fact that this diagnosis

22 HPAC, F 147/66.

23 Karl Leonhard et al., *Individualtherapie der Neurosen* (Jena: Gustav Fischer Verlag, 1963).

24 Parallels are found particularly in the treatment of obsessional disorders (exposure and response prevention). Malach, "Die Individualtherapie Karl Leonhards—Rekonstruktion und Vergleich mit verhaltenstherapeutischen Methoden der 50er und 60er Jahre," 90, 100.

25 According to the terminology used by Leonhard and his team, a neurosis is "ideohypochondriac" (*ideohypochondrisch*) "when the disorder is in the idea, the fear, the conviction" and it is "psychohypochondriac" (*sensohypochondrisch*) "when it is accompanied by biased and subjective feelings." Karl Leonhard, "Unterscheidung der ideohypochondrischen und der sensohypochondrischen Neurose," in *Individualtherapie der Neurosen*, ed. Karl Leonhard et al. (Jena: Gustav Fischer Verlag, 1963), 117.

26 "Ideohypochondrische Entwicklung unter dem Bilde zahlreicher Phobien bei einer ängstl.[ichen]-anankastischen Persönlichkeit mit erhöhter vegetativer Erregbarkeit." HPAC, F 147/66, Epikrise, December 6, 1963.

contained a characterization of the patient's personality can be explained by the conception of neurosis defended by Leonhard. According to him, the form of neurosis a patient suffered was usually determined by their "internal structure," more than by external events.[27]

This conception is part of a classical tradition in the field of psychiatry, one that dated back to the late nineteenth century and which placed increased emphasis on endogenous factors in the genesis of psychological and mental disorders. According to this approach, individuals who suffer from such disorders exhibit a "predisposition," a hereditary "terrain," that can explain the emergence of a neurosis or psychosis. Thus, the possible external causes become secondary factors. Leonhard argued that the individual's *personality* played a decisive role in the genesis of neurosis and that, consequently, the therapist must identify and understand it before being able to establish an accurate diagnosis and implement a therapy plan. Furthermore, the use of the concept of personality was part of an overall trend in the psychiatry of the 1960s that aimed to extend its scope of action: beyond the illness, which could be episodic, the psychiatrist could examine the patient's personality, which by definition is a lasting feature.[28] This diagnosis fits within a historical continuity—well beyond the creation of the GDR—while being representative of a trend in the field of psychiatry that was found on both sides of the Iron Curtain.

According to the precepts of individualized therapy, Hannelore E. should have gradually confronted the situations that triggered anxiety in her (taking care of children, talking with strangers, crossing bridges, etc.). Along with these practical exercises, therapeutic interviews were conducted with the patient to discuss in more detail the conflictual relationship she had with her husband. Below is an excerpt from her file, dated October 11, 1963. The notes were taken after she had spent a few days at home:

---

27 Karl Leonhard "Abgrenzung der neurotischen Grundformen" in *Individualtherapie der Neurosen*, ed. Karl Leonhard et al. (Jena: Gustav Fischer Verlag, 1963), 11.

28 As highlighted by historian Benoit Majerus regarding the Belgian psychiatrist Paul Sivadon, "with the concept of "personality," he extends the scope of investigation of the psychiatrist who can then examine not only the disease, the pathology, which is episodic, but also more long-term aspects." ("Avec le concept de "personnalité"; il étend le champ d'investigation du psychiatre qui s'intéresse dès lors non seulement à la maladie, à la pathologie qui est épisodique, mais également à des éléments plus durables.") This analysis can easily be applied to the explanatory model proposed by Karl Leonhard, in which the patient's personality plays a central role in the emergence and development of the disease. Majerus, *Parmi les fous*, 191.

> We note, however, that she was always worse off after spending time at home. She explained, in this regard, that she had no symptoms when she left the clinic to go home, but that all her fears and anxieties, and particularly headaches, came back the minute she was back at home. It then became apparent that the two spouses had truly disconnected from each other, as a result of differences in political views. The husband showed great zeal for politics, spent almost all his evenings in all kinds of meetings, without notifying his wife that he was going. He tried, quite awkwardly, to convince his wife to share his political ideas. As for the patient herself, she proved impervious to his words.[29]

The patient mentioned those particular tensions at the end of her stay at the clinic and contradicted what she had claimed after being admitted about having a "harmonious relationship" with her husband. Thus, it was only after spending several weeks in the clinic that the patient confided that she and her husband had political differences that caused them to drift apart. In the context of a nondemocratic regime, like that of the GDR, where contradicting the official discourse was not tolerated, these differences bore a particular significance. Given that the only authorized meetings were those whose participants toed the official political line (meetings of the Communist Party or of mass organizations supposed to spread its ideological message), it can be deduced that the patient's husband was particularly zealous and that he defended the point of view of the authorities, whereas she lacked his interest in and enthusiasm for the subject. By admitting to disagreements with her husband, Hannelore E. admitted that she held views not in accordance with the official political line. The interviews with the therapist seem to have provided a context that was conducive to such confidences. Moreover, immediately after this passage and in the same paragraph, mention is made of the lack of sexual "harmony" between the spouses. Thus, politics and sexuality did constitute the main motives for disagreement between the spouses. (In addition, her husband's homosexual past, which she

29 "Es fiel jedoch auf, daß sie stets wieder verschlechtert von ihren Besuchen zu Hause zurückkam. Sie äußerte sich dazu, daß sie auf der Hinfahrt noch beschwerdefrei sei, jedoch alle Befürchtungen und Beklemmungen und insb. die Kopfschmerzen wieder sofort da seien, wenn sie die Wohnungstür hinter sich geschlossen hat. Es stellte sich nun heraus, daß die beiden Eheleute sich recht auseinandergelebt hatten, weil politische unterschiedliche Ansichten bestanden. Der Mann ist politisch eifrig tätig, fast immer ist er abends zu irgendeiner Sitzung, ohne seiner Frau etwas davon zu sagen. Er versucht nicht gerade in zugewandter Art seine Frau von seinen politischen Ansichten zu überzeugen. Die Pat. wiederum zeigt sich in seinen Reden gegenüber unzugänglich." HPAC, F 147/66, Krankengeschichte, October 11, 1963.

found out about only after they were married, was clearly a painful situation for the patient as well.)

In the case of Hannelore E., political tensions were but one factor of conflict between her husband and herself, but they appeared to have a much more significant effect on the relationship between patient Helmut E. and his wife.[30] Following his admission into the psychotherapy unit in 1966, during the anamnesis, the patient provided new information about his relationship with his ex-wife. Below is an excerpt from the file in which the issue is mentioned:

> Until 1964 the marriage was happy enough. His wife did not work. She started working in 1964. Prior to this, differences in political views had already led to serious rows between them. The patient complains about his wife's excessive enthusiasm for politics, about her defending the party's point of view, about her putting society before family and neglecting the children. A nine-year-old son and five-year-old daughter were born of this marriage. His wife was about to become a multifunction civil servant.[31]

The patient's file also shows that these conflicts resulted in a divorce pronounced about a month before Helmut E.'s admission into the clinic where he was treated for cardiac phobia. Although Helmut E. was himself a member of the party, he clearly did not support his wife's enthusiasm for politics, even though his profession—he was a prosecutor in the military (*Militärstaatsanwalt*)—required that he devote himself to the cause of the state and, therefore, to the construction of a socialist society. During the anamnesis, he had informed the doctor that, because of his wife's political and professional activities, he often had to take care of the children (although he had resumed his studies), "which weighed heavily on him."[32] In this case, the doctor's position on the subject is reflected throughout the file, and in

30 HPAC, M 337/66.

31 "Bis 1964 war dann die Ehe halbwegs ugt [gut]. Seine Frau war nicht berufstätig, nahm 1964 ein Arbeitsverhältnis auf. Schon vorher hatten unterschiedliche politische Auffassungen zu ernsthaften Streitereien geführt. Der Pat wirft seiner Frau vor, sie sei politisch vernarrt, vertrete den Standpunkt, erst die Gesellschaft und dann die Familie und würde die Kinder vernachlässigen. Aus der Ehe gingen 1 9 jähr Sohn und eine 5 jähr Tochter hervor. Sei Frau sei im Begriff, Multifunktionärin zu werden." HPAC, M 337/66, Krankengeschichte, Anamnese (nach Angaben des Pat.), Soz. Entwicklung, June 13, 1966.

32 HPAC, M 337/66, Krankengeschichte, Anamnese (nach Angaben des Pat.), Jetzige Beschwerden und ihre Entwicklung.

his final report, he describes as "extreme" the conception of life of the patient's wife.[33]

For both men, giving priority to one's political career at the expense of one's family responsibilities did not seem to be the path a woman should take. Here we find a traditional view of gender roles in the home, which also corresponded to the dominant representations in the GDR. Although male/female equality was an objective of the socialist project—which was to be realized through work—matters pertaining to domestic life fell within the responsibility of the female members of households.[34] Although, in the GDR, women benefited from a policy that promoted their integration into the labor market, which contributed undoubtedly to their emancipation, "socialist marriage" was far from equalitarian, and women still performed most domestic tasks.[35] As shown in the case of this couple, the wife's political engagement—because it undermined the traditional division of roles in the household—could give rise to marital discord, even though, given his profession and membership in the party, the husband would have been expected to support her investment in serving the socialist society. While the nature of the disagreements between Helmut E. and his wife was clearly mentioned in the *Krankengeschichte,* which was a document for internal use only, it was merely alluded to in another document in the file; a file which could be read by actors outside the clinic.

Indeed, in the expert assessment requested by the patient's employer (in this case the attorney general of the GDR), the physician simply mentioned "extreme differences between the husband's and wife's conceptions of life" or a "nonharmonious marital relationship"[36] as sources of tension in Helmut E.'s life. No mention was made, at any time, of the political nature of the disputes between Helmut E. and his wife. This elision can be explained by the fact that this document could be read outside the boundaries of the clinic, in this case a representative of the GDR authorities who might possibly frown at the critical eye with which Helmut E. regarded his ex-wife's political engagement. Thus, the function of the *Krankengeschichte,* as well as the fact that it was reserved for internal use, allowed its author more freedom to record the precise details divulged by the patient.

33 HPAC, M 337/66, Epikrise, September 8, 1966.

34 Harsch, *Revenge of the Domestic: Women, the Family and Communism in the German Democratic Republic.*

35 Ibid., 292–3.

36 HPAC M 337/66, psychiatrisches Gutachten, November 2, 1966.

Is Education Necessarily Socialist?

As evidenced by the patients' records, "political disagreements" between the spouses could become particularly virulent when the children's education was discussed. The above-mentioned case of Gisela R., where ideological views clashed with religious beliefs, is a good example of this. With regard to Gisela R., it is interesting to note that, according to the patient, it was the fact that she exercised a professional activity that helped her gain self-confidence and therefore that empowered her to "take control" of her children's education.[37] Gisela R.'s case supports the view that, in the 1960s, women in the GDR perceived themselves as having gained self-confidence and autonomy.[38] In this particular case, we find that the policy pursued by the East German authorities and intended to promote female employment resulted in an outcome that was quite contrary to the intention behind the project of constructing a socialist society. Pursuing a profession outside the home helped Gisela R. gain enough self-confidence to make herself heard on private matters; and in doing so she opposed the views of both her husband and the state. This is, among other things, what led her to secretly send her children to catechism classes, as she explained to the director of the clinic. According to the file, the patient's husband was advised to be more tolerant regarding the religious education of their children. Yet, the doctor in charge of Gisela R., who spoke with the husband and wrote the medical record, was probably a member of the Communist Party.[39] In the 1960s, only a minority of the clinic's physicians were members of the SED (the Socialist Unity Party of Germany). Overall, because of their social origin, their generally conservative political stance, and their distrust of the regime's policy for the restructuring of the healthcare system, the doctors tended to keep their distance from the communist regime.[40] Until the construction of the Berlin Wall, this occupational group was strongly represented among the masses of people who immigrated to the West. Thus, the doctor who took care of

37 HPAC, F 373a/72, Krankengeschichte, Anamnese, Zur Persönlichkeit.

38 Harsch, *Revenge of the Domestic*, 302.

39 His name appears in the reports of the Group of the Party dated 1964. It can be assumed that in 1962, though he was not a full member, he was at least party candidate or about to be. LAB [Landesarchiv Berlin], C REP 904-225 Nr. 4, Minutes of the meeting, November 25, 1964.

40 With regard to the situation of medical physicians in the GDR, see Ernst, *"Die beste Prophylaxe ist der Sozialismus". Ärzte und medizinische Hochschullehrer in der SBZ/DDR 1945–1961*; Müller, "Die Ärzteschaft im staatlichen Gesundheitswesen der SBZ und der DDR 1945–1989."

Gisela R. was among a minority of doctors who were also communist comrades. His advice to the patient's husband is in contradiction with the claim made by his clinic's comrades, in a report dated December 1964, that "in their medical decisions [...], doctors defend the interests of the state."[41] In this specific case, the doctor, although he was a party comrade (or was about to become one), placed secondary emphasis on ideology, taking a position that went against educational precepts imposed by the communist authorities. The clinic provided a space that allowed one to somewhat deviate from the official doctrine, even when the therapist was in the ranks of the party.

The type of tension that Gisela R. experienced was not uncommon in the GDR. According to sources of legal data concerning divorce cases, ideological conflicts between spouses often resulted from the attachment of one of them to religion.[42] In 1962, when patient Ruth R. discussed the conflicts she believed were responsible for her illness, she mentioned, first and foremost, the education she received from her parents, which was in complete contradiction with the position defended by her husband, be it political or religious.[43] During her stay in the psychiatric unit, in the summer of 1962, Sabine E. also mentioned such conflicts. According to her file, this thirty-six-year-old teacher suffered from "reactive depression." Her illness was seen as a reaction to one or more difficult experiences. Although her condition appeared to result primarily from her separation from her husband, Sabine E. mentioned, while she was being treated, a second source of torment: "the ideological education of her son and her own stance on the subject."[44] We then learn that her ex-husband was a party official who, according to her, forced her to join the party when they were married, which, given her confessional education, resulted in her suffering from internal tensions. Choosing the type of education Sabine E. and her husband wanted for their children led to a resurgence of ideological clashes between them. According to the record:

> She [Sabine E.] now fears that he [her husband] will influence the child; this is why she never wants to leave her child alone with his father. She does not really know either what ideological orientation the child's education should take.

41 LAB, C REP 904–225 Nr. 13, Einschätzung der ideologischen Situation an der Nervenklinik, December 8, 1964.

42 Betts, *Within Walls: Private Life in the German Democratic Republic*, 106.

43 HPAC, F 598/64, Krankengeschichte, January 21, 1961.

44 HPAC, F 385/62, Krankengeschichte, July 9, 1962.

Thus, Sabine E. was faced with a difficult choice: should she follow the official guidelines—defended by her ex-husband—or rather give her child an education based on religious principles, similar to the education she, herself, received? Compromise seemed difficult in that the two "ideological orientation[s]" were in total contradiction to each other, the Marxist–Leninist ideology considering religion to be an instrument of manipulation and domination by the ruling classes. According to the official guidelines, Sabine E. should stand by her husband's side on the subject. Yet, again, according to the file, the doctor does not seem to have reminded the patient of the normative discourse disseminated by the authorities. He let Sabine E. decide for herself what she must undertake in the future. At the end of her stay, the physician noted the following in the file:

> In the course of several interviews, we managed to help Mrs. E. to somewhat distance herself from thoughts linked to her ex-husband, which until now, determined her day-to-day experience of life, and to concentrate on future problems related to her own role in life and to the education of her child.[45]

Though Sabine E. was apparently invited to think about the education of her son, nothing was said in the file about any recommendation from the doctor concerning the educational path she should choose. Let us recall that her doctor belonged to a professional category that was particularly attached to religious values and their transmission.[46] This extract from the file suggests that the normative message disseminated outside of the clinic's boundaries did not necessarily have any authority. Unlike the judiciary, which, when dealing with marital disagreements, relayed the official discourse on socialist morals,[47] the psychiatric institution appears here to have been a space in which one could adopt a pragmatic approach to, or even distance oneself

45 "Im Verlaufe mehrere Gespräche wurde doch erreicht, dass sich Frau R. von dem bisher ihren ganzen Alltag bestimmenden Gedanken an ihren geschiedenen Ehemann etwas distanzierte und sich mehr den zukünftigen Problemen ihrer eigenen Rolle im Leben und dem der Erziehung ihres Kindes zuwandte." HPAC F 385/62, Krankengeschichte, July 27, 1962.

46 Thus, the tacit obligation to participate in the *Jugendweihe* (youth consecration) was one of the reasons why physicians sought to leave the GDR in the 1950s. Ernst, *"Die beste Prophylaxe ist der Sozialismus,"* 63–4.

47 For more the subject, see Jane Freeland's ongoing thesis project on domestic violence in the GDR: *Negotiating a Space for Women in the State: Domestic Violence in East Germany, 1971–1990* (Carleton University, Ottawa, Canada). See also Freeland, "Morals on Trial: State-Making and Domestic Violence in the East German Courtroom."

from, the official guideline. Although both doctors and judges attempted to participate in the management of family conflicts, they did not follow the same logic.

Thus, the sources I have used show that, in the 1960s, the marital conflicts experienced by East German families could take a political hue. Those discords developed along similar lines of conflict as those experienced in Western families: the role of women in the home, the sharing of tasks, the question of transmission (of religious values in particular). The particularity of the GDR lies in the fact that these lines of tension, within the context of that era, could assume a political and ideological dimension, which contributed to exacerbating them. In a context where the family home was meant to foster the all-round development of the "socialist personality," these interpersonal tensions were all the more significant as they pointed, more or less directly, to the fact that one or the other protagonist distanced him- or herself from the socialist project. And it so happens that the perspective of the East German authorities was characterized by a binary logic according to which an individual who did not fully support the development of a socialist society could only be considered as an opponent to the regime. This Manichean perspective explains why family conflicts with political undertones could be particularly delicate situations, and this at a time when the family garnered renewed interest from the state. A therapeutic conversation, then, could be a chance to address such issues—however sensitive they might be—with the doctor or psychologist. When a medical recommendation was called for, it does not appear to have strictly followed the behavioral norms set by the official discourse; and the therapist could appear as an alternative authority figure. An examination of the file of patient Elsa G. confirms this hypothesis and shows the complex interaction between family conflict and geopolitical events in the context of the GDR. The third part of this study is devoted to the detailed analysis of this patient's file.

Family, Politics, and "Jeu d'Échelles" (Game of Scales)

Elsa G. was admitted on July 27, 1961, into a psychotherapy unit of the clinic. She was sent there from the outpatient clinic unit (polyclinic), and she complained of cardiac pain and headaches, among other problems. After being admitted, and while her medical history was being taken, the patient, aged forty-six, described her family situation and the tensions she experienced. Below are some of the doctor's notes on the subject:

> Her husband has been retired for two years; works in the morning until noon—as a volunteer at the party office. In the afternoon, he is at home, peering into all the cooking pots. She feels anxious and oppressed, but only when she sees him. He is selfish, lives for politics alone, would like to educate his whole family according to his political beliefs. Patient believes that they should also have fun sometimes; for example, his oldest daughter is not allowed to listen to *Schlager der Woche* [Hits of the Week][48] or to watch the shows broadcast on the West German TV channel.

Sexually, he has not yet satisfied her, unlike her first husband. He invests himself but then can read the newspaper.

> She has two children with her current husband; has a daughter with her former partner; she is already married and has left home. Her sixteen-year-old daughter does not care much about her father, and the fourteen-year-old son "knows how to handle him" when they're talking about politics.[49]

According to the patient's statement, as it was transcribed in her file, "politics" was indeed a source of tensions in her family circle, between her husband and herself, and between him and their daughter. He was retired, but he pursued political activities in the party, where he worked as a volunteer every morning. His political engagement went beyond the party's office and extended into the family sphere, where he tried to impose his views. In doing so, he performed his duties as a party comrade, such as they were formu-

48 A weekly radio show broadcast on RIAS (Rundfunk im amerikanischen Sektor) radio, whose head office is located in West Berlin.

49 "Em. ist seit 2 Jahren berentet, arbeitet vormittags bis 12 Uhr—ehrenamtlich im Parteibüro—nachmittags ist er zu Hause, guckt in alle Töpfe. Sie bekommt Beklemmungen und Angst, wenn sie ihn nur sieht. Er ist egoistisch, lebt nur für seine Politik, möchte seine ganze Familie auch in diesem Sinne erziehen. Pat meint, dass es auch mal etwas Lustiges geben müsse, so darf ihre grössere Tochter z. B. keinen "Schlager der Woche" hören, nicht das Programm des westlichen Fernsehens einschalten. Sexuell sei sie von ihm noch nie befriedigt worden, ganz im Gegensatz zu ihrem ersten Mann. Er sei wohl bei der Sache dabei, könne aber anschliessend Zeitung lesen. Sie habe mit dem jetzigen Em. noch zwei Kinder, ihre Tochter aus erste Ehe sei schon verheiratet und aus dem Haus. Ihr 16–jähriges Mädchen halte gar nichts vom Vater, wogegen der 14–jährige Junge "den Vater so richtig zu nehmen versteht, in bezug auf die Politik," HPAC F 448/61, Krankengeschichte, Anamnese, Familiäre Situation.

lated in the statutes of the SED, and according to which each member must "behave as a role model in his or her professional and political activities and private life."[50] These statutes date back to 1950, but from the 1960s onward the private lives of party members started to play an increasing role in the party's relationship with its members.[51] The members were formally prohibited from watching or listening to the West German media. Allowing his daughter to watch a program broadcast by West German television would have conflicted with the partisan commitment of this man, and could have resulted in sanctions against him.

The doctor's notes in the patient's file show a degree of skepticism on his part. Following the notes on the patient's medical history, the doctor wrote that "for every piece of information provided by the patient, you always get a sense that it does not correspond to the truth."[52] The therapist definitely doubted the veracity of the patient's declaration and saw the emphasis she placed on her family problems as an attempt to attract attention to herself ("the patient understands, from the doctor's tone and words, that she's failing to attract enough attention by describing her ills; so she minimizes them to some degree and places primary emphasis on her family situation"[53]). This doubt regarding the patient's claims points to a diagnosis of hysteria—such as it was understood in Europe at the time—according to which the subject did not want to be ill but yet wanted to be recognized as a suffering subject.[54] Let us note that Karl Leonhard seems to have had a different understanding—which remained influenced by past notions—of this diagnosis since, in 1964, he wrote that "hysterics *want* to be sick."[55] This diagnosis was confirmed, a few days later, following the visit of the clinic's director.

50 "Das Parteimitglied ist verpflichtet, [...] in seiner politischen und beruflichen Tätigkeit und im persönlichen Leben Vorbild zu sein." Socialist Unity Party of Germany statutes, 1950.

51 On the subject, see Christian, "Le parti et la vie privée de ses membres en RDA."

52 "Bei allen Angaben der Pat. hat man immer das Gefühl, dass sie nicht der Wahrheit entsprechen.... Da Pat aus dem Tonfall und der Unterhaltung des Untersuchers entnimmt, dass sie durch eine Schilderung ihrer Beschwerden keine genügende Zuwendung finden würde, verniedlicht sie diese bis zu einem gewissen Maße und legt das Hauptgewicht auf ihre familiäre Situation." HPAC, F 448/61, Krankengeschichte, Befund, Psychisch.

53 Ibid.

54 "Der Hysteriker will als Leidender gelten, es wäre jedoch falsch zu behaupten, er wolle krank sein." Claus Haring and Karl Heinz Leickert, *Wörterbuch der Psychiatrie und ihrer Grenzgebiete* (Stuttgart: F.K. Schattauer Verlag, 1968), 298.

55 "Hysteriker wollen krank sein, Hypochonder fürchten es zu sein." Leonhard, *Differenzierte Diagnostik*, 85.

A few days after the patient's admission and before the final diagnosis was made, as was customary within the unit, the husband was interviewed by the therapist, who questioned him about possible disputes between the spouses. According to Elsa G.'s husband, there was no political disagreement between his wife and himself: "His wife gets mad because she is not allowed to watch Western TV."[56] As for their sex life, he thought it was fairly satisfactory. Again, sexuality seems to have been discussed in parallel with politics. Furthermore, the patient and her husband expressed very different perceptions of the degree of harmony that prevailed in the household. We find here one of the peculiarities of the *Krankengeschichte*, a source in which the voices of the patient and of their relatives intermingle, confront, and are superimposed on each other through the medical filter. Following this conversation with the husband, the spouses were invited to talk with each other in the presence of the doctor. Below are some notes on the subject:

> The confrontation between the spouses indicates that the current conflict between mother–daughter and father–son continues. Mother and daughter compete with the son for the husband's favor (politically), yet feel ousted by the son. The girl likes light music, likes to dress well, likes watching Western TV, and gets full approval from her mother, but both fail to stand up against the father, who despite his rather soft way of heading the family, is intolerant when it comes to politics.

Patient finally says categorically that the doctor should advise her husband to allow them to watch the West [German] TV program.[57]

56 "Auf die Frage, welche Differenzen zwischen ihm und Pat. bestünden, meint er, dass sie in politischer Hinsicht keine hätten, dass die Ehefrau sich nur darüber aufregt, dass sie keinen Westsender sehen dürfe. Zum Sexuellen meint er, dass sie ca. 1 x in der Woche noch GV haben, dass die Pat. auch meist glücklich dabei sei." HPAC, F 448/61, Krankengeschichte, Verlauf, Aussprache mit dem Ehemann der Pat., July 31, 1961.

57 "Aus einer Gegenüberstellung des Ehepaares wird deutlich, dass der momentane Konflikt zwischen Mutter-Tochter und Vater-Sohn besteht. Mutter-Tochter r[i]valisieren mit dem Sohn, um die Gunst des Mannes (in politischer Hinsicht), fühlen sich jedoch von dem Sohn aus dem Felde geschlagen. Tochter liebt leichte Musik, kleidet sich gerne gut, sieht gern West-Fernseh, worin sie völlige Zustimmung der Mutter findet, sich beide jedoch dem Vater gegenüber nicht durchsetzen können, der trotz seiner weichen führbaren Art in politischer Hinsicht intolerant ist. Pat. erklärt abschliessend kategorisch, dass Ärztin Em. befehlen möchte, dass sie und ihre Tochter den Westsender sehen dürfen." HPAC, F 448/61, Krankengeschichte, Verlauf, Aussprache mit dem Ehemann der Pat., July 31, 1961.

According to these notes, in order to make her husband yield (he was described by the author of the report as "intolerant when it comes to politics"), the patient sought the support of the medical team, and in so doing assigned to the latter the role of alternative authority figure. The doctor in question does not seem to have directly complied with the patient's request. However, in a subsequent interview with the husband, he was advised to "regain the confidence of his children by responding more sympathetically to their needs, especially their questions."[58] Thus, the doctor invited Elsa G.'s husband to show more flexibility in his demands regarding politics, as a clearly zealous member of the party. Thus, the medical authority somewhat distanced itself from the official line, such as it was dictated by the party.

Mention was made in the record—dated August 19, 1961—of the advice given to the patient's husband; and in addition to this, the clinic's director, during one of his visits to the unit a few days later, made a diagnosis (*hysterische Reaktion bei Debilität*), and expressed the view that, as far as patient Elsa G. was concerned, "the current situation in Berlin will help resolve the conflict."[59] Leonhard believed that the closing off of the last crossing point from East to West, which had taken place ten days earlier, during the night of August 12 to 13, 1961, would help resolve the family conflicts experienced by the patient. The construction of the Berlin Wall was clearly perceived as a way of keeping Western influences out of East Germany, influences that were a key factor in the tensions between father and daughter. Thus, the doctor was of the opinion that this geopolitical event would help improve harmony in the family, remarking that the geopolitical paradigm of the Cold War would intermingle with family life. The East German society does seem to be characterized by this "game of scales" (*jeu d'échelles*),[60] in which personal destinies and the greater history intersect; this intermingling being particularly significant for the population of the city of East Berlin, which sat at the heart of the confrontation between the two blocs.

58 "Inzwischen hatten wir Gelegenheit mit dem Em. der Pat zu sprechen. Dieser leidet sehr darunter, dass seine Gattin seine Interessen den Kindern gegenüber nicht mit vertritt. Er gibt zu, dass er bisher nicht verstanden hat, die mangelhafte gesellschaftspolitische Erziehung in der Schule durch seinen Einfluss zu ergänzen. Wir berieten ihn, sich das Vertrauen der Kinder durch verständnisvolles Eingehen auf deren Belange und besonders auf deren Fragen zurückzugewinnen." HPAC, F 448/61, Krankengeschichte, Verlauf, August 19, 1961.

59 HPAC, F 448/61, Krankengeschichte, Verlauf, Chefvisite, August 24, 1961.

60 Revel, "Présentation."

However, Leonhard's prognosis seems to have been incorrect. Indeed, as the patient's records show, the construction of the Berlin Wall did nothing to alleviate the tensions between the patient and her husband. Discharged on August 25, 1961, Elsa G. returned to the clinic in early September for a follow-up visit. The closing of the borders brought no improvement to the family situation. Contrary to what the clinic's director had hoped, the Berlin Wall did not end the disputes that separated Elsa G. and her husband. Although the Wall physically closed off the last crossing point to the West, it could never stop the population of the GDR from keeping in contact with the other Germany (thanks, in particular, to television airwaves, which could still cross borders). Nevertheless, the prognosis made by the psychiatrist, according to which this geopolitical event would resolve the conflicts affecting the patient's family, shows the extent to which geopolitical paradigms and personal destinies were intertwined in the representations of the East German society.

As we come to the close of this study, it must be concluded that analyzing patients' records makes it possible to approach the relationship between psychiatry and the socialist state from a new perspective. According to information traces found in these sources, the psychiatric realm can be a space that not only allows for some freedom of political speech—for patients—but also allows healthcare professionals to somewhat distance themselves from the official ideological line. Several possible explanations can be found for this situation, explanations that pertain first of all to the context of the GDR, but also to the specific situation of the Charité. As stated previously, medical professionals in East German society could maintain a relative distance from the political regime, which may explain a degree of openness when listening to patients as well as the nature of the recommendations given to the latter. The director's personality, which far from corresponded to the "socialist professor" model and whose authority strongly influenced the day-to-day running of the clinic, could also have been a factor. As for the type of therapy practiced (*Individualtherapie*), it was based on individual interviews with the therapist, which encouraged the patient to speak more freely.

Be that as it may, and although these elements must be taken into account, this "liberation speech" seems to have been primarily related to the status given to the patient's speech in the field of psychiatry. Thus, beyond the specific context of the Charité or of the GDR, there is a paradigm inherent in the psychiatric realm. Indeed, in the field of psychiatry, the patient's speech is the only means of identifying the ills of the patient, and it is therefore well received by psychiatrists or psychologists, who, through a specific interpretation grid, use it to make a diagnosis. As stated by historian Benoît Majerus, the "words [of patients] are locked in a diagnostic circularity: they are a further sign of their illness and their illness is a reason to not consider their words."[61] It is indeed the status given to those words that explains the relative freedom of expression the patients were granted in their interaction with the therapist. It is because they were psychiatric or psychotherapy patients, and because their words were perceived as signs that could help make a diagnosis, that patients could discuss sensitive issues in the context of the East German society, such as the political conflicts that affected their families.

Finally, it is the logic inherent in psychiatric reasoning—the search for a diagnosis is paramount here—that explains why the patients were allowed to speak (and why their words were written down by the doctor). The idea of "diagnostic circularity" takes a special dimension in the context of the GDR dictatorial regime. The therapeutic conversation appears, in the said context, as an interaction in which both patients and doctor (or psychologists) were given some leeway. The traces of this interaction, recorded in the patients' records, enable the historian not only to reconstruct individual experiences—which are generally not mentioned—but also to ponder on how the healthcare professional interpreted those experiences.[62] The psychiatric clinic was neither an instrument of repression of political opponents, nor was it a place of active resistance to the Marxist–Leninist ideology; thus it seems to have been a place that reveals the diversity and complexity of the relationships between individuals—be they patients or therapists—and the project of social transformation, driven by the socialist state.

61 "Leurs mots sont enfermés dans une circularité diagnostique: ils sont un signe supplémentaire de leur maladie et leur maladie est une raison pour ne pas prendre en compte leurs paroles." Majerus, *Parmi les fous*, 24.

62 For more on the subject, see two studies based on the same type of sources: Le Bonhomme, "Au croisement des logiques politiques et medicales: les 'patients-camarades' des services psychiatriques de la Charites (Berlin-Est, Republique democratique allemande, 1959–1964)"; idem, "Viols en temps de guerre, psychiatrie et temporalités enchevêtrées. Expériences de femmes violées par les soldats de l'Armée Rouge entre la fin de la Seconde Guerre mondiale et le début de la période de paix (République démocratique allemande, 1958–1968)."

CHAPTER X

Turning Women into Alcoholics: The Politics of Alcohol in Late Socialist Czechoslovakia[1]

Esther Wahlen

In October 1971, a team of Czech psychiatrists inaugurated a remarkable new facility. In a castle near Prague, they set up the first institution in Czechoslovakia—and one of the first in Europe—offering treatment exclusively for female alcoholics.[2] The treatment program for women was part of a broader network of institutions with which Czech and Slovak psychiatrists strove to improve the provision for alcoholics. Besides gender-specific treatment, they offered short-term interventions for inebriated troublemakers, outpatient programs for alcoholics and their families, long-term inpatient treatment, and aftercare clubs to guide and encourage former patients in their new, sober life.

If with this elaborate network of treatment institutions, Czechoslovakian alcohol expertise was in line with international developments, the professional approach to alcohol problems might seem odd for a socialist country. In states known for their idealistic view on social order, alcohol problems had for a long time figured as symptoms of socioeconomic difficulties or bourgeois legacy. However, the various initiatives to treat alcoholism did not target the material or sociocultural conditions of alcohol problems. Instead, psychiatrists approached these problems on an individualized level,

1 The present chapter is part of my dissertation *The Politics of Alcohol in Late Socialist Romania and Czechoslovakia*, defended in January 2017 at the European University Institute, Florence, Italy.

2 F. Kukal, "Rok ženské léčebny v Lojovicích," *Zápisy z Apolináře* 25.3–4 (1973).

by offering better services to a small number of people diagnosed with the *disease* of alcoholism. How can we account for this pathological approach to alcohol problems in late socialist Czechoslovakia? While historians of alcohol and drug history have delineated a general trend toward the professionalization and pathologization of alcohol problems, they have so far concentrated on the United States and the United Kingdom, often presenting these trends as a gold standard of Western liberal democracies.[3] Alcohol policies in non-Western states, to the contrary, usually appear as either overly ideological, ignorant toward alcoholics, or belated in their reactions to rapidly rising numbers of alcoholics in the second half of the twentieth century.[4] These assumptions are not only factually incorrect, but also insinuate that the pathologization was a logical solution to alcohol problems and not a theory informed by time-specific ideas about social diseases.

In this chapter, I aim to approach the pathological reading of alcohol problems from a different angle and investigate why, in the 1970s, it gained ground in many countries, what made it convincing as a tool to analyze social problems, and what effects it had on the provision of social deviancy. In particular, I focus on the professionalization of alcohol policies in late socialist Czechoslovakia. Picking up on the argumentation of the preceding chapters, I attempt to relocate East-Central European alcohol politics within a broader European framework of tackling social problems. To analyze the trend in alcohol politics, I follow Eszter Varsa and Fanny LeBonhomme and focus on the objects of medical health provision, in this case on changes in the category of the alcoholic patient in late socialist Czechoslovakia. Based on background analyses of the Health Ministry, reports and discussions about treatment practices in local expert journals on alcohol addiction, and interviews with former psychiatrists, I will first reconstruct the growing importance of medical treatment for the politics of alcohol. Secondly, I investigate why and how this interest in the pathological moments of alcohol problems made women visible as patients. Lastly, I link

3 For the most influential works on the history of alcohol and substance policy, see Levine, "The Discovery of Addiction: Changing Conceptions of Habitual Drunkenness in America"; Berridge and Edwards, *Opium and the People: Opiate Use in Nineteenth-Century England*; Nicholls, *The Politics of Alcohol: A History of the Drink Question in England*.

4 For example, in the "International Encyclopedia" on alcohol history, the otherwise well-informed Hasso Spode claims that the German Democratic Republic, in its politics of alcohol, "virtually returned to the eighteenth century." Spode, "Germany," in *Alcohol and Temperance in Modern History*.

the pathologization of alcohol problems to a new line of social policy and argue that it reflected a depoliticized reading of social problems.

By relating state-socialist health politics to presocialist legacies as well as domestic and global sociocultural transformations, I investigate different scales of discussing alcohol problems. Pointing out parallels and differences in Eastern and Western European countries, I aim to reach a more balanced perspective on how states, beyond bloc affiliation, interpreted and approached social problems in the "late modern" period.

From Solution to Management: The "Alcohol Question" in Czechoslovakia

Historians have located the onset of "modern" politics on alcoholism in the eighteenth and nineteenth centuries. In this period, politicians and social movements all over the world started conceptualizing occurrences of excessive drinking as a coherent problem and turned alcohol problems into a matter of public concern and dedicated political action.[5] The territories of East-Central Europe were no exception in the international preoccupation with alcohol problems. Anti-alcohol activism emerged mainly in big cities throughout the empire. Researchers and activists participated in international conferences and were usually not restrained by later geopolitical ideas about Eastern and Western belonging.[6]

As we can see in the first and second part of the book, nation-building aspirations proved a catalyst for health and social policy measures in the region. The "alcohol question," too, experienced an upsurge in the wake of nation building in the early twentieth century. In the territories that were to form the independent state of Czechoslovakia, the later presidents Tomáš G. Masaryk and Edvard Beneš were among many other nation builders who used the "alcohol question" to bring up matters of the nation and to convey concerns about civic consciousness. In this period, the medical provision for alcoholics was not in the limelight of national alcohol politics. Presenting temperance as a question of commitment and strong will, policy makers

5 See Courtwright, *Forces of Habit: Drugs and the Making of the Modern World*, 174–6; Berridge, *Temperance: Its History and Impact on Current and Future Alcohol Policy.*

6 Consider, for example, the research and activism in turn of the century Transylvania: Marius Rotar, "Probatoriul unei istorii a alcoolismului in Romania secolelor XIX-XX," *Brukenthal Acta Musei Sibiu* 2.1 (2007).

and activists did not approach alcoholics as *patients*, but as *citizens* who were considered responsible for as well as capable of restraining themselves. The means of choice to cure drunkards was not prison or medical treatment, but lectures, publications, and other forms of popular enlightenment.[7]

In the 1930s and 1940s, the focus on civic education was superseded by sociobiological readings of social problems. In many countries, policy makers and scientists popularized ideas about the degenerative potential of alcohol consumption for the biological and moral quality of the national collective. Particularly in countries with strong fascist movements, concern about national degeneration produced a repressive attitude toward alcoholics, who were considered biologically and morally inferior. The repressive stance found its most radical expression in Germany, where National Socialists banned "chronic alcoholics" from marrying and procreating, and with the 1933 Law for the Prevention of Genetically Diseased Offspring induced the sterilization of thousands of "chronic alcoholics."[8] Under the German occupation of Bohemia and Moravia, the activists of the Czech Abstinent Association cooperated with German organizations, but they did not advocate similarly repressive measures against alcoholics. More than anything else, they reduced their activities.[9]

After the Second World War, alcohol politics lost its radical moments in many countries. However, in both Eastern and Western Europe, policy makers still clung to the idea that alcohol problems could be successfully fought. In the Czechoslovak Socialist Republic, where the Communist Party had taken over absolute state power in 1948, the "fight against alcoholism" became a political endeavor. In line with the new political mainstream, anti-alcohol advocates described alcoholism as a "bourgeois vestige"[10] that could be eradi-

7 For the writings of Masaryk and Beneš on the "alcohol question," see Tomáš G. Masaryk, *O alkoholismu: Předneseno v Dělnickém domě na Vsetíně dne 11. září 1905*, 2nd ed. (Prague: Tiskařské a nakladatelské družstvo Pokrok, 1908); Edvard Beneš, *Problém alkoholové výroby a abstinence* (Prague: Otakar Janáček, 1915). For a focus on civic consciousness, see for example the speeches presented at a national gathering about the "alcohol question" in *1922. Republikánská liga pro mravní obrodu národa a Československý abstinentní svaz, Alkoholismus a zájmy života: Anketa pořádana v Praze dne 6. ledna 1922* (Prague: Československý Kompas, 1922).

8 See Proctor, *The Nazi War on Cancer*, 141–53.

9 Also the general tone of the publications did not change significantly. See, for example, Ctibor Bezděk, "Mravnost a práce—toť zdraví a život," *Vyšší národ* 23.4 (1943).

10 Cover of the journal *Zdravý lid* 28.7/9 (1949). Československý abstinentní svaz, Týden střízlivosti I, 7, March 14, 1949. Národní archiv České republiky (hereafter NAČR), fond Ministerstvo práce a sociální péče, Boj proti soc. chorobám (proti nikotinismu a alkoholismu). Inv. č. 1298, sign. 1620, ka 640.

cated by transforming socioeconomic structures. In Western European countries, the anti-alcohol rhetoric was less ambitious, but also here, policy makers still advocated education campaigns in the countryside and incisive cuts on the supply side in the 1950s. The medical provision of alcoholics, to the contrary, presented only a marginal aspect of alcohol politics.[11] People who displayed alcohol-related problems were placed in mental hospitals or left in the care of their families or general practitioners. Only in bigger cities like Chicago or London could one find a small number of specialized treatment programs, but none of them amounted to a systematic policy approach.[12]

If large-scale endeavors to change people's consumption habits and consciousness had been appropriate answers in the 1950s, they failed to address the questions asked in the 1970s. At the turn of the 1960s and 1970s, alcohol problems received renewed attention in many countries. In both Eastern and Western Europe, social scientists, doctors, nutritionists, journalists, psychologists, criminologists, traffic experts, economists, family counselors, and many others raised alarm about a recent upsurge in alcohol consumption and its consequences on health, demography, accident rate, criminality rate, and so on. Their worries did not result in a common approach, however. To the contrary, the solutions to alcohol problems were compartmentalized. Rather than developing a unified political solution to alcohol problems, the various experts identified problem areas that they aimed to study and tackle as problems in their own right. Notably, and in contrast to the preceding periods, neither social policy makers nor experts promised to successfully solve alcohol problems. With short-term interventions, they instead strove to manage the most pressing and visible expressions of these issues.

The Disease Theory of Alcohol

In Czechoslovakia, the shift in alcohol politics occurred during a period of social policy reorganization. In 1968, Warsaw Pact troops had invaded the country to end what they saw as a "counterrevolution," that is, a period of

11 For postwar alcohol politics in France, see Bohling, "The Sober Revolution: The Political and Moral Economy of Alcohol in Modern France, 1954–1976"; for England, see Nicholls, *The Politics of Alcohol.*

12 For the development of alcoholism treatment in the United Kingdom and the United States, see White, *Slaying the Dragon: The History of Addiction Treatment and Recovery in America,* 216; Thom and Berridge, "'Special Units for Common Problems': The Birth of Alcohol Treatment Units in England."

economic, political, and cultural experimentation of which the Soviet Communist Party had not approved. After the invasion, a more loyal leadership came to power, which struggled to reclaim legitimacy. In the ensuing period of "normalization," they proved aware of widespread political disillusion and accordingly desisted from revolutionary language and practices. At its official meeting in 1971, the Czechoslovakian Communist Party consolidated a new focus on social policy measures. With better social and health services, the government tried to foster citizens' feelings of social security. Paulina Bren has outlined how this new line of social policy nurtured a turn to "the private," a depoliticized life where the domestic sphere became the "favored site for acting out citizenship."[13]

It was in this context that the Czech and Slovak health ministers updated the national politics of alcohol. With a new decree, issued in the spring of 1973, they did not radically alter existing regulations, but markedly shifted the focus of alcohol politics from an emphasis on educational measures to a pronounced concern for "improving ambulant and inpatient anti-alcohol treatment."[14] In the following years, the new Czechoslovak alcohol decree gave rise to the best-organized system of medical provision for alcoholics in the Soviet bloc. In this system, several types of institutions fulfilled complementary tasks for dealing with different types and phases of alcohol problems. To start with, "sobering-up stations" were responsible for establishing control over drinkers who had rioted in the streets or otherwise disturbed the public peace. Although most people were brought to these stations by police forces, the main function of the stations was not to punish them; there would have been easier ways to do so. Sobering-up stations were run by medical personnel who tried to pacify the troublemakers and cater for their physical well-being.[15] The second element in the Czechoslovak treatment system consisted of anti-alcohol counseling centers. Besides registering the

13 For the quote, see Bren, *The Greengrocer and His TV: The Culture of Communism after the 1968 Prague Spring*, 159. On the political reorganization in Czechoslovakia, see Milan Otáhal, *Normalizace, 1969–1989: Příspěvek ke stavu bádání* (Prague: Ústav pro Soudobé Dějiny AV ČR, 2002). For social policy under normalization, see Lenka Kalinová, *Konec nadějím a nová očekávání: K dějinám české společnosti v letech 1969–1993* (Prague: Academia, 2012).

14 "Zpráva o návrhy opatření k řešení problematiky alkoholismu a jiných toxikománií. Usnesení 70. schůze předsednictva ÚV KSČ," 20 April 1973. NAČR, Předsednictvo ÚV KSČ 1971–1976, sv. 77, ar. j. 74, 6.

15 Jaroslav Skála and Irena Hrodková, "Protialkoholní záchytné stanice ve světě a u nás," in *Ochrana společnosti před alkoholismem a jinými toxikomániemi*, ed. Jaroslav Skála (Prague: Avicenum. Zdravotnické nakladatelství, 1982), 65–71.

patients' data, the counseling centers diagnosed the patients' needs and coordinated the treatment process. They suggested outpatient treatment—administered by the employees of the counseling centers—or, in more serious cases, advised the alcoholics to undergo inpatient treatment.[16] The inpatient treatment institutions were the third pillar of the treatment system, offering a dedicated treatment program for alcoholics. In most cases, it lasted three months and was fully covered by the national health insurance.[17]

The upsurge of medical and counseling programs for alcohol problems was driven by a theory that had its origin in the United States. In the 1940s—that is, shortly after the US government had given up on the idea of a large-scale national prohibition—E. M. Jellinek and his colleagues at the department for Applied Physiology at Yale succeeded in popularizing the "disease model," according to which alcoholism is characterized by pathological (addictive) drinking habits. Adherents of the disease model did not promote abstinence as a political ideal. It offered a depoliticized view of alcohol problems, targeting only those drinkers who were *addicted* to alcohol and suggesting appropriate treatment programs to cure them of this addiction.[18] Starting in the 1960s, the disease model gained currency on a global scale and decisively shaped the professional and popular understanding of alcohol problems and the associated political programs. In all of Czechoslovakia's neighboring states, both to the East and to the West, new health acts codified the treatment of alcoholics and induced the establishment of separate wards for the treatment of alcoholics in the 1970s and 1980s.[19]

16 The official guidelines for outpatient treatment were updated in 1969. Věstník Ministerstva zdravotnictví České socialistické republiky, "Zřizování a činnost protialkoholních poraden, částka 7–8, ročník XVII," September 30, 1969, reprinted in *Zápisy z Apolináře* 3–4 (1969): 73–88. For a practical interpretation of these tasks, see Arnoštka Maťová, "Úkoly sociálních pracovnic v protialkoh. zařízeních," *Zápisy z Apolináře* 3–4 (1973): 55–6.

17 For the history of specialized treatment facilities for alcoholics, see Jaroslav Skála, *... až na dno? Fakta o alkoholu, pijáctví a alkoholismu*, 3rd ed. (Prague: Avicenum. Zdravotnické nakladatelství, 1977), 83–4.

18 Elvin Morton Jellinek, *The Disease Concept of Alcoholism* (New Haven: Hillhouse Press, 1960). See also Levine, "The Discovery of Addiction."

19 For Hungary and Poland, see the contributions of Zsuzsanna Elekes and Jacek Morawski in Hunt, Takala, and Klingemann (eds.), *Cure, Care, or Control: Alcoholism Treatment in Sixteen Countries*, 27 and 43; for the German Democratic Republic, see Unger, *Alkoholismus in der DDR: Die Geschichte des Umganges mit alkoholkranken Menschen in der ehemaligen DDR im Zeitraum 1949 bis 1989*, chapter 5; for Austria, Eisenbach-Stangl, *Eine Gesellschaftsgeschichte des Alkohols: Produktion, Konsum und soziale Kontrolle alkoholischer Rausch- und Genussmittel in Österreich 1918–1984*, 262–70; for the Federal Republic of Germany, Wienemann, "Hundert Jahre betriebliche Suchtprävention: Visionen und Wirken der Mäßigkeitsbewegung in der Arbeitswelt."

The Advent of Female Alcoholics

The disease model of alcoholism did not simply complement other, more structural approaches to alcohol problems. It expressed a qualitative shift in the politics of alcohol, offering pathological interpretations of alcohol problems *at the expense of other readings*. In Czechoslovakia, as well as in other countries, the pathological reading of alcohol problems translated on the one hand into a growing number of institutions and service programs for alcoholics; on the other hand, it distinctly affected the way alcoholics were treated and eventually also *who* was treated as an alcoholic. Until the mid-twentieth century, problematic drinking habits were usually assigned to men. Starting in the 1960s, however, doctors and policy makers all over the world discerned women as a new "risk group" of alcoholism. Also in Czechoslovakia, psychiatrists exhibited growing concern about the phenomenon of female drinking and conducted studies in order to understand the particularities of women's drinking.[20]

With their new interest in female drinkers, psychiatrists did justice, to some extent, to the rising numbers of women in alcohol treatment institutions. Sobering-up stations, counseling centers, and treatment institutions had all reported an increase in female patients from the mid-1960s onward—a trend that was in line with international developments. There are no conclusive data on the development of female drinking behavior, but many studies from different countries have confirmed that in this period women drank more in public than they used to.[21] However, the mounting interest in female alcoholism cannot only be explained by external factors. First of all, women *had* been drinking before. By the beginning of the twentieth century, anti-alcohol activists had occasionally brought up female drinking, describing in gruesome details the effects of a mother's alcohol

20 For the international context, see Keith Martin and Cincinnati Family Service Agency, *Alcoholism in Women: Identification, Its Relevance in Predisposition* (Northampton: Smith College School for Social Work, 1974). For Czechoslovakia, see, for example, A. Brzek and R. Müllerová, "Příspěvek k zvláštnostem ženského alkoholismu," *Protialkoholický obzor* 10.1 (1975); A. Marcinková and D. Hunáková, "K výskytu alkoholických psychóz u žien," *Protialkoholický obzor* 11.3 (1976); E. Uhravá and G. Jurčiová, "Vývojové trendy v populácii alkoholičiek liečených v protialkoholickej poradni v Bratislave," *Protialkoholický obzor* 20.3 (1985): 157–60.

21 Thom, *Dealing with Drink: Alcohol and Social Policy: From Treatment to Management*, chapter 8. For a study on drinking patterns in Czechoslovakia, see Marcinková and Hunáková, "K výskytu alkoholických psychóz u žien."

consumption on her children and family life. What seems to have been a relatively widespread phenomenon, particularly in rural regions and in Slovakia, did not receive too much attention before the late socialist period.[22] Second, while increased, women's numbers were still comparatively low in the late socialist period. Even at their peak, from 1969 to 1972, women hovered at around five percent of all patients in sobering-up stations. In psychiatric hospitals, the relative numbers of female alcoholics were higher, but still low compared to men. In the late 1970s, there was only one woman for every ten male alcoholism patients.[23] In all of their institutions, Czech and Slovak alcohol experts were still faced with a vast majority of male drinkers.

The preoccupation with female alcoholism was thus not simply a logical reaction to a new phenomenon. More than that, it reflected the changing interpretation of alcohol problems in the late socialist state. In earlier decades, alcohol problems were considered a national question, a structural problem, or a problem of public order—in any case, a problem of political importance that was by definition publicly visible through acts like brawling, rioting, delinquent activities, and immoral behavior. As long as alcohol problems were characterized by their public consequences, those whose drinking was unobtrusive did not form an important part of the problem. As women tended to confine their drinking to their home, visible only to those in their individual environments, they were typically not in the picture.[24] In this way, the new politics of alcohol fell into line with a new direction of social politics. As we have seen, in the 1970s the "private" became an important arena of social policy. The concern about women alcoholics fit into a new concern about family life, which aimed at restoring traditional family values and thus nurtured a critical engagement with gender roles.

The disparity between women and men in sobering-up stations (1:20) and in psychiatric treatment institutions (1:10) confirms this interpretation.

22 "Quido Mann (za Ochranu matek a kojenců)," in *Alkoholismus a zájmy života: Anketa pořádana v Praze dne 6. ledna 1922*, ed. Republikánská liga pro mravní obrodu národa a Československý abstinentní svaz (Prague: Československý Kompas, 1922); see also J. Hraše, *Eugenické a kulturní úkoly ženy* (Prague: Nakladatelství J. Otto, 1928).

23 "Alkoholismus u žen v ČSSR," *Zápisy z Apolináře* 26.1–2 (1977). Due to different standards in evidencing alcoholics, the ratio of male to female drinkers is hard to compare across countries. Beth Thom reports the balance between male and female drinkers in counseling services in England to have been more balanced, roughly 1:3. Thom, *Dealing with Drink*, 160.

24 For an interpretation of gendered patterns of drinking in Czechoslovakia, see Karel Nešpor, "Ústavní léčba žen závislých na alkoholu," *Protialkoholický obzor* 23.1 (1988): 45–52; Jaroslav Skála, D. Janýnšková, and Jiří Heller, "Alkoholismus u žen v ČSSR a příklad jejich léčby," *Zápisy z Apolináře* 29.1–3 (1980).

Women were, according to the data, a lot less likely to riot in public than male drinkers, and also less often constrained to take up treatment as a result of being involved in traffic accidents or engaging in public drunkenness or delinquency. Although in medical treatment programs, too, women were underrepresented, their relative numbers were much higher.[25] As in the 1970s the medical aspects of alcohol problems became more important than their public consequences, women's drinking became more visible. Psychiatrists in treatment institutions proved more sensitive to "hidden" forms of alcoholism and added to a growing body of research on the specificities of female drinking.[26] More aware of subtle expressions of drinking problems, they were also more likely to detect women's drinking and encourage them to undergo treatment. In the late 1950s, only seven percent of patients in inpatient treatment institutions had been hospitalized due to doctors' recommendations. In the early 1970s, this number had risen to twelve percent, and by the mid 1980s, 40 percent of all female alcoholism patients reported to have followed a doctor's recommendation.[27]

The intimate relation between the disease model and female alcoholism resulted in a number of particularities. In both research and treatment methods, psychiatrists paid attention to the psychopathology of their female patients to a much larger extent than in studies on male alcoholics. They argued that as alcohol drinking was less socially acceptable in women than in men, women were more likely to drink alone and very often did so in reaction to personal crises, which were usually linked to family problems. Men, on the contrary, tended to develop their addiction out of a social habit. Studies confirmed that more often than male patients, female patients had a prehistory of suicide attempts and psychiatric hospitalization and were more likely to suffer from depression and family problems. As a result, women's drinking would comparatively often result in social isolation, neuroses, and psychotic illnesses.[28]

25 Nešpor, "Ústavní léčba žen závislých na alkoholu."

26 For the phenomenon of "hidden" alcoholism, see P. Riesel, "Identifikace skrytých alkoholiků a lejich léčba," *Protialkoholický obzor* 11.2 (1976): 44–7.

27 E. Uhravá and G. Jurčiová, "Vývojové trendy v populácii alkoholičiek liečených v protialkoholickej poradni v Bratislave," *Protialkoholický obzor* 20.3 (1985): 157–60.

28 Jiří Heller, "Odlišnost syndromu závislosti na alkoholu u žen," *Zápisy z Apolináře* 28.2–4 (1979): 56–9; also see P. Pokorná and L. Šrutová, "Faktory ovlivňující vznik závislosti na alkoholu a jiných drogách u žen," *Protialkoholický obzor* 11.5 (1976): 139–41; Nešpor, "Ústavní léčba žen závislých na alkoholu."

Furthermore, psychiatrists observed women to display forms of addiction that differed from what was known for men. Women reportedly had a tendency to combine excessive drinking with an overuse of medical drugs. Like in other countries, the mass production of psychotropic drugs was a relatively new phenomenon in Czechoslovakia, and psychiatrists had just started to discover the dangers associated with their unregulated consumption.[29] As medical drugs were easily accessible and their consumption could be better concealed than excessive drinking, they seemed to have a particular appeal to women, with female addicts being reportedly very careful to not make their substance use habits visible. Indeed, psychiatrists observed that, on average, people addicted to psychotropic drugs were younger and more likely to be female than alcoholics. In the new Prague Center for Drug Addiction, there was one woman for every three male substance users. In institutions for alcoholics, the ratio was usually one woman for ten or more men.[30]

In the early 1970s, psychiatrist Jiří Heller criticized that despite the different experiences and habits of substance users, most doctors still used the same methods for female and male alcoholics. In order to find more appropriate answers to female alcoholism, Heller and his team reorganized the anti-alcoholic ward in Lojovice Castle near Prague. Starting in 1971, Lojovice provided thirty-two places exclusively for women. In the years to follow, Lojovice remained the only specialized treatment institution for women in Czechoslovakia; however, many psychiatric hospitals and psychiatrists introduced special treatment programs for women in their wards for alcohol treatment. With these initiatives, Czechoslovak alcohol treatment followed a recent international trend of setting up gender-specific treatment. Jaroslav Skála, the most renowned Czech alcohol expert, claimed that the inspiration for this institution derived from a treatment facility in southwestern Germany.[31]

29 A. Marcinková and D. Hunáková, "Prispevok k toxikománii žien, hospitalizovaných na psychiatrickom oddelení v Nitre," *Protialkoholický obzor* 10.6 (1975): 169–70.

30 Jaroslav Skála, "Abúzuz a závislost u mužů a žen—některé rozdíly," in Člověk a alkohol, ed. Josef Kvapilík (Prague: Avicenum. Zdravotnické nakladatelství, 1985).

31 See Skála, *Lékařův maraton: Ber a dávej*, 57–8; Heller, "Odlišnost syndromu závislosti na alkoholu u žen." Interview with Jiří Heller and Olga Pecinovská, January 24, 2014. For the international context, see Thom, *Dealing with Drink*, 158–9. For Austria, Eisenbach-Stangl, "Treatment-Seeking and Treatment-Reluctant Alcoholics: A Two-Class Alcohol-Treatment System in Austria," 179; for Poland and Yugoslavia, Jaroslav Skála, "Úvodní řeč 13 září 1977 při zahájení I. Kongresu socialistických zemí pro prevenci a terapii alkoholismu a jiných toxikomanií," *Zápisy z Apolináře* 26.3–6 (1977).

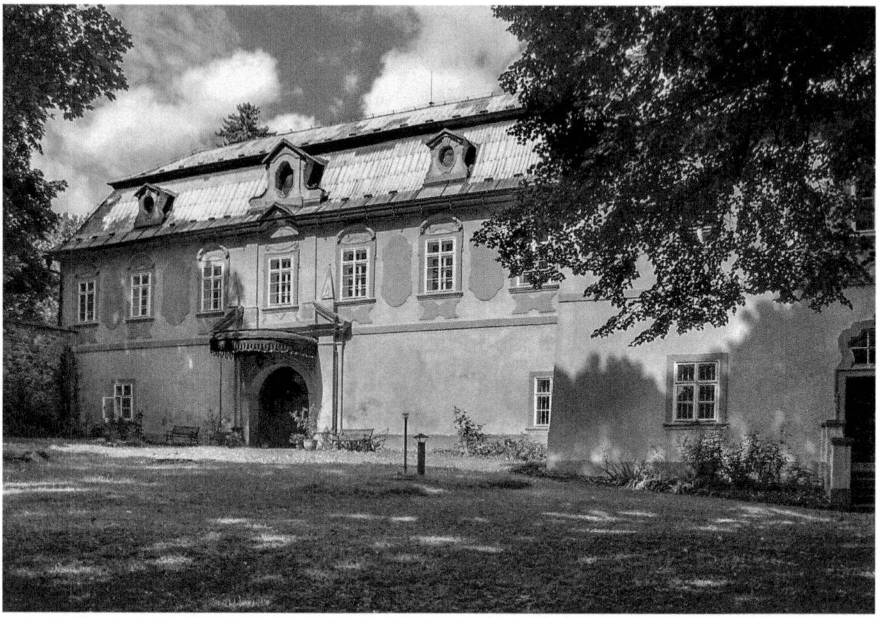

Figure 10.1: *The castle of Lojovice.* In: Czech Wikipedia user Packa, Baroque castle in Lojovice, part of Velké Popovice, Czech Republic, August 18, 2008, own work, CC BY-SA 3.0, https://commons.wikimedia.org/w/index.php?curid=4612588 [last accessed: April 21, 2017].

Explanation of Figure 10.1: Before being a home to female alcoholics, the castle belonged to Franz Ringhoffer, founder of the famous Velkopopvický brewery. After the Second World War, Ringhofer's property was nationalized and since 1958 used for anti-alcohol treatment. In 1971, psychiatrists moved the male patients of Lojovice to another facility in South Bohemia and started the first women-only treatment facility in the country. Today, the castle has been restituted.

While the new concern for female alcoholics also reflected societal fears about changing gender roles, it is worth noting that the idea to introduce gender-specific treatment did not (only) result from essentialist assumptions about gender differences. Psychiatrists stressed that the experiences of female alcoholics differed systematically from their male counterparts due to different societal standards, with women experiencing more social pressure and their drinking being more stigmatized. In Lojovice and elsewhere, the program for female alcoholics was therefore designed to meet the specific needs of female drinkers. With secluded treatment programs, psychiatrists aimed to create a space for female addicts, in which they could speak about their experiences more freely, without the restraints of a societal structure that was often perceived as hostile, that had aggravated their disease, or was at least not considered conducive to their condition.[32]

Inner Struggles, Therapeutic Revolutions, and "A Lot of Space Where Nobody Asked Too Much"

In the treatment of women, the alcohol experts of Lojovice placed particular importance on a qualitative therapeutic atmosphere. The use of psychotherapeutic elements was a relatively new phenomenon in the treatment of male and female alcoholics alike. Not only in Czechoslovakia, but also in England, the United States, and many other states east and west of the Iron Curtain, alcohol treatment before the 1970s had combined some form of medical intervention to alleviate the physical symptoms of drinking problems (gastric problems, for example) with deconditioning programs such as aversion training. In the latter, alcoholics were made to ingest their preferred alcoholic beverage together with an emetic, a combination which was supposed to trigger nausea and in the long run condition aversion to the beverage. As a form of conditioning, aversion therapy was in line with official Soviet therapeutic approaches, which mainly followed Ivan Pavlov's behaviorist approach.[33] In nonsocialist countries, too, aversion therapy was a common treatment element and could be found in many European countries well until the 1970s.[34]

In the 1960s and 1970s, hospital programs in both Eastern and Western Europe enriched the treatment for alcoholics with psychotherapeutic elements.[35] In Czechoslovakia, alcohol experts showed a growing interest for neuroses and psychoses as the cause of their patients' disease.[36] Besides ad-

32 Interview with Jiří Heller and Olga Pecinovská, 24 January 2014; on motivations for gender-specific treatment in England, see Thom, *Dealing with Drink*, 160–1.

33 Ėtkind, *Eros of the Impossible: The History of Psychoanalysis in Russia.*

34 For treatment methods in England, see Thom, *Dealing with Drink*, 42–63, 136; for the United States, see White, *Slaying the Dragon*, 216–20. For aversion therapy in several European countries, see Skála,... až na dno? 83–4.

35 For the growing importance of psychotherapeutic elements in alcohol treatment in England, see Thom, *Dealing with Drink*, 136; for the United States, White, *Slaying the Dragon*, 216–20; for Sweden, Rosenqvist and Kurube, "Dissolving the Swedish Alcohol-Treatment System"; for the GDR, Kochan, *Blauer Würger: So trank die DDR.*

36 This can be traced from articles in the bi-monthly journal *Anti-Alcohol Horizon* [*Protialkoholický obzor*]; see for example D. Junasová, V. Novotný, and E. Kolibáš, "Kazuistický príspevok ku klasifikácii alkoho-

ministering medication for the physiological side of the disease of alcoholism, they encouraged their patients to understand their own drinking problems as a psychological disease. To help patients assess and articulate their internal conflicts, psychiatrists encouraged methods such as diary writing, individual counseling sessions, and collective meetings in which patients were urged to reflect upon their habits and the underlying problems.[37] Depending on capacities, institutions offered to hospitalize the alcoholics' family members for up to one week. Considered an integral part of the treatment program, spouses received sickness benefits during this period.[38] All of these approaches enforced a psychopathological reading of alcohol problems, which located the root of the problems within the individual and his or her intimate surroundings and had to be understood by analyzing personal conflicts and pathological behavior and relationships.

In research and reports on counseling sessions, we can furthermore observe an interesting upsurge in psychoanalytical language and practice. Psychoanalytical research had flourished in interwar Czechoslovakia.[39] However, under Stalinism, leading psychiatrists in the Soviet Union had denounced the theories of Sigmund Freud as bourgeois and individualistic.[40] In the 1970s, psychoanalytical thought and practice experienced a clandestine revival in several socialist countries.[41] In Czechoslovakia, psychiatrists were still careful not to make direct references to Freud, but they managed to revive his theories and adapt them for their purposes.[42] The popularity of psychoanalysis reflected a new fascination with individual pathologies and their effect on society. By introducing psychological counseling

lických psychóz," *Protialkoholický obzor* 11.4 (1976); R. Károlyiová, E. Medvecká and J. Medvecký, "Alkoholické psychózy," *Protialkoholický obzor* 12.4 (1977), 20.

37 Skála, *... až na dno?* 83–4.

38 P. Kucek, "Efect psychoterapie na manželského partnera liečeného alkoholika," *Protialkoholický obzor* 15.1 (1980): 37–8; interview with former patient F. and his wife J., January 16, 2014.

39 Marks, "From Experimental Psychosis to Resolving Traumatic Pasts: Psychedelic Research in Communist Czechoslovakia, 1954–1974."

40 Ėtkind, *Eros of the Impossible*. In the Soviet Union, psychiatrists similarly revitalized Freudian theories in the late 1970s, making use of even more intricate methods to masquerade their interest. See Miller, *Freud and the Bolsheviks: Psychoanalysis in Imperial Russia and the Soviet Union*, 120, 126, 146.

41 Recent studies have suggested that to a greater or lesser extent, psychoanalytic elements found entry in psychiatric treatment in the German Democratic Republic, Hungary, and most strongly in Yugoslavia. For Yugoslavia, see Savelli, "The Peculiar Prosperity of Psychoanalysis in Socialist Yugoslavia"; for the GDR, Leuenberger, "Socialist Psychotherapy and Its Dissidents"; for Hungary: Buda et al., "Psychotherapy in Hungary during the Socialist Era and the Socialist Dictatorship."

42 Marks, "From Experimental Psychosis to Resolving Traumatic Pasts."

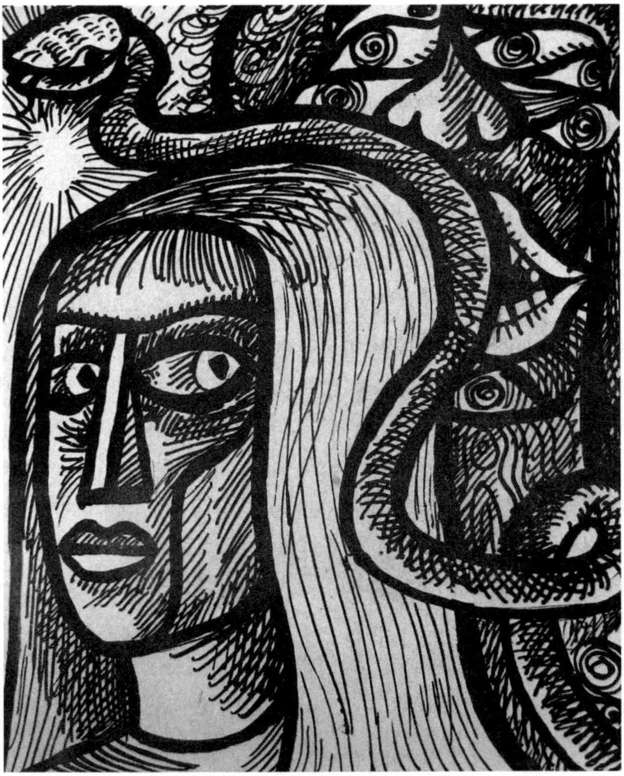

Figure 10.2: *Psychological approaches to the disease of alcoholism.*
In: *Zápisy z Apolináre* 24, no. 3–4 (1975), 74.

Explanation of Figure 10.2: In the 1970s, the programs in anti-alcohol departments encouraged patients to find new ways of expressing themselves. Besides diary writings, many patients took to painting, drawing, and other artistic measures to express their understanding of their disease. The results were occassionally published in internal journals of the facilities.[43]

into the treatment programs, alcohol experts did not mainly target inebriated people who made trouble on the streets or committed crimes under the influence of alcohol. Instead of addressing the visible and violent consequences of alcoholism, they focused on the patients' inner conflicts and

43 I would like to thank Petr Popov, head of the Clinic of Addictology of the Charles University Prague and custodian of the *Zápisy* archives, for the permission to reprint the above image. Despite thorough investigations not all possible copyright owners could be identified. In case I have by any chance and involuntarily infringed any copyright, I hereby declare that the use of the images is entirely non-commercial and solely serves educational purposes. Therefore, I claim that the use of the images meets the requirements of the fair use statute.

tried to discern the underlying, subconscious reasons for their addiction.[44] With this individualized approach to the patients' drinking, psychiatrists contributed to a depoliticized understanding of alcohol problems. The reasons for drinking lay within the individual, and there seemed to be no significant relation between drinking problems and social factors. Alcohol addiction could affect everyone, and it did not distinguish between managers and factory workers or between men and women.

Psychoanalytic methods and psychotherapeutic counseling were of particular interest in the treatment of female alcoholics. While the treatment for men, too, became more differentiated and began to include counseling for individuals and their families, the programs in Lojovice showed an even more pronounced focus on psychotherapy. In order to create a qualitative therapeutic atmosphere, the hospitalization period for women was lengthened to seventeen weeks, in comparison to thirteen for men. In line with the disease model of alcoholism, the psychotherapeutic methods were designed to analyze individual experiences of the patients and reveal their inner struggles and pathological relations to their intimate environment (mainly their family). Experts thus located the roots of alcohol problems within the alcoholic patient and less in the broader socioeconomic conditions. Understanding the subconscious motivation for their drinking and its various pathological expressions, the therapeutic program was to help the patient develop strategies to cope with conflicts without resorting to addictive habits.[45]

The psychological reading of alcohol problems was no isolated movement. In the decades after the Second World War, social policy programs in many states became less visionary. After the war, governments in both East and West had been eager to build and consolidate the conditions for economic and social prospering. The intensity of economic restructuring had differed vastly both across Europe and within political blocs. All over Europe, however, the hopes connected to social and economic progress stifled in the 1970s and called for a new orientation. In this period, social policy makers refrained from promising successful solutions to social deviance, like juvenile delinquency or alcoholism. Instead, they strove to eradicate the

44 Levine, "The Discovery of Addiction."

45 For a similar argumentation, see Savelli, "The Peculiar Prosperity of Psychoanalysis in Socialist Yugoslavia," 287.

most visible excesses of these deviances and consolidate social order. To justify this unambitious approach, policy programs addressed these "excesses" not as social woes, but as individual failures induced by a low level of education, parental incompetence, bad environmental influence, and inner conflicts.[46] Families and individuals who struggled to live up to societal standards were offered help on the basis of individualized casework. Referring to the United States, Martin Halliwell has outlined a "therapeutic revolution" after the Second World War, which he argues induced a more individual interpretation of phenomena that had previously been conceptualized as social problems. As Halliwell points out, this shift in medical practice was not a culture-free development; it stemmed from a fundamental reinterpretation of social normality and affected all areas of private and public life.[47]

Also in late socialist Czechoslovakia, the reinterpretation of social diseases was shaped by political circumstances. The disease theory gained ground when the Czechoslovak government struggled for legitimacy and desisted from idealistic promises for a better future. Instead, social policy makers settled for feasible programs of social provision. This does not mean that the disease model was the result of a top-down social policy program; it was not a *political* redefinition of alcohol problems: instead, politicians acknowledged the psychiatrists' authority in the field of alcoholism and enforced their solutions. Psychiatrists who practiced during the socialist period have described the official stance as a tolerant negligence, opening up "a lot of space where nobody asked too much,"[48] and thereby leaving room for considerable agency. For example, while it was well-known to the psychiatrists that informers of the Czechoslovak Secret Service participated in training programs or group meetings of patients, alcohol experts could carry out most initiatives. According to the psychiatrist Jiří Heller, the pioneer of Czech alcohol treatment Jaroslav Skála "was diligent and started working without asking if he was allowed to. And when the action or activity was already going on, then the officials just took it like it was, and did not ask too much. The worst was to ask for permission. Nothing was permitted."[49]

46 For the context of the United States, see Gordon, *Heroes of Their Own Lives: The Politics and History of Family Violence: Boston, 1880–1960*, 23–6.

47 Halliwell, *Therapeutic Revolutions: Medicine, Psychiatry, and American Culture, 1945–1970*, 10–14.

48 Interview with Olga Pecinovská, January 24, 2014.

49 Interview with Jiří Heller, January 24, 2014.

This formulation—"the officials just took it like it was, and did not ask too much"—suggests that health policy makers in late socialist Czechoslovakia were well aware of the treatment practices. Accordingly, they did not simply "fail" to regulate the field of medical provision, and the scope of action left to psychiatric experts was no accident. Based on the example of state-socialist Yugoslavia, Mat Savelli has similarly argued that psychiatrists gained authority in defining diseases and developing treatment plans because the government proved reluctant to develop its own solutions.[50] Neither in Czechoslovakia nor in Yugoslavia did health ministries simply neglect to provide more politically appropriate interpretations of social diseases. The ministers granted space to medical experts because they deemed them responsible for problems that were outside of the political realm. The strong role of the medical profession in defining social diseases and treatment approaches was thus the result of a depoliticized view on alcoholism and other problems. Alcohol experts did not have to be politically strictly in line to serve the new line of social policy. Often, they transgressed the "binaries of either overt dissidence or conformity."[51] For example, Skála and other influential alcohol experts were not party members, but they proved willing to cooperate with representatives of the KSČ. These in turn were not averse to integrate new initiatives into the official approach to alcohol problems in the country.[52]

Conclusion

The policy measures of the early 1970s were not the first attempts to tackle alcohol problems in Czechoslovakia. What is more, the regulations did not distinguish from earlier initiatives by being more successful. Not only in Czechoslovakia but also in other countries did alcohol consumption further increase in the following years and new habits of drug use spread. But as other chapters of this book have shown, the success of public health state programs is not the same as their social impact. Public health policy measures may not always solve social problems, but they reliably reveal and

50 Savelli, "The Peculiar Prosperity of Psychoanalysis in Socialist Yugoslavia," 287.

51 Marks, "From Experimental Psychosis to Resolving Traumatic Pasts."

52 Skála had been a party member for four years. In 1953, he was excluded for voting against the currency reform. On Skála's political career, see Skála, *Lékařův maraton*, 49–50.

shape sociocultural concepts about social order, categories of social provision, and visions for social betterment. The 1970s alcohol decrees embodied a new approach toward alcohol problems. All over the world, states embraced a psychopathological reading of alcoholism, pinning down the problem to a relatively small group of people who were declared in need of specialized treatment.

Focusing on the inclusion of women in the category of patient provision, I have argued that the new gender-specific treatment programs were neither a mere reaction to the upsurge in drinking—which was, however, a reality—nor did they present the only logical solution to women's excessive drinking. Female alcoholism started to attract attention because alcohol problems were redefined from a public nuisance into a disease, and drinkers turned from troublemakers into patients. Female drinkers, who had been less present as troublemakers in sobering-up stations, became increasingly visible as drinkers in a period when excessive drinking was considered to reflect psychopathological problems and disturbed family relations.[53] The feminization of the drinker thus confirmed the trend to depoliticize social problems and locate them within the individual drinker and his or her intimate surroundings.

By advancing a psychopathological interpretation of alcohol problems, socialist Czechoslovakia joined an international trend supported by the World Health Organization and adopted by states as diverse as the United States, Great Britain, France, Austria, Hungary, and Yugoslavia, to name only a few.[54] While there were differences between countries, bloc affiliation did not play a decisive role in shaping national alcohol politics. Sure enough, international travel was more difficult to arrange for alcohol experts from state-socialist countries, but psychiatrists from Czechoslovakia were acquainted with current research in Western states, too. They sought interna-

53 The "feminization" of alcohol treatment was also reflected in popular representations of alcohol problems. Several TV screenings testify to this development, for example the "Televizní klub mladých: Diagnosa 303," Československá televize, early 1980s (exact date unknown). In 1980, Czechoslovak television screened a documentary about the treatment of female alcoholics in Lojovice, "Lékař a vy: Žena a alkohol," Československá televize, January 9, 1980. AČT, database PROVYS.

54 For the United States, see White, *Slaying the Dragon*; for Great Britain, Thom, *Dealing with Drink*; for France, Mossé, "The Rise of Alcohology in France: A Monopolistic Competition"; for Austria, Eisenbach-Stangl, "Treatment-Seeking and Treatment-Reluctant Alcoholics"; for Hungary, Elekes, "The Development of an Alcohol-Treatment System in Hungary"; for Yugoslavia, Lang and Srdar, "Therapeutic Communities and Aftercare Clubs in Yugoslavia."

tional cooperation, presented local approaches at conferences abroad whenever they could, and published in international journals.[55] As Sarah Marks has argued for the field of psychiatry in general, international scientific events showed a relative convergence in research trends, and the experts' "solidarity with this community outweighed any commitment to local ideological particularisms."[56] Alcohol experts in Prague were better connected to their Western German colleagues than to those in Romania, for example, and the disease model was more contested in Italy than in Czechoslovakia.[57] Dismissing state-socialist programs as overly ideological would simplify a complex reality that was shaped by international entanglements, domestic legacies, and recent political and economic developments.

I would thus like to pick up on the hypothesis of this volume and suggest relocating state-socialist social politics within a broader "late modern" European framework of approaching social problems. The disease theory of alcoholism gained ground in the sociopolitical atmosphere in the 1970s in liberal democracies and state-socialist countries alike because it offered a depoliticized reading of social problems. Instead of ascribing alcohol problems to structural societal wrongs, it explained them as individual shortcomings that could be alleviated by means of professionalized interventions. In a more general perspective, the pathologization of alcohol problems thus reflects how policy makers came to gradually accept social deviance as a social reality. During a crisis of state legitimacy, the depoliticized approach toward social problems presented an attempt to reestablish control over social order. This individualized and pragmatic attitude toward social problems was eventually embraced by many states, both east and west of the Iron Curtain, and may therefore be considered a common parameter of "late modern" statehood.

55 On international conference participations, see for example the autobiography of Jaroslav Skála, *Lékařův maraton*, 58–80.

56 Marks, "From Experimental Psychosis to Resolving Traumatic Pasts: Psychedelic Research in Communist Czechoslovakia, 1954–1974."

57 For Romania, I refer to research for my dissertation; see footnote 1. See also Doina Constantinescu, *Cotribuţii la studiul de tratament în alcoolismul cronic* (PhD diss., Institut de Medicină şi Farmacie Bucureşti, 1990). For Italy, see Poldrugo and Urizzi, "The Italian Paradox: Treatment Initiatives and Falling Alcohol Consumption."

CHAPTER XI

"The Gypsy Population Is Constantly Growing": Roma and the Politics of Reproduction in Cold War Hungary

Eszter Varsa

INTRODUCTION[1]

This chapter deals with state interference in population and individual health through the examination of reproductive policies and practices in state-socialist Hungary. The politics of reproduction is central to understanding how new regimes construct the state, especially after systemic changes; how (bio)politics is being reshaped; and what the relationship between the state and its citizens is like.[2] From direct involvement by banning abortions to more indirect methods of family support and welfare policies, the official politics of reproduction in Cold War Eastern and Southeastern Europe was pronatalist.[3] This fitted the long-term tradition of concern about

1 I would like to thank the Ervin Szabó Library in Budapest for the permission to reprint the images in this article. Despite thorough investigations not all possible copyright owners could be identified. In case I have by any chance and involuntarily infringed any copyright, I hereby declare that the use of the images solely serves educational purposes. Therefore, I claim that the use of the images meets the requirements of the fair use statute.

2 Gal and Kligman, "Reproduction as Politics."

3 Pronatalism manifested itself in a variety of policies, especially after the legalization of abortion in most state-socialist countries following the Soviet example, where the decree of 1936 outlawing abortion was repealed in 1955. Pronatalist measures between the mid-1960s and the end of the 1980s included family- and child-welfare policies, such as extended child allowances and maternity benefits, in Poland, East Germany, Hungary, and Bulgaria. In numerous countries this was accompanied by a limited increase in the number of places in nurseries and kindergartens. At the same time, abortion legislation also became more restrictive, most of all in Ceaușescu's Romania, where it was banned again in 1966.

the "dying of the nation" that was characteristic of imperial politics and nation-state–building processes in different European regions throughout the twentieth century. This chapter investigates continuities in reproductive and population control discourses across the systemic divide between the decades prior to and following the onset of state socialism in Hungary, specifically the reappearance of eugenics from the 1950s onward. Through an examination of reproductive policies and ensuing practices with reference to Romani and majority Hungarian populations between the 1950s and 1980s, it discusses mechanisms of inclusion and exclusion along the intersections of gender and race/ethnicity that were embedded in the regulation of health in state-socialist Hungary. The chapter relies on the qualitative analysis of medical journal articles, publications by the Hungarian Red Cross, and local council and ministerial documents on birth control, family planning, and the "Gypsy question,"[4] and devotes specific attention to Szabolcs-Szatmár County in the northeastern region of Hungary, where the density of the Romani population in the discussed period was higher (five percent) than the national average (three percent).[5]

The Historiography of Reproductive Politics in State-Socialist Eastern and Southeastern Europe

The politics of reproduction in state-socialist Eastern and Southeastern Europe has been analyzed primarily from a gender perspective, in regards to the negative effects of restrictive population control tools on the lives of women. Feminist researchers paid particular attention to the Stalinist repressive approach to reproductive issues, including the ban of abortion in

4 I use both Roma and "Gypsy" in order to highlight that there is a difference between those persons authorities identified as "Gypsies" and those who would identify themselves as Roma. While in Hungary, Roma also self-identify using the word "Gypsy," I use Roma whenever I refer to members of this ethnic group. I retained, however, the term "Gypsy" in accordance with the primary sources used for this chapter, such as in the name of the organization "Coordination Committee for Gypsy Affairs." Except in case of collocations, such as the "Gypsy question," I do not use inverted commas around the term "Gypsy" for the sake of readability.

5 The first representative survey on the Romani population in state-socialist Hungary was conducted by members of the Research Institute for Sociology at the Hungarian Academy of Sciences in 1971. Counting as "Gypsy" those who were identified as such "by their non-Gypsy environment," the survey established that most Roma (75,000 to 80,000) lived in the eastern region of Hungary, including the counties of Szabolcs-Szatmár, Hajdú-Bihar, and Békés. István Kemény (ed.), *Beszámoló a magyarországi cigányok helyzetével foglalkozó 1971-ben végzett kutatásról* (Budapest: MTA Szociológiai Kutató Intézete, 1976).

the early 1950s in the wider region as well as in the case of Ceauşescu's Romania following the mid-1960s.[6] Studies emphasize the burdens women bore as a result of the intrusive nature of state control in the private lives and bodies of women, and women's techniques of resistance in the face of totalitarian power.[7] Another strand of research draws attention to the increasing importance women's roles as mothers gained, especially following de-Stalinization and the parallel fading away of equalization discourse in the People's Democracies of the region.[8]

While approaching state-socialist policy making and ensuing practice in the field of welfare from a critical gender perspective, the above literature reflects only marginally on the extent to which reproductive policies affected different groups of women differently. Reproductive discourses encourage or pressure some groups of women to give birth, while at the same time they discourage and restrict others from doing so.[9] An intersectional perspective taking into account both gender and racial/ethnic differentiation, such as Gisela Bock's important study on population control in National Socialist Germany, can qualify statements made on the basis of a homogenizing approach to women as a social group, as well as amend a critical stand on racism by including the differential effects of racist policies on men and women. Contrary to the general assumption about the predominantly pronatalist character of National Socialism in Germany, Bock stated that pronatalism targeted German women of Aryan origin only. Women of "inferior quality," including women of Jewish origin, were instead targets of antinatalist policies.[10]

While there is a rapidly growing body of literature on eugenics and racism with regard to pronatalism in interwar and Second World War East and Southeast European societies, intertwined with a politics of nation-state building in the region, a systematic exploration of continuities in eugenics, including gender and race/ethnicity intersections, in the postwar and Cold

6 Kligman, "Political Demography: The Banning of Abortion in Ceausescu's Romania."

7 Pető and Kossuth, "Women's Rights in Stalinist Hungary: The Abortion Trials of 1952–53."

8 Fidelis, "A Nation's Strength Lies Not in Numbers: De-Stalinization, Pronatalism, and the Abortion Law of 1956 in Poland." Lynne Haney and Mária Adamik drew similar conclusions in the case of Hungary, although not in direct reference to reproductive politics. See Haney, *Inventing the Needy: Gender and the Politics of Welfare in Hungary*; and Adamik, "Az államszocializmus és a 'nőkérdés': A legnagyobb ígéret—a legnagyobb megaláztatás."

9 Yuval-Davis, *Gender and Nation.*

10 Bock, "Equality and Difference in National Socialist Racism."

War decades is still lacking.[11] A notable exception is Vera Sokolova's study of sterilization in state-socialist Czechoslovakia, in which she described how an ethnically neutral law in the 1970s, limiting the use of sterilization to certain categories of "deviancy," was racialized at local-level practice, leading to the forced sterilization of large numbers of Romani women.[12] Concerning population control in state-socialist Hungary, Attila Melegh drew attention to the selective nature of Hungarian pronatalist discourses in the 1970s and antinatalism with respect to marginalized social groups, including Roma. Placing the Hungarian case in a comparative global perspective, he pointed to the appearance of neo-Malthusian population control discourses regarding families with many children in the economic crisis of the 1970s.[13]

Bringing a local-level focus into the investigation of reproductive discourses and practices with regard to both Romani and non-Romani populations in state-socialist Hungary, my research shows that medical professionals' concern about increasing abortion rates among women was coupled with eugenic concern about the future of the Hungarian nation, from as early as the 1956 legalization of abortion. County committee reports of the party and reports by organizations such as the local branches of the Hungarian Red Cross and the Coordination Committee for Gypsy Affairs,[14] as well as discourse by local physicians demonstrate that pronatalism was directed only at selective groups of Hungarian women. Parallel to a general pronatalist discourse across the four decades of state socialism in Hungary, Romani women were targeted by varying degrees and forms of antinatalist discourses and practices.

In what follows, I will first summarize the major population policies and the main characteristics of how the "Gypsy question" was handled in state-socialist Hungary, placing the period between the 1950s and the 1980s in a longer, twentieth-century perspective. Next, I will show that prona-

11 Bucur, *Eugenics and Modernization in Interwar Romania*; Turda, "In Pursuit of Greater Hungary: Eugenic Ideas of Social and Biological Improvement, 1940–1941"; Szikra, "A szociálpolitika másik arca: Fajvédelem és produktív szociálpolitika az 1940-es évek Magyarországán."

12 Sokolova, "Planned Parenthood behind the Iron Curtain: Sterilization of Romani Women."

13 Melegh, "Living to Ourselves: Localising Global Hierarchies in State-Socialist Hungary in the 1970s and 1980s," and *On the East/West Slope: Globalization, Nationalism, Racism and Discourses on Eastern Europe.*

14 The Coordination Committee for Gypsy Affairs was an administrative unit responsible for transmitting to county-level institutions and coordinating the execution of national directives concerning the Gypsy population. The coordination committees submitted regular reports to the Council of Ministers covering issues of employment, living, health, and social conditions.

talism targeting young, better-to-do women went hand-in-hand with anti-natalism directed at less well-to-do, mostly Gypsy women. While focusing on the alarming trends in decreasing birth rates among the majority population, Hungarian medical professionals highlighted the high infant mortality rates and the continuous increase in birth among Gypsies. In particular, in the 1960s the Ministry of Health encouraged doctors to propagate abortion free of charge as a means of fertility control among Romani women. Following the introduction of the population policy program of 1973, discourse and practices aiming to increase not simply quantitative but qualitative reproduction entailed the prevention of "unwanted birth." In general, this was aimed at a decrease of abortion as a means of fertility control among women. Conscious family planning to increase the birth of healthy infants in the 1970s and the 1980s targeted the better-educated layers of Hungarian society, while health education among the lower-qualified and poorer layers of society, especially Roma, aimed at a decrease of birth rates. Medical journals also contributed to the stigmatization of Roma with references to the inborn, negative characteristics of Romani men and women affecting their fertility and mortality rates. The identification of the reproduction of Roma in terms of the burden they posed on the Hungarian state and society was part of the prewar and wartime eugenic discourse in relation to the Gypsy population, perceived to be undeserving of social support, an argument that resurfaced at local levels immediately following the legalization of abortion in Hungary. At the same time, the philosophy of population control identifying rapid population growth as a primary cause of development problems, such as poverty, was characteristic of post-1945 international population politics in relation to the global "third world." This parallel demonstrates that the assumption that birth control leads to the improvement of impoverished living conditions was not specific to state-socialist or Hungarian minority politics.

The Politics of Reproduction and the "Gypsy Question" in Twentieth-Century Hungary

Reproductive discourses and practices in late-nineteenth- and early-twentieth-century Eastern and Southeastern Europe, like in Western European and North American imperial powers in the eighteenth and nineteenth centuries, were tied to modernization and nation-building projects. The breakup of the Habsburg Monarchy and the rearrangement of national borders following the end of the First World War in Eastern Europe gave a special salience to nationalisms and nation-building efforts in the region, including Hungary.[15] Reproductive discourses and policy-making were important elements of these processes. Concerns about the "dying of the Hungarian nation" emerged in the early 1920s, intertwined with the nationalist and eugenic movements of the time, resulting in pronatalist reproductive politics.[16] By the 1940s, these discourses gained a racist content. Marius Turda and Paul Weindling's extensive research on the social history of health and medicine in interwar East and Southeast Europe demonstrated that the radicalization of national politics went hand-in-hand with a eugenic program mixed with racial thought.[17] Concerning Romania, for example, scholarship has established the link between eugenics and the development of anti-Roma policy in the late 1930s and early 1940s, and the role eugenics played in the deportation of Roma to Transnistria in 1942.[18] The combination of nationalism, eugenics, and racism in the government activity in Hungary during the Second World War contributed to the racial othering of "Jews," who were considered inferior and dangerous to the nation's health.[19] Gypsies became the second most undesired minority group to whom the health problems of the country were attributed.[20] Central to the nationalist and racialized eugenic program in 1930s and 1940s Hungary were health and welfare measures aiming to encourage birth among the Christian peasant population, identified as the source of national strength.[21] Positive eugenics was accompanied by negative eugenic measures, such as Act 15 of 1941 prohibiting marriage between Jews and non-Jews, aimed at the elimination of the racially and biologically unworthy from the body of the nation, and thereby at the improvement of the biological stock of Hungarians.[22]

15 Trencsényi et al., *Nation-Building and Contested Identities: Romanian and Hungarian Case Studies*; Turda and Weindling (ed.), *Blood and Homeland: Eugenics and Racial Nationalism in Central and Southeast Europe, 1900–1940*.

16 Szikra, "A szociálpolitika másik arca."

17 Turda and Weindling, *Blood and Homeland*.

18 Thorne, "Assimilation, Invisibility, and the Eugenic Turn in the 'Gypsy Question' in Romanian Society, 1938–1942"; Turda, "'To End the Degeneration of a Nation;'" idem, "The Nation as Object: Race, Blood, and Biopolitics in Interwar Romania"; Ioanid, *The Holocaust in Romania*.

19 Turda, "In Pursuit of Greater Hungary."

20 Baran and Gazdag, "The Fate of the Hungarian Psychiatric Patients during World War II."

21 Ibid., and Szikra, "A szociálpolitika másik arca."

22 Turda, "In Pursuit of Greater Hungary," 561.

A variety of welfare incentives, as well as forced measures to influence birth rates, characterized twentieth-century Hungarian reproductive policy-making. For example, abortion had been illegal in Hungary since the nineteenth century. Customary legal practice, however, was permissive of abortion in the interwar period when the pregnancy endangered the health of the mother. Following the end of the Second World War, abortion regulations were quickly liberalized with reference to the sexual violence committed against women during the war. Besides the regulation of abortion, family-oriented social benefits such as child allowances and child-care leaves, social insurance measures like maternity benefits, and a network of nurseries and kindergartens had been made available to specific groups of employed women since the late nineteenth century.[23]

The onset of state socialism brought about a restrictive turn in reproductive politics in Eastern and Southeastern Europe. In Hungary in 1953, in the framework of the social protection of mothers and infants, legislation concerning the punishment of abortion was strengthened.[24] This so-called "Ratkó Act" established medical committees to decide upon abortion requests and introduced special taxes for the childless.[25] These committees followed strict guidelines that limited abortion to serious health endangerment of women. Abortions were practically banned, and physicians, obstetricians, as well as women accused of self-administering abortions received heavy punishments. In this year, abortion-related court cases and punishments doubled in comparison to previous years. At the same time, the decree extended the social support of employed mothers by a one-time maternity grant and the provision of baby clothes after birth. While the birth rate shortly increased as a result of the abortion ban, the number of illegal abortions, unwanted pregnancies, premature births, as well as the number of children placed in children's homes also grew.[26]

In 1954, following de-Stalinization and the Thaw, the Ministry of Justice revised the guidelines to be followed by abortion committees to allow

23 Inglot, Szikra, and Rat, "Continuity and Change in Family Policies of the New European Democracies: A Comparison of Poland, Hungary and Romania," 20–2.

24 Decree 1004/1953 (II.8.) of the Council of Ministers on the Protection of Mothers and Infants, in *Törvények és rendeletek* (Budapest: Jogi- és Államigazgatási Könyv- és Folyóiratkiadó, 1953).

25 The restrictive measure introduced in 1953 was not a law but a decree, which in common usage was labeled the Ratkó Act, after Anna Ratkó, who was the minister of health at the time.

26 András Klinger and István Monigl, "Népesedés és népesedéspolitika Magyarországon az 1970-es és az 1980-as évtizedben," *Demográfia* 4 (1981).

health endangerment, as well as social and familial grounds, to be taken into consideration when making decisions. Finally, in the summer of 1956, abortion was legalized.[27] While maintaining the system of abortion committees in decision-making about abortion requests whose members were made up of both medical professionals and local council representatives, Decree 1047/1956 of the Council of Ministers placed the right of the final decision with the women who filed a request. In consequence of the liberalized policy as well as the lack of contraceptives, the yearly number of abortions performed rocketed in the next decade.[28] At the same time, fertility rates dropped, and in the early 1960s Hungarian birth rates were among the lowest in the world.[29] A decrease in birth rates, however, was not just a Hungarian phenomenon, but characterized all Eastern European societies, from Poland to East Germany, which embarked on catch-up industrialization and urbanization with the large-scale involvement of women in the labor force after 1945.[30] Moreover, this tendency fitted a general, global trend in fertility decline, which accompanied economic development in Western Europe and North America, and other regions of the so-called "first world" in the twentieth century.[31]

Reports produced by the Central Committee of the party in Hungary in the 1960s concerning the population question focused on the alarming decrease in birth rates. Part of the proposed incentives to increase birth rates addressed the regulation of abortion. A frequently named problem was the high number of abortions requested by and performed on young, single women, endangering their future fertility. By the mid-1960s, the strengthening of the preconditions for the performance of abortion was already on the

27 Decree 1047/1956 (VI.3.) of the Council of Ministers on the Regulation of Questions Related to the Termination of Pregnancies and the Punishment of Abortion, in *Törvények és rendeletek*, 1957.

28 From more than 123,300 registered pregnancy terminations in 1957, the number of abortions reached almost 207,000 in 1969. Ferenc Kamarás, "Terhességmegszakítások Magyarországon," Data archive of TÁRKI Social Research Institute, http://www.tarki.hu/adatbank-h/nok/szerepvalt/Kamaras-99.html [last accessed: April 24, 2017].

29 The birth rate fell by close to 100,000, that is by nearly 50 percent, between 1954 and 1962, from 23 births per 1,000 to 12.3, and fertility dropped below replacement level in the same period, decreasing from 3 to 1.8. Ferenc Kamarás, "Születési mozgalom és termékenység az elmúlt 125 évben,"*Statisztikai szemle* 74 (1996): 668.

30 Haney, *Inventing the Needy*, 92.

31 Melegh draws attention to the contradictory expectation by Hungarian demographers concerning fertility, namely that it would increase with economic development in a socialist society. Melegh, "Localising Global Hierarchies," 274–5.

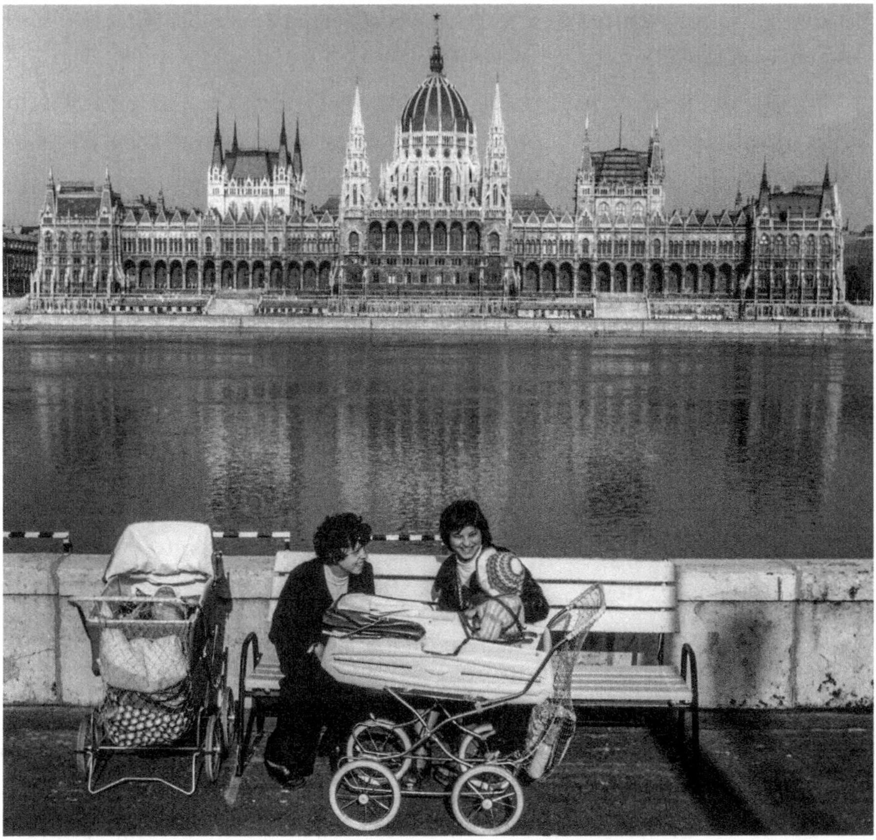

Figure 11.1: *Young mothers taking a rest; in the background the Hungarian Parliament* [Pihenő kismamák gyerekeikkel, háttérben a Parlament], Budapest, 1976. Photo by Albert Kozák, MTI, from The Photographic Collection of the Hungarian National Museum.

agenda of the Central Committee. Fearing public uproar, however, the Politburo refrained from tightening the preconditions for the performance of abortion until the early 1970s. In the meantime, in 1967 the government introduced a generous maternity benefit (GYES) that allowed mothers with a year of employment to receive the equivalent of their salary for six month and added to this a flat-rate grant for up to two more years.[32] In 1969, the grant was extended to up to three years. This measure spear-

32 Decree 3/1967 (I.29.) of the Ministry of Labor, in *Törvények és rendeletek* (Budapest: Közgazdasági és Jogi Könyvkiadó, 1968), 289. In other state-socialist countries, comparable maternity leave measures provided much shorter amounts of paid leave. See Haney, *Inventing the Needy*, 297.

headed a maternalist turn in welfare politics that was closely linked with pronatalist intentions.[33]

Finally, in an effort to increase birth rates, in 1973 the Council of Ministers introduced a decree that, besides a variety of welfare incentives supporting families with children, also entailed compulsory marriage counseling, the expansion of the institutional network of family and women protection counseling centers, and the restriction of the abortion decree of 1956.[34] Abortion committees gained in authority and agreed to requests only in cases where the pregnant women were above forty, they were single or separated, they (or their husband) did not own an apartment, they had had three or more births or had two live children and another obstetrical event, or the pregnancy was the result of a criminal act. This reproductive policy program also introduced the eugenic concept of "qualitative reproduction," which defined the desired number of children to be born into a Hungarian family at three, and emphasized the importance of giving birth to healthy children.[35]

In the 1980s, a final turn in the reproductive policy program of state-socialist Hungary was characterized by an openly selective pronatalist measure, in order to encourage the middle class to have more children. In 1985, the flat-rate GYES was amended by an income-differentiated child-care grant (GYED), following detailed analyses of GYES recipient patterns that showed that the maternity benefit was primarily used by working-class women in the lower-earning categories.[36] The introduction of GYED was in fact partly a response to an influential group of populist writers, pushing from the early 1970s onward for a "quality selection" in reproductive policy measures.[37] Public debate around the issue of birth rates and fertility in the early 1980s, however, contained clearly eugenic undertones, including the

33 In fact, the issue of the restriction of abortion was the subject of intense debate in the meetings of the Politburo in 1966. While agreeing that the legislation of 1956 was "too liberal," they also refrained from implementing restrictive legislation, such as those applied in Ceaușescu's Romania. The introduction of GYES came as a "compromise" pronatalist measure. For a detailed discussion of the introduction of GYES, see Inglot, Szikra, and Rat, "Continuity and Change," 26–8; and Haney, *Inventing the Needy*, 101–9.

34 Decree 1040/1973 (X.18.) of the Council of Ministers on Population Political Tasks, in *Törvények és rendeletek*, 1974.

35 On the larger global social-economic context of this turn in Hungarian reproductive politics in the 1970s, see Melegh, "Living to Ourselves," and *On the East/West Slope*.

36 Haney, *Inventing the Needy*, 177.

37 Ibid., 178; Inglot, Szikra, and Rat, "Continuity and Change," 31.

accusation that well-situated women were "on a birth strike" as well as occasional racist arguments regarding the Gypsy population.[38]

In numerous East and Southeast European countries with a substantial Romani population, this was the first time in the state-socialist period that the "Gypsy question" was addressed by a series of specifically targeted policy frameworks and actions, aiming at the improvement of their employment, educational, and housing conditions.[39] Importantly, the first party resolution on the situation of Roma in Hungary in 1961 declared the Gypsy population not an ethnic group, but a "backward social layer" to be assimilated into working-class Hungarian society.[40] In the second half of the eighteenth century, the Habsburg emperors Maria Theresa and Joseph II had attempted to assimilate Roma into the Hungarian peasantry by prohibiting them from traveling, wearing traditional clothes, and speaking their language, by putting pressure on Roma to take up certain occupations, as well as through the removal of Romani children from the care of their parents.[41] Following a lack of success, however, the Gypsy question largely remained a punitive, police, and administrative issue in the nineteenth and early twentieth centuries in the Monarchy and the interwar Hungarian state.[42] The persecution of Roma during the Second World War did not reach the same levels of organization, institutionalization, and execution as in Germany and Austria, but there were numerous advocates of the "final solution of the Gypsy question," including medical professionals using racialized eugenic arguments.[43] The state-socialist government initiated a clear break with the stigmatizing approach toward Roma characteristic of the previous political

38 Heller, Némedi, and Rényi, "Népesedési viták Magyarországon 1960–1986," 67–8, 172.

39 Apor, "Cigányok tere: Kísérlet a kommunista romapolitika közép-kelet-európai összehasonlító elemzésére, 1945–1961." In some countries (Hungary, Czechoslovakia, Bulgaria, or Romania), there were a series of specific policies targeted at "the Gypsy population," while in other state-socialist countries (Yugoslavia and, with the exception of a decree on compulsory sedentarization, Poland), the assimilation of Roma was foreseen to take place through policies aimed at the whole population.

40 Stewart, "Communist Roma Policy, 1945–1989 as Seen through the Hungarian Case," in *Between Past and Future: The Roma of Central and Eastern Europe*; Majtényi and Majtényi, *A Contemporary History of Exclusion: The Roma Issue in Hungary from 1945 to 2015*; "Tasks Related to the Improvement of the Situation of the Gypsy Population," Decree by the Politburo of the Hungarian Socialist Workers' Party's Central Committee, June 20, 1961, in *A magyarországi cigánykérdés dokumentumokban, 1422–1985*, ed. Barna Mezey (Budapest: Kossuth, 1986), 240–2.

41 Barany, *The East European Gypsies: Regime Change, Marginality, and Ethnopolitics*, 93–4.

42 Pomogyi, *Cigánykérdés és cigányügyi igazgatás a polgári Magyarországon.*

43 Gyula Purcsi Barna, *A cigánykérdés "gyökeres és végleges megoldása": Tanulmányok a XX. századi "cigánykérdés" történetéből* (Debrecen: Csokonai Kiadó, 2004).

regime. The practical realization of policies that were meant to improve the situation of Roma, however, was affected by the prewar and wartime habits of thinking about "the Gypsies." Two characteristic examples were the introduction of separate color identification cards for Roma between 1953 and 1961, in order to identify the "work shy" endangering Hungarian society, and, in the field of healthcare, the continued practice of forced bathing, carried out with support of the police by local medical staff between the 1940s and the 1980s.[44] The discourses and practices related to the issue of birth rates and reproduction between the second half of the 1950s and the 1980s in Hungary discussed below, provide examples of the continuation of eugenic thought and practices as well as the stigmatization and at times racial othering of Roma in the state-socialist context.

Abortions in the 1960s: Too Many and Not Enough

Following the legalization of abortion in 1956 and throughout the 1960s, there was mounting concern among medical professionals and policy makers about the falling birth rates in Hungary. This concern, however, was selective in terms of gender, class, and ethnicity. A problem that physicians who protested against the legalization of abortion in 1956 frequently named was the high number of abortions requested by and performed on young, single, well-situated women. In Békés County in Southeast Hungary, for example, several physicians and hospitals denied the performance of abortion with reference to a lack of personnel and adequate conditions to carry out the sudden increase in abortion requests. They drew attention to the dramatic increase in the number of abortions, especially among women without children or with two or less children. The lead physician of Békés County went as far as issuing a decree to all regional and municipal physicians of the county in November 1956 to restrict consent to abortion requests. Contrary to the content of the decree of 1956, which placed the fi-

44 Ibid., and Gábor Bernáth (ed.), *Kényszermosdatások a cigánytelepeken, 1940–1985* (Budapest: Roma Sajtóközpont, 2002). Roma, especially so-called "wandering Gypsies," accused of spreading epidemics such as typhus were exposed to forced bathing when such epidemics broke out during the interwar period. This practice continued during and following the Second World War into the state-socialist period, when it was regularly used by local authorities to implement hygienic measures, including delousing. Gypsy settlements were surrounded by police forces, and people were not only obliged to take a bath in the mobile bath wagons transported to site, but also, as part of delousing, all their body hair was cut. Toxic chemical powders, such as DDT, were also used well into the 1960s.

nal decision with the women who filed an abortion request, the presidents of abortion committees in the county were to consent to abortion only in case of health endangerment of the mother or on so-called social grounds, to be testified by the local social secretary and district nurse. The underlying nation-based argumentation that characterized the resistance of physicians to the new abortion decree manifested in a discussion by the leading medical and social professionals of the county in early 1957. Dr. Károly Magyar, director of the maternal clinic of the town of Szarvas, claimed that the decree of 1956 "violated the interests of the Hungarian nation."[45] Several doctors refused to carry out abortions, and emphasized that the decree was opposed to the "Hungarian position" and "foreign to the interests of the nation" when it allowed women to decide whether or not they wanted an abortion: "What would happen when the male members of society were to decide themselves whether they went down to the mines or not, stood by the workbench or not, entered the military or not, offered their life to their country or not? Women undoubtedly suffer much during childbirth ([but] have much joy in their children later), but they owe this to society," stated Dr. Balázs Szendi, county district lead obstetrician.[46] He formulated his concerns, when he opposed the decree in a clearly gendered framework, because it allowed women to disregard their obligations as vessels of the nation.

When obstetricians, social secretaries, and district nurses urged a tightening of the preconditions for the performance of abortions, fearing a dramatic drop in birth rates, they were especially critical about the refusal of young women to give birth, as their financial conditions, they argued, were not bad: "Women in a difficult social situation need to be helped, especially when they already have three children. But when they simply say, 'I will not carry out my pregnancy, because I want to buy kitchen furniture,' or 'It is uncomfortable and my belly loses its shape,' this is unacceptable as a ground. This is appalling," argued Dr. Szendi. Professionals also claimed that women living in cities with less than three children were requesting more abortions than women in the countryside: "It is usually not the mothers with many children who request an abortion but those who are lazy and

45 Minutes of the meeting of the Health Department of the Central Committee of Council of Békés County, January 7, 1957, Hungarian National Archives (MOL), XIX-C-2-d. 16.d. 1957.

46 Ibid.

the well-situated."[47] In order to keep the so-called "comfort category" of young women from terminating their pregnancies, the county lead physician recommended a national policy amendment in line with the practice he had introduced at county level to the Ministry of Health in 1957.[48]

Documents produced at the local level also reveal the ethnically selective nature of pronatalism in state-socialist Hungary. At the same time as medical and social professionals worried about decreasing birth rates among young, well-to-do women, they also expressed their dissatisfaction with the fact that "Gypsies" and "those with a reduced mental capacity" were not requesting abortions. This kind of language was not unusual. The social referent of Orosháza, for example, stated: "Gypsies and the degenerate did not request the termination of their pregnancies." This comment is an example of the casual use of a racialized eugenic vocabulary in this period that recalled widespread racial hygienic concerns during the 1930s and the Second World War about social groups who were not to reproduce.[49] The argument that the increasing fertility rate of Roma composed a threat and a burden to the state was an element of the prewar and wartime eugenic discourse in relation to the Gypsy population in Hungary. Identifying "Gypsyness" with "work-shyness," advocates of this position warned against the growing number of unproductive members of the population and the spreading of the "unproductive gene" that, especially in the case of intermarriage between Gypsy and non-Gypsy, composed a eugenic threat in the form of national degeneration.

Concern about the increasing number of children born into Romani families and the perception of this phenomenon as a burden on the state reappeared in the state-socialist context. It formed part of an antinatalist argument directed at Roma that manifested not only in local discussions, but was also formulated in the Ministry of Health in the early 1960s. While raising attention to the alarming trends in decreasing birth rates among the majority population, the Ministry of Health requested doctors to propagate abortion free of charge as a means of fertility control among Romani women.[50] The ministerial directive followed one of the investigations regarding

47 Ibid.

48 The ministry rejected the proposal.

49 Minutes, MOL, XIX-C-2-d. 16.d. 1957.

50 Directive 94.662/1962 by the Ministry of Health on the improvement of the situation of the Gypsy population, MOL, XIX-C-2-i 20.d. 1963.

the "situation of the Gypsy population" conducted by the Hungarian Socialist Workers' Party in 1962.[51] The party referent in charge of the investigation informed the ministry that the "question of abortion" needed special attention with regard to "families with many children." Based on local-level information emerging from the results of the investigation in Heves County in northeast Hungary, the party referent stated that there were families with five to six or "even ten children," who lived in extreme poverty. Equating such families with Romani families, he established that "due to fear, most Gypsy women did not consult abortion committees to terminate their pregnancies." His policy recommendation to the ministry encouraged the more widespread application of abortion among poor women, and especially Romani women with many children, as a form of birth control. Accordingly, women who due to financial reasons did not make use of abortion to terminate their pregnancies were to have abortions free of charge or receive financial support to cover the fee. As a result, in the summer of 1962, the Mother, Infant, and Child Protection Department, in consultation with the Social Policy Department of the Ministry of Health, issued a directive instructing all county- and city-level lead physicians to intensify the education of the Gypsy population concerning "the rights secured by the decree of 1956" that legalized abortion.[52] Physicians were to ensure that the Gypsy population was well informed about abortion.

The directive identified the continuous increase in the birth rate and the high fertility rate of Roma (in comparison to the majority Hungarians) as a burden on the state:

> Women living in Gypsy settlements did not make use of their right to abortion and gave birth to a child each year. They could not support these children, who survived only as a result of social provisions. Gypsy women were partly afraid of and partly could not cover the costs of an abortion. As a result, it was not uncommon that Gypsy families had five, six, or even more children. A new child in such families was a further burden on parents already living in difficult circumstances.[53]

51 "A Note to Comrade Simonovits." Letter by Zoltán Vadas, Head of the Mother, Infant and Child Protection Department of the Ministry of Health, to István Simonovits, Deputy Minister of Health, June 19, 1962. MOL, XIX-C-2-i 20.d. 1963.

52 Directive 94.662/1962, MOL, XIX-C-2-i 20.d. 1963.

53 Ibid.

Besides intensifying the spread of information about abortion among Roma, the directive also requested "the immediate remission" of abortion-related fees "in case Gypsy women refused to have an abortion, because they were unable to cover the costs."[54]

An inquiry from a county head physician in 1963 to the Ministry of Health regarding the application of the directive furthermore suggests that while abortion also emerged as a birth control method among non-Gypsy mothers in poor social conditions, "families with many children" in practice were equated with Gypsy families.[55] The physician addressed the ministry with the question whether "non-Gypsy mothers in similar or even worse social conditions than Gypsy mothers" were also covered by the directive and could have abortions free of charge, claiming that "the present practice often disadvantaged non-Gypsy mothers."[56] The referent in charge at the ministry gave a positive answer and stated that there was no regulation in place that discriminated between Gypsy and non-Gypsy patients with regard to the costs of their hospital treatment. This exchange reveals that while the directive was intended to decrease birth among all those considered to be unable to support their children and thus a burden on the state, in daily medical practice the inability to provide for their family and the burdensome increase of birth was associated with Gypsyness. In other words, despite the intention of policy makers in everyday practice, the social category of poverty was ethnicized.

These documents represent the selective nature of pronatalism in state-socialist Hungary, which guaranteed the exclusion of those considered to be a burden on the state by not being able to take financial responsibility for their children. The ministerial directive, however, also reveals that by the early 1960s, when the "Gypsy question" was addressed at a national level by special policies, it was largely conceived of as a problem of reproductive control. The antinatalist recommendation of the directive specifically targeted Gypsy women with many children, in an otherwise critical context concerned with anti-Gypsyism and the resulting disadvantages suffered by the Gypsy population in the field of health. The regularly conducted surveys

54 Ibid.

55 "The remission of abortion-related costs." Letter of inquiry from the Health Department of the Executive Committee of the Council of Fejér County to the Ministry of Health, April 19, 1963. MOL, XIX-C-2-i 20.d. 1963.

56 Ibid.

and resulting reports about the situation of the Gypsy population since 1961 assessed the improvements as well as the failures in the living, employment, health, and educational-cultural conditions of Roma. The new directive, resulting from an earlier survey, followed a similar pattern when it concluded that it was a problem that in several localities in the country, Gypsy children were left out of compulsory vaccination and health-education initiatives. The directive urged physicians to improve the health conditions (especially the supply of clean water) at Gypsy settlements. It also criticized the fact that Gypsy women were often excluded from the gift-set of baby clothes provided to mothers of newborns in Hungary since the early 1950s, and that healthcare provision for the inhabitants of Gypsy settlements was unsatisfactory. Regarding the protection of mothers and children, the directive nevertheless established that Gypsy women did not have enough abortions and gave birth to too many children. This approach by policy makers in the Ministry of Health implies that improving the situation of Roma in state-socialist Hungary was, from the very beginning, coupled with the idea of reducing the size of the Romani population.

This idea was, however, not unique to the state-socialist context or to Hungary. The belief that reducing the birth rate among Roma would contribute to an improvement of their living standards shows parallels with the philosophy behind post-1945 international reproductive politics in relation to the size of the population in the global "Third World." Specifically, as Betsy Hartmann has pointed out, intervention by population organizations and international aid agencies in Asia, Latin America, and Africa, "as well as among ethnic minorities and poor communities in many parts of the industrialized world," was motivated by the assumption that population growth was the primary cause of problems, such as poverty, hunger, economic stagnation, and political instability in these regions and among these population groups.[57] Similar motivations and the goal to improve population quality lay behind the introduction of the one-child policy in state-socialist China in 1978.[58] These Western organizations and leaderships promoted birth control and tried to persuade as well as force the populations in question to give birth to fewer children, without trying to improve their economic and social conditions.

57 Hartmann, *Reproductive Rights and Wrongs: The Global Politics of Population Control*, xix.

58 Anagnost, "A Surfeit of Bodies: Population and the Rationality of the State in Post-Mao China."

Hartmann drew attention to the fundamental flaws behind this philosophy, rooted in a Malthusian orthodoxy about the threats of global overpopulation coupled with Western ethnocentrism. Applied selectively to the poor of the Third World and ethnic minorities in the West, this philosophy left unaddressed the role of industrialized countries in contributing to poverty and low productivity. Since the early twentieth century, Western middle-class fears of high fertility rates among the poor, whose expanding numbers they perceived as threatening to their own well-being, have mixed with eugenic and racially differentiated discourses, policies, and practices in the United States and Europe. In the United States, for example, blaming "racially subordinate groups" for threatening quality population development resulted, for example, in the use of sterilization as a birth control measure among African-American women as late as the 1970s.[59] Concerning state-socialist Hungary, Attila Melegh has shown that with the gradual dismantling of the country's welfare system, beginning with the economic crisis in the 1970s, the idea of "supporting only 'quality' population" strengthened. In what follows, I will show that the introduction of the concept of qualitative reproduction in 1973 contributed to an increasing identification of Gypsies, and the fertility of Gypsy women, with poor quality reproduction and "unwanted birth."

Qualitative Reproduction and Controlling "Unwanted Birth" in the 1970s and the 1980s

In 1973, Hungary's reproductive policy program introduced the concept of "qualitative" reproduction, which entailed the improvement of perinatal care in order to "secure the birth of healthy infants." As a result, emphasis in both national and local-level practices shifted to the propagation of health education and conscious family planning. In fact, family planning and healthy birth aimed at an increase of the number of healthy children born into educated, better-to-do Hungarian families, in order to reach an average family size of three children. One of the leading representatives of the qualitative reproduction program, the geneticist Endre Czeizel, formulated it as follows:

59 Melegh, *On the East/West Slope*, 53–5. On the connection between race and reproductive politics in the USA, see, among many others, Roberts, *Killing the Black Body: Race, Reproduction and the Meaning of Liberty*.

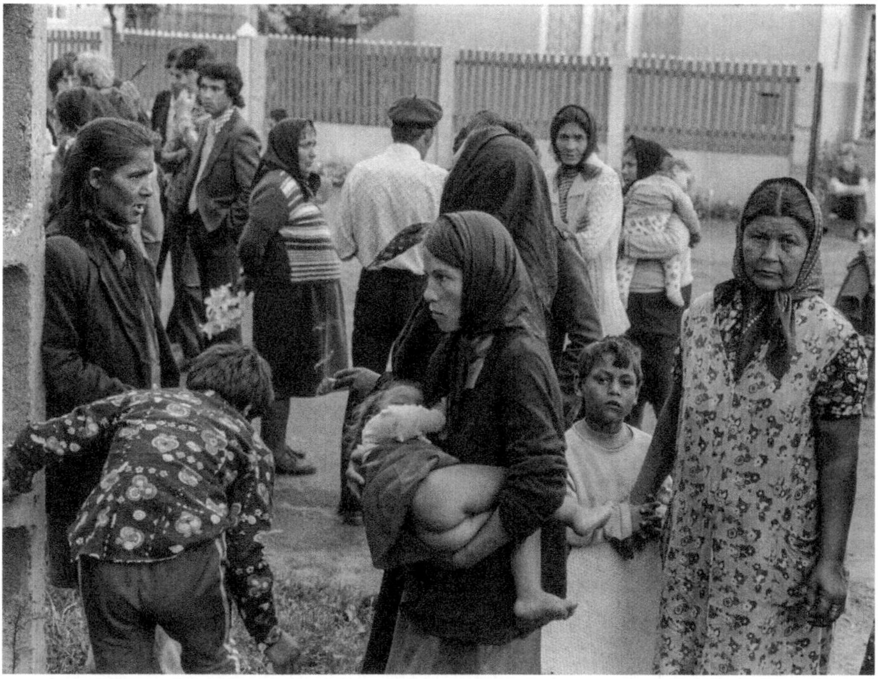

Figure 11.2: *Gypsies at Nyírlugos* [Cigányok Nyírlugoson], 1987. Photo by Gábor Demszky, The Photographic Collection of the Hungarian National Museum.

The relationship between the number of children born into a family and the educational status of the mother reveals serious shortcomings in our family planning. Three and more children are primarily born into families where the mother has not completed her primary school education, in other words to mothers having a worse economic and social background. Despite substantial social support, the per capita income in such families is too low, which seriously hinders the development of the child's talents. Our goal is to reach an equilibrium in family planning, which means that families with a better educational background and from average and better-to-do families, who form the majority of our society, would be ready to have two to four children, while less-educated families having a lower standard of living would make use of modern contraceptive methods and above a certain number of children would responsibly regulate the birth of their children.[60]

60 Endre Czeizel, *A gyermekvárás felelőssége: Képes útmutató családtervezéshez* (Budapest: Medicina Kiadó, 1977).

The program was thus explicitly eugenic in character, as the regulation of birth and fertility rates reflected a biopolitics in which the economic and social background of families was equated with the healthy development of children and in consequence a healthier society.

As a variety of health and health-education related documents and publications of representatives of local councils, the Coordination Committee for Gypsy Affairs, Red Cross activists, and medical professionals demonstrate, the translation of the policy program into practice with regard to Romani families meant the propagation of the use of contraceptives to decrease birth rates on eugenic grounds. Reproductive practices in the 1970s and 1980s reinforced an equation of Gypsyness with a disadvantaged economic and social context, endangering the healthy development of Hungarian society. A recurrent subject was the demographic situation of the Gypsy population, emphasizing the continuous growth in the number of births and family size. In its 1969 report the Coordination Committee of Szabolcs-Szatmár County stated that 12.9 percent of live births "were Gypsies."[61] It added that in the past five years, this figure had grown: "We note that the size of the Gypsy population of the county is constantly growing, and contrary to official figures, their number is around 32,000, making up six percent of the county's total population." The report expressed concern about the growing size of the Gypsy population, their living conditions, as well as the ensuing social-political questions, including the fact that "one-third of social welfare payments were given to Gypsies." In her 1979 report to the department on family politics at the Ministry of Labor, the national secretary of the Coordination Committee for Gypsy Affairs drew attention to the larger average family size of "Gypsy families" as compared to "Hungarian families."[62] While one- and two-member households made up 40 percent of "Hungarian households," they only made up 20 percent of "Gypsy households." However, five-member and larger households made up about 15 percent of the total Hungarian households, while among Gypsy households this was 37 percent. The report concluded with the "happy fact" that increasing urbanization and changes in lifestyle led to a fall in the birth rate "among Gypsies, too."

61 "Information report on the situation of the Gypsy population," July 16, 1969, MOL, XIX-A-28.f. 8.d.

62 Documents of the Coordination Committee for Gypsy Affairs in Szabolcs-Szatmár County. MOL, XIX-A-28.f.8.d.

In the case of Roma, conscious family planning translated in a decrease in family size and the number of births. A decree proposed by the City Council of Mátészalka in northeastern Hungary in 1977 emphasized the importance of health education among the Gypsy population, especially regarding "conscious family planning and appropriate lifestyle that characterized the socialist type of person."[63] The social referent of Szabolcs-Szatmár County claimed that "conscious family planning" and continuous health education brought about good results: "The use of modern contraceptives was spreading (40 to 48 percent) among families with many children. As a result the number of births fell."[64] A report from the Council of Nagyecsed, a small town in Szabolcs-Szatmár County, stated that mother and infant protection and "the realization of conscious family planning required great efforts from medical professionals." They provided monthly health education seminars, but most effective, they said, were individual conversations. "Unfortunately, these did not bring about expected results either. While the number of births slowly decreased in comparison to the Hungarian population, it was still higher than ten years ago."[65] The Szabolcs-Szatmár County division of the Hungarian Red Cross reported to the national directorate about their activities among the Gypsy population in 1975, devoting special attention to family planning and the prevention of "unwanted birth." Red Cross voluntary activists helped the local health services in directing women's attention to the prevention of unwanted birth. Health education among pregnant Gypsy women carried out by the physicians and medical professionals of maternity clinics had the "utmost importance," the report stated.[66]

The notion of a high number of births among the Gypsy population as a burden on the state remained a central part of antinatalist practices in the framework of family planning and health education directed at Roma.

63 "Decree proposal: Decree by the Central Committee of the City Council of Mátészalka on the execution of decrees related to the improvement of the conditions of the Gypsy population, September 23, 1977." MOL, XIX-A-28.f. 8.d.

64 "Report about the situation of the Gypsy population in the county and the execution of the tasks for the year of 1978," György Miklovich, referent for social policy, April 17, 1979. MOL, XIX-A-28.f. 8.d.

65 "Report about the effect of the party and government decrees and local measures in the interest of backward social groups on the integration of the Gypsy population, changes in their family structure and relations to other social layers," by the president of the Council of Nagyecsed, March 31 1979. MOL, XIX-A-28.f. 8.d.

66 "Report by the directorate of the Hungarian Red Cross in Szabolcs-Szatmár County about the situation of the Gypsy population and the methods and opportunities for their health education," February 28, 1975. MOL, P2130 282.d. 124.t.

The vice president of the City Council of Mátészalka presented his concern about the increasing birth rate among the Gypsy population in 1977 to the county council, claiming that "the largest problem" was the increase in the number of families with six or seven and not infrequently ten children.[67] An "even more serious problem" was that there were three, four, or more children in such families, too, where both parents were unemployed and "lived only from social welfare benefits," without entitlement to family support. The report concluded that "regular and continuous health education concerning family planning and the prevention of unwanted birth should therefore become a central part of healthcare. The goal should be to have in each family only as many children as parents could support without difficulties." Red Cross activists took part in propagating family planning and contraceptive devices among Roma across the country. A report from Borsod-Abaúj-Zemplén County in northeast Hungary drew similar conclusions about the goal of family planning, stating that the assumption that "all Gyspy families had many children was false":

> Regarding the average family size, especially concerning the future, we have the following fundamental statement: "Among families at a higher cultural niveau, it can sometimes already be observed, that they give birth to as many children as they can support in normal and acceptable conditions. Furthermore, an increasing number of women ask for the termination of their pregnancies, even in case of a first-time pregnancy! [sic] A substantial number of women, especially young women, demand Infecundin, while elder women with many children demand intrauterine contraceptives." In Borsod County the percentage of these women is up to 30 percent of all women of childbearing age.[68]

Such a comment on the termination of a first-time pregnancy is especially striking because in the case of non-Romani women, physicians warned against the danger of infertility in relation to pregnancy termination, and this argument formed one of the backbones of debates around the renewed restriction of abortion.

67 "Report to the Executive Committee about the execution of the decrees concerning the improvement of the living conditions of the Gypsy population," Lajos Kövendy, vice president of the City Council of Mátészalka, September 12, 1977. MOL, XIX-A-28.f. 8.d.

68 Untitled excerpt from a report from Borsod-Abaúj-Zemplén County, n.d. MOL, XIX-A-28.f. 3.d. Infecundin was an oral contraceptive produced in Hungary from 1967.

Antinatalism directed at Roma furthermore included direct interventionist measures. As in the 1960s, local authorities not only propagated the use of contraceptives among Roma, but also introduced special differentiated measures by making them free of charge for "Gypsy mothers," in order to decrease the number of "Gypsy births." The district general practitioner, a gynecologist in the small town of Nagyecsed, served as an exemplary case in a Red Cross report on their activities among the Gypsy population in Szabolcs-Szatmár County. He provided free pregnancy screenings for Gypsy women on a weekly basis to "filter out those unwanted pregnancies, where the necessary conditions for the raising of a further child were not available."[69] Furthermore, as part of an organized medical action plan, the council provided free oral contraceptives to Gypsy mothers who were not covered by the state-provided social insurance.[70] After a countywide investigation, the Coordination Committee of Szabolcs-Szatmár County called the decrease in Gypsy births "an outstandingly successful outcome,"[71] attributing it to their "enormous efforts" to "increase the more widespread availability and use of contraceptives." The council went as far as financing these efforts from its own budget: "We provided 50,000 forints' worth of free contraceptives to Gypsy mothers. At the same time, the use of intrauterine devices was spreading. It was welcome news that the number of Gypsy women using the pregnancy counseling services and health-education seminars was steadily growing."[72]

Meanwhile, medical professionals reinforced the association between low mental capacity and the "primitivism" of Roma. For example, the Red Cross report of 1975 stressed the importance of the spread of intrauterine contraceptives among Romani women by claiming that they were incapable of taking the pill regularly: "Experience showed that oral contraceptives were not always applicable in their case, because they were unreliable and did not take the medicament on a regular basis."[73] A 1979 report from

69 "Report by the directorate of the Hungarian Red Cross in Szabolcs-Szatmár County about the situation of the Gypsy population and the methods and opportunities for their health education," February 28, 1975. MOL, P2130 282.d. 124.t.

70 Social insurance was tied to employment. This reference means not only that that these women had no access to free health-care services, but also that they were unemployed.

71 "Report on the results of the improvement of the situation and integration of the Gypsy population," March 15, 1976. MOL, XIX-A-28.f. 8.d.

72 Ibid.

73 "Report by the directorate of the Hungarian Red Cross in Szabolcs-Szatmár County." MOL, P2130

Szabolcs-Szatmár County described that family protection, one of the main tasks of the Red Cross, was especially difficult among Gypsies. "Since their knowledge about food and cooking and their habits are very primitive, our activists provide them with useful advice in this terrain as well as in budgeting their income and planning family life. The results of the latter are tangible from the increase in the number of Gypsy women, who used contraceptives to prevent unwanted pregnancy and attended family counseling."[74]

Medical journals also contributed to the stigmatization and at times racialization of the fertility and health practices of Roma. Based on a survey conducted on birth control practices among "an especially backward and uncultured layer among the Gypsies," one article claimed that there was no relationship between the number of planned and actual pregnancies among mothers from this group.[75] The authors argued that this phenomenon had to do either with "certain characteristics (habits, superstitions)" of the mothers or "with such a degree of primitivism that [made] the existence of individual will unrealistic." They agreed on "the elemental force of increasing family size affecting [this] primitive population."[76] Another article described Roma as people "living at a lower form of social organization, characterized by a short increase in tolerance and activity levels followed by a longer downward period."[77] The author claimed that "an inability for regular life was typical of population groups whose socialization did not meet the requirements of developed societies and humanized living, where there was no need any more for the sudden mobilization of psychological forces (to fight in case of danger) and only rarely was a there a chance for complete relaxation."[78] A physician from a public health and epidemic station in western Hungary went as far as defining "Gypsyness" as belonging to "a layer in society whose traditions, lifestyle, and values differed at times extremely and in a negative direction from those of the majority."[79] While advocating

282.d. 124.t. Intrauterine devices were preferred by physicians because they assured long-term birth control, releasing hormones directly into the uterus without having to rely on the women in question.

74 "Red Cross activism among the Gypsy population and the backward social layers," May 21, 1979. MOL, P2130 282.d. 126.t.

75 Dr. György Seregély, Dr. Miksa Almásy and Ildikó Höffner, "Elmaradott lakosságcsoport magatartása a születésszabályozás terén," *Egészségügyi felvilágosítás* 8 (1967).

76 Ibid., 112.

77 Attila Elekes, "Egészségnevelés a cigánylakosság körében," *Egészségügyi felvilágosítás* 16 (1975).

78 Ibid., 153–4.

79 Pál Kneffel, "Cigánytelepeink higiénés helyzete és az egészségnevelés," *Egészségügyi felvilágosítás* 16 (1975).

the necessity of education to improve the hygienic conditions in Gypsy settlements, the author urged the collection of "objective" information on the "genetic features" of Gypsy children, suggesting a "biological foundation" behind the difficulties of Gypsies to assimilate.[80] Rejecting the accusation of discrimination, the author also recommended the use of "healthy coercion" in order to force Gypsies living in "shabby-house conditions" to work, and the use of police force to carry out hygienic measures, such as delousing. This vocabulary is reminiscent of the discourse applied by medical professionals on the "[final] solution of the Gypsy question" in Hungary during the Second World War.

Finally, the eugenic character of the reproductive politics of the 1970s and 1980s was also reflected in the formulation of antinatalism directed at Romani mothers and children as a measure of health improvement. Health education, pregnancy counseling, and contraceptives were not only to lead directly to a decreasing birth rate among Roma, but the elimination of "too early, too late, and too frequent" birth among Roma was to contribute to a healthier society. Proposals formulated by the vice president of the Council of Szabolcs-Szatmár County regarding the improvement of the situation of the Gypsy population in 1973 and 1974 urged for "measures as a result of which the number of [Gypsy] women giving birth under the age of eighteen" would decrease: "We find that a very high percentage of Gypsy women become pregnant under eighteen, a phenomenon that is definitely harmful." The report gave exact percentages for the regions with the highest birth rate for under eighteens among Roma.[81] Physicians also provided their own research data to prove that premature birth, likely to lead to children's physical and mental disability, was overrepresented among the Gypsy population, putting it in direct relation with the "too early, too late and too frequent" pregnancies of Gypsy women. Among the causes, some listed women's irresponsibility and lack of mental capacity to control their pregnancies.

A brochure published for Red Cross activists in 1986 exemplifies several of the above-mentioned elements of the eugenic reproductive politics of the 1970s and the 1980s.[82] Aiming at the health education of Roma,

---

80 Ibid., 250.

81 "Proposal to the Executive Committee about the situation of the Gypsy population and future tasks," from the vice president of the Council of Szabolcs-Szatmár County, 1973. MOL, XIX-A-28.f. 8.d.

82 Dr. Lajos Gaál, *Útmutató a cigánycsaládokat gondozó Vöröskeresztes aktivisták részére* (Budapest: Magyar Vöröskereszt OVB és a Cigány Koordinációs Bizottság, 1986).

it connected antinatalism with improving the health conditions and securing the good health of the future generations of Romani children. The brochure was a joint publication of the Red Cross and the Coordination Committee for Gypsy Affairs, bearing the subtitle *For the Health of Our Children.* Written by a physician who published extensively on the Gypsy question in medical journals, it addressed its imagined readership both in Hungarian and Romani. Turning to Romani parents as a friendly advisor, Dr. Gaál emphasized their personal responsibility in having a healthy family. "Remember," he called out to parents, "what kind of shanty houses you lived in just a couple of years ago, and you did not attend to your health and cared badly for your infants."[83] Concerning pregnancy and the care of newborn babies, Dr. Gaál warned that after giving birth women were to wait at least a year before getting pregnant again, otherwise the birth weight of the next child would be low. He also drew attention to contraceptives that allowed women to have "desired pregnancies." The brochure advised Romani women about the relationship between personal hygiene and a healthy child: "Living in bad conditions, drinking alcohol, smoking, and having an unsatisfactory diet" during pregnancy, it said, frequently led to miscarriage or premature, underweight children with an increased risk of infant mortality.[84] Premature children often had a physical or mental disability, and ended up in special schools. Infants not only needed a separate bed, but also had to be washed daily. "Clean infants were not only healthier but also more beautiful," claimed the booklet, showing the picture of a smiling baby dressed in white.[85] Accompanied by photos that juxtaposed a bad (dirty, unclean, unhealthy) living environment and behavior with an exemplary one (clean, hygienic, and healthy), a section bearing the title "In the Interest of Our Children" contrasted a picture of a Romani family with five and another with two children.[86]

The first photo, showing the family from a distance, stated that "It was difficult to support such a large family," while the second, depicting two smiling parents from up close, was titled: "In the interest of our children."[87] The accompanying text in Romani and Hungarian listed a number of ways

83 Ibid., 2.

84 Ibid., 40.

85 Ibid., 42.

86 See acknowledgement in footnote 1 in this article.

87 Ibid., 48–9.

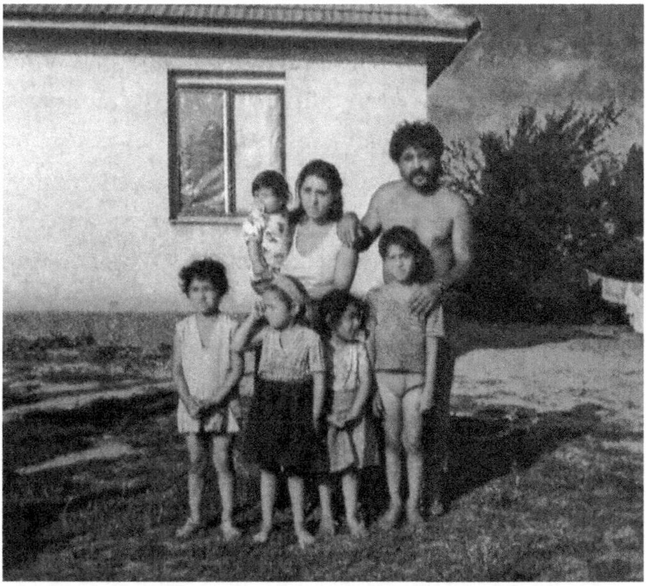

Figure 11.3: *It is difficult to support such a large family* [Az ilyen nagy családot nehéz eltartani. Kászávé báré csáládosz phároj té linkrén]. Photo by Lajos Gaál. In: Lajos Gaál, *Útmutató a cigánycsaládokat gondozó Vöröskeresztes aktivisták részére* (Budapest: Magyar Vöröskereszt OVB és a Cigány Koordinációs Bizottság, 1986), 48.

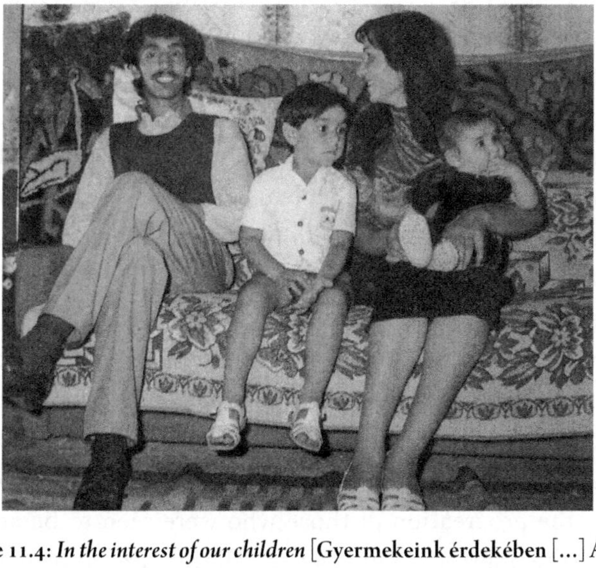

Figure 11.4: *In the interest of our children* [Gyermekeink érdekében [...] Ámáré sávoréngé szásztyipészté]. Photo by Lajos Gaál. In: Lajos Gaál, *Útmutató a cigánycsaládokat gondozó Vöröskeresztes aktivisták részére* (Budapest: Magyar Vöröskereszt OVB és a Cigány Koordinációs Bizottság, 1986), 49.

in which parents could ensure a better future for their children. Besides the importance of being employed and providing a good parental example of cleanliness, it also explicitly referred to having a large family as financially problematic: "It is not hard to calculate that it is easier to support a four- or five-member family than to provide food for six or seven hungry mouths."[88] The final sentences used the first person plural to express an earnest desire for change in the interest of the young generation: "While retaining *our* nice traditions (singing, dancing, music, and mother tongue) *we* must alter *our* lives so that the world of shanty housing remains only a bad memory." Placing the responsibility for better living and the better future of Romani children with their parents, the brochure clearly delineated the responsibility of Romani women in the field of family planning. When they wanted to secure a healthy future for their children, Romani women were to give birth to no more than two or three children.

Conclusion

This article examined state interference into population and individual health through an analysis of reproductive discourses, policy making, and practices in Hungary between the 1950s and the 1980s. While state socialism has been overwhelmingly conceived of in terms of a rupture in relation to political, economic, and social structures, a focus on the regulation of reproduction—constituting a central element of the building of public health—revealed specific continuities. Following the legalization of abortion in 1956, eugenic discourses that had been widespread in interwar Eastern and Southeastern Europe, including the racial hygienic vocabulary in use during the Second World War, reappeared. Representatives in the field of medicine and public health advocated a selective form of pronatalism that was directed at increasing the birth rate among educated and better-to-do women, while women with less fortunate educational and economic backgrounds were targeted by antinatalist discourses and practices. This reflected eugenic efforts to improve the collective health of the population by encouraging the procreation of those who were seen to be able to secure the birth and the upbringing of healthy children. From the early 1970s on-

88 Ibid., 48.

ward, it constituted the reproductive policy program of the state under the heading "qualitative reproduction." Medical professionals were important agents in this arena, involved in the popularization and execution of eugenic ideas at the national and local level. A comparison of these two levels reveals discrepancies between policies, such as the access to abortion, and their practical implementation. At the same time, it highlights the centrality of public health and its representatives in shaping mechanisms of social inclusion and exclusion in a state-socialist society. Eugenically selective pronatalism was connected to the shaping of the "Gypsy question" in state-socialist Hungary. This happened through the frequent, automatic equation of Gypsyness with the inability of Gypsies to provide for their children. The reproduction and "constantly growing size" of those defined as Gypsies was in turn considered a burden on the state and a danger to the "quality" of the population. Furthermore, while generally supporting the need to educate Roma in the field of health and hygienic practices as a way toward improving their health status, medical professionals also voiced their belief in the inborn negative characteristics of Gypsies, hindering this process.

CHAPTER XII

Underimplementing the Law: Social Work, Bureaucratic Error, and the Politics of Distribution in Postsocialist Serbia

Andre Thiemann

In late summer 2013, at noontime, an old Lada Niva wound its way through the Central Serbian countryside. Inside the hot and creaky chassis, the driver, Bogdan,[1] regaled his passengers with stories about "social cases" living along the road. Bogdan (born in 1950), who lived in a neighboring village, worked for the area's Center for Social Work (CSW) since 1997. Next to him sat the psychologist Siniša (born in 1974), an urbanite from Moravac. Siniša, who was in his sixth year of temporary employment at the CSW, listened with a mixture of interest and amusement. During the more imaginative passages of Bogdan's talk, Siniša turned around, winked at me, and smiled. He had indicated earlier that the driver was a good source of gossip about the people cared for by the CSW. Important for the subsequent discussion of bureaucratic error, Bogdan told us the open secret that the Milović family, to whom we were headed, lived quite decently from selling dried mushrooms and wild herbs in Moravac.

We arrived in the center of Gornje Selo and parked near the location of the local council (*mesna zajednica*), opposite the recently whitewashed Stari Voćar building,[2] the home of the Milović family. "Ah, that [whitewash-

1 Toponyms and personal names have been anonymized to guarantee the confidentiality of my informants. Exceptions pertain to interviews with fellow social scientists. Translations from Serbian are mine.

2 "Stari Voćar" means "Old Fruit-Grower." The spacious, two-story building was made of dressed granite. Defunct for two decades, it was draughty and the roof leaked. Until the 1990s, the fruit-growing sec-

ing] has been done for the recent Rakijada [yearly show of fruit brandies] by the local council," assumed Siniša. As we stepped into the sun, Siniša exclaimed: "See, what fresh air they have up here?!" Rajko Milović (born in 1951), wearing jeans and a faded red baseball cap, awaited us at the gate and asked us in. There were cold firesides in the courtyard; the rest was tilled with paprika plants. Bogdan stayed outside, while Rajko, Siniša, and I climbed up the external staircase. There was no handrail, and one stone was loose. The small patio/kitchen was a bit foul smelling and not very neat, but freshly washed grapes lay on a clean plate. Rajko was quick to tell Siniša that there was enough food in their home, revealing a big sack of flour. We went into the living room, where Ranko (born in 1999), a dark, squint-eyed boy, slim and smallish for his age, sat on the couch and watched the reality soap *Farma* (The Farm). The bed in front of him was made, but in a corner of the room sat a heap of dirty laundry. Siniša asked the boy how he was and how he was doing at school, while Ranko stared at the screen and answered in monosyllables. Siniša wanted to know from Ranko why he was not in school today, and the latter replied, "I took a day off" (this answer amused Siniša, back in the car). Yet, for now, Siniša reminded Rajko that his son needed to attend school. Rajko replied: "Of course, what needs to be done will be done, no worries."

We descended the stairs and stepped back on the street. With a nod to the roof, Rajko said that he had been asked to renovate it, but the local council told him that this was not necessary any more. Rajko then recounted how he had recently visited the mayor in Moravac, who had promised him two spare containers to be converted into a dwelling. The containers were left over after an earthquake in the neighboring municipality. These containers would soon be installed on the hill where Rajko's paternal house once stood, a kilometer from here. Bogdan the driver told Rajko: "Put both containers together, let the craftsman make a hole between them for you," but the concrete bases for the containers had already been cast by a village craftsman. Siniša added: "Keep the new place in order." Rajko: "For sure." Bogdan: "Don't let them fool you; climb on their roof if they don't give you what they

---

tion of the municipal PIK (Agro-Industrial Combine) had operated such buying-up and storage stations throughout the municipality. For the political economy of the field, see Thiemann, "'It Was the Least Painful to Go into Greenhouse Production': The Moral Appreciation of Social Security in Post-Socialist Serbia."

promised!" Rajko replied that the city had already meant to build the containers by now, but since it was a church holiday he could wait another couple of days. He continued to tell us how he planned to raise sheep, a goat, and chicken on the hill. After a small pause, Siniša summed up the day's finding: "Food is there"—flipping a finger on Rajko's belly—"and money is there, too"—pointing to the pack of cigarettes in Rajko's front pocket. Rajko, lighting a cigarette, replied: "Well, better smoking than drinking." Bogdan interjected: "It's a pain for you right now that there are no mushrooms, eh?" (*Jebe te sad da nema pečurke, e?*). Rajko: "Whatever" (*Jebiga*). I wanted to know from Rajko how he earned his money now, and he said: "I do day labor in agriculture, and dig graves in the village, which is €40 directly into my pocket." As we left, Siniša told us in amazement: "You couldn't make up such a character!" (*Takav mora da se rodi!*), indicating that he saw Rajko as a person of rough edges and bravado, although not quite trustworthy and with doubtful parenting resources.[3]

In this vignette I represented a routine check-up on a family of "users" (*korisnik, ~ci*) of the CSW by the psychologist of the "child and adolescent protection team" in postsocialist Serbia. Routine check-ups were performed yearly, but in urgent cases more frequently. The psychologist expressed the generalized self-perception by the CSW's employees when he characterized their professional approach as "primarily humanistic work" (*u glavnom humanistički rad*).[4] In this chapter, I analyze what the social workers subsumed under this statement, and how this shaped their local politics of distribution. I focus on the emerging long-term, complex welfare state relation between the Milović family and the CSW, in order to explore how the social situation was influenced by professional debates in the CSW dating back to the late socialist period until 2010.[5]

Analyzing how social workers mediated the growing social insecurity during postsocialism, I add to the discussion of grassroots policy formation by local health and welfare professionals (see, e.g., Bernasconi, Le

3 Diary notes, September 13, 2013.

4 Diary note about Siniša, November 9, 2009.

5 For lack of space I leave aside the fascinating recent counsel and control actions addressed to the Milovići's parenting style by a network of actants, including the local council, the municipality, the school, the police, neighbors, journalists, and local philanthropists. These processes are discussed in my dissertation thesis entitled "State Relations: Local State and Social Security in Central Serbia" (Martin-Luther University Halle/Saale 2016). I thank the Max Planck Institute for Social Anthropology and the Volkswagen Foundation for funding.

Bonhomme, Wahlen, and Varsa in this volume). In my ethnographic case study,[6] the responsible professionals, particularly the Milovići's long-term social worker Ana (born in 1951), veered the increasingly exclusionary central state law on social protection in order to help those whom they evaluated as needy. The social workers pushed their professional discretion in a contradictory process that I call "bureaucratic error." Regarding "error," I follow recent theorizing that takes the "shifting and incompatible meanings of erring as a starting point to explore the critical potentials and risks of embracing error, randomness, failure, and non-teleological temporalities."[7] By "bureaucratic," I mean rule-based, documented action in a social collective (bureaucracy) "designed to unify and control individuals." In an ideal-typical bureaucratic organization, a person "who causes things to happen without writing or being written about" is seen as "improper at best, corrupt at worst."[8] Stopping short of not writing, social workers manipulated the written accounts to satisfy both the necessities of documentation and their professional values. This was because in practice, street-level bureaucracies like the CSW work both on bureaucratic and professional rationales. This causes the typical street-level bureaucracy's dilemma:

> [P]rofessional norms of behavior toward clients provide a measure of resistance to bureaucratization. Street-level bureaucrats' claims of professional status imply a commitment that clients' interests will guide them in providing service. The implicit bargain between the professions and society is that in exchange for self-regulation they will act in clients' interest without regard for personal gain and without compromising their advocacy.[9]

Thus, my concept of bureaucratic error describes the open-ended negotiation of professional and bureaucratic norms within street-level bureaucracies. During my participant observation, I found that this bureaucratic error was directed both at the local poor and at fellow social workers. First, for the lo-

6 The ethnographic method and the anthropology of public health are discussed in Hahn and Inhorn, "Introduction," in *Anthropology and Public Health: Bridging Differences in Culture and Society*.

7 ICI, "Project Description: Core Project 'Errans,'" Berlin Institute for Cultural Inquiry, 2016 https://www.ici-berlin.org/projects/errans/ [last accessed: April 11, 2017].

8 Matthew S. Hull, *Government of Paper: The Materiality of Bureaucracy in Urban Pakistan* (Berkeley: University of California Press, 2012), 129, 130.

9 Lipsky, *Street-Level Bureaucracy: Dilemmas of the Individual in Public Services*, 189.

cal citizens in whose interest social workers pushed their professional discretion, the process was ambivalent. They received, as it were, favors that were granted flexibly, which they would have preferred to be inalienable rights.[10] Second, the users and the social workers alike tended to evaluate such processes through a kind of normative dualism, according to which they expected the state to fail its broad responsibilities, while they were hopeful (but not assured) that the family could provide for needs.[11] Third, concerning the internal dynamics of the CSW, social workers explained to me individually and collectively that they chose to work in a humanist profession and that they were not willing to compromise their ethics. Their professional self-understanding was formed at the complex intersection of personal dispositions, professional education, and ongoing socialization in an institution.[12] While I concentrate on practices in and around the CSW, I contend that the allusion to humanism was linked to (though not determined by) the professional education of social workers since late socialism. The standard textbook on social policy by Professor Dušan Lakićević, required reading for the elder generation of social workers, contained the following definition:

> The realization of the principle of humanism in social policy is inextricably linked to the general humanization of society. Because the meaning of the essence of socialism is the liberation of man [sic] and the humanization of society, only socialist humanism can be comprehensive and real humanism. In [capitalist] class society [...] humanism can only be partial.[13]

Over countless cups of Turkish coffee, the social workers not only discussed their cases, but through them also how the larger social transformations impacted their professional self-understanding as humanist workers. By the time of my initial fieldwork (2009–2010), the CSW's employees had thus developed a fairly standardized discretionary procedure that is best characterized as an "implementation deficit" of exclusionary laws.[14] This meant

10 Brković, "Management of Ambiguity: Favours and Flexibility in Bosnia and Herzegovina."

11 See Thelen, Thiemann, and Roth, "State Kinning and Kinning the State in Serbian Elder Care Programs."

12 See Oberfield, *Becoming Bureaucrats: Socialization at the Front Lines of Government Service*, 19.

13 Dušan Lakićević, *Socijalna Politika*, 5th ed. (Belgrade: Savremena administracija, 1991), 36.

14 See Bergen and While, "'Implementation Deficit' and 'Street-Level Bureaucracy': Policy, Practice and Change in the Development of Community Nursing Issues."

that social workers extended social aid to families when the eligibility of the recipients was in doubt, although it became increasingly not strictly legal to do so. I want to stress that this policy innovation was less the result of pre-existing moral economic relations with the poor, than a generalized feeling of responsibility for an inclusive politics of distribution actualized in concrete situations.

The social workers acted out their inclusive distribution in a number of tensions. One was the possible contradiction between children's individual and the families' collective needs, also addressed by Friederike Kind-Kovács (in this volume). Another factor were new forms of bureaucratic organization and paperwork introduced by 2008, which were intended to decrease the street-level bureaucrats' professional discretion and which were enforced by the director. Like all policy, the local politics of distribution in the CSW was "never a completed project. Indeed, [...] policy is always subject to revisions and inflections, which open up a politics of translation in which there are always possibilities at stake. Policy, then, is necessarily unfinished."[15] My contribution to the literature is to document how despite all odds, legal norms could be underimplemented by social workers, drawing on their professional humanism in the interest of the population. Highlighting how resources that were formed during socialism shaped (and were transformed by) capitalism, I complicate the dominant narrative of international donors. The latter construct their "right to intervene" by "denying, or paying lip service to, earlier welfare assemblages in the pre-1991 socialist period, during which Yugoslavia developed social welfare policies often seen as 'between' those of an imagined 'West' and 'East.'"[16] In sum, I argue that continuing a trend since late socialism, the CSW remained an important local arena for the negotiation of state responsibility.

The chapter is structured as follows. First, I show how the assemblage of the Yugoslav welfare state was historically coproduced by international, national, and local actors translating socialist, social democratic, and liberal welfare traditions. Second, I follow how from 1991 onward, legal principles and organizational regulations increasingly excluded the rural poor, and I portray one social worker's critical reading of the situation. Third, I use the

15 Clarke et al., *Making Policy Move: Towards a Politics of Translation and Assemblage*, 15–16.

16 Stubbs, "Performing Reform in South East Europe: Consultancy, Translation and Flexible Agency," in *Making Policy Move: Towards a Politics of Translation and Assemblage*, 72.

case study of the Milovići family to demonstrate how social workers underimplemented the new legal strictures and produced their "politics of distribution," highlighting two moments of bureaucratic error. Fourth, I represent the arguments with which the director of the CSW legitimated her curtailing of these innovations.

The History of the Centers for Social Work

Rather than trying to provide a comprehensive history of the post-Yugoslav welfare system, I focus on one significant local institution, the CSW, in order to understand the processes of local social policy formation under socialism and capitalism.

Transnational translation processes were paramount in the formation of what became late socialist Yugoslavia's "rather generous welfare system based on the principles of solidarity and equality."[17] In the wake of the Second World War, the need for state provision of social security was accepted by the new socialist authorities to address health and welfare problems like poverty, rural–urban migration, and what had been diagnosed around 1945 (and quickly silenced) as "Partisan's war neurosis."[18] Initially, the "administrative workers" and "social protection officers" worked in the Women's Antifascist Front (AFŽ), the Communist Party, and the larger communities.[19]

Early on, Yugoslavia also adopted Soviet welfare principles of social security provision based on the workplace.[20] After the break between Tito and Stalin in 1948, and "in accordance with the trends towards international cooperation with the Western countries, schools for social workers were founded in Yugoslavia. The first school was founded in Croatia in 1952, [...] the second in Slovenia in 1955 and later, in 1958, schools were opened in Belgrade, Sarajevo and Skopje."[21] The generalized introduction of social work

17 Marija Stambolieva, "Conclusion: The Post-Yugoslav Welfare States: From Legacies to Actor Shaped Transformations," in *Welfare States in Transition: 20 Years after the Yugoslav Welfare Model*, ed. Marija Stambolieva and Stefan Dehnert (Sofia: Friedrich Ebert Foundation, 2011), 350.

18 See Karge, in this volume.

19 Zaviršek, "Engendering Social Work Education under State Socialism in Yugoslavia," 736; Ivana Dobrivojević, *Selo i Grad: Transformacija Agrarnog Društva Srbije 1945–1955* (Belgrade: Institut za savremenu istoriju, 2013), chapter 3.

20 See Thelen and Read, "Introduction: Social Security and Care after Socialism: Reconfigurations of Public and Private," 7–8.

21 Ajduković and Branica, "Some Reflections on Social Work in Croatia (1945–1989)," 258–9.

curricula and of social insurance schemes in the 1950s was supported by US advisors and influenced by trips to Sweden and UN exchange programs in the 1960s.[22] The establishment of CSWs throughout the country proceeded in parallel.[23] As a result, the Yugoslav welfare state "was [one of] the first socialist states that professionalized social work" beyond the family and the workplace.[24] For instance, it preceded the advanced Hungarian welfare state of the 1960s[25] by a decade.

The drive to professionalize the welfare system continued, and by the early 1970s it led to the establishment of university degree programs of social work. At Belgrade University, a Diploma of Social Work could be acquired at the Faculty of Political Sciences since 1974.[26] The curriculum included courses on social work and social policy.[27] Professor Dušan Lakićević, who influenced the emerging socialist humanist policy, had already lectured at Belgrade's High School for Social Work.[28] Later, at the university department, he authored the standard textbook cited above, which was recommended to me by his student Ana Čekerevac, a former social worker and presently professor of social policy and social work in Belgrade and Podgorica (Montenegro). Professor Čekerevac maintained that while the practice of social work had not always been up to its own standards, the Yugoslav theory was very progressive.[29]

Besides social work, other disciplines producing employees for the CSWs included psychology, child pedagogy, *defektologija*,[30] gerontology, and sociology. Historians of health have only just begun to research the

22 Zaviršek, "Engendering Social Work"; Leskošek, "Social Policy in Yugoslavia between Socialism and Capitalism," 240.

23 See Zaviršek, "Engendering Social Work," 738.

24 Leskošek, "Social Policy in Yugoslavia," 239.

25 See Haney, "'But We Are Still Mothers': Gender, the State, and the Construction of Need in Postsocialist Hungary," in *Uncertain Transition: Ethnographies of Change in the Postsocialist World*, 153–4.

26 According to an urban legend, initial plans to embed the institute within the Philosophy department failed because the latter's socialist humanist 'Praxis School' had fallen into political disfavor by then (personal communication, Marina Blagojević, May 4, 2016).

27 Interview with Dr. Biljana Sikimić, July 12, 2009.

28 See Zorka Erčić, Dušan Lakićević, and Milorad Milovanović, *Socijalni Rad i Socijalni Radnici: Zbornik Radova Povodom Desetogodišnjice Više škole za Socijalne Radnike u Beogradu (1957–1967)* (Belgrade: Visoka škola za socijalne radnike, 1967).

29 Interview with Ana Čekerevac, October 23, 2009. Her statement valorized the efforts by a preceding generation of social policy scholars to translate a unique Yugoslav welfare approach out of socialist, liberal, and social-democratic influences. At the same time, it can be read as a critical comment on contemporary, neoliberal social policy tendencies (see footnote 16).

30 *Defektologija* translates roughly as "special education."

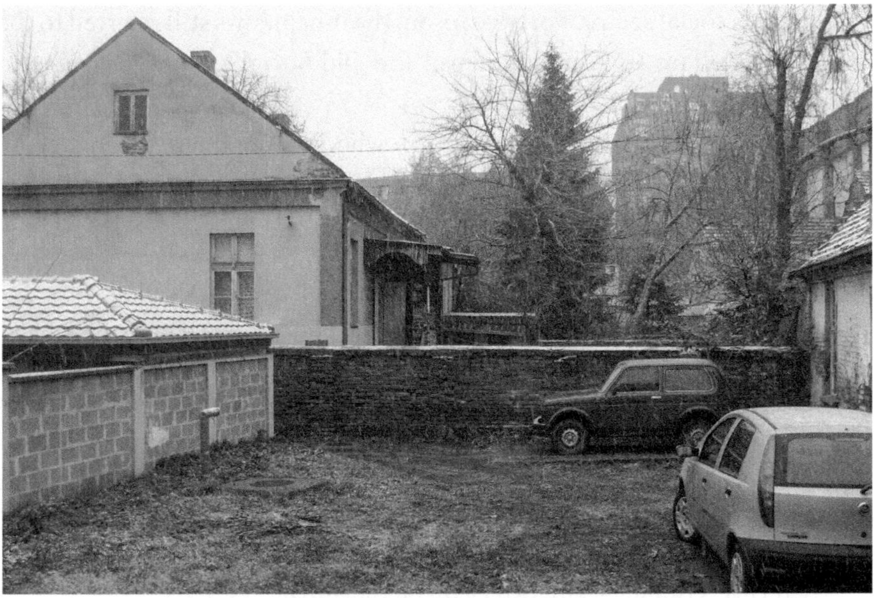

Figure 12.1: *Center for Social Work courtyard with car park.*
Picture by Andre Thiemann, Serbia, December 14, 2009.

complex history and "proliferation" of psychoanalysis, psychology, and psychiatry in Yugoslavia, which "encouraged a more humanistic (as opposed to mechanistic) conception of mental illness."[31] In any case, Siniša, whom we met in the opening vignette, studied family systems psychology in Belgrade in the late 1990s and early 2000s. The CSW in Moravac, Siniša's present workplace, had been founded in 1960 and was initially "linked to The Health (*Zdravstvo*)."[32] At the outset, it had operated in nearby Varošica then the center of a rural municipality. At some point in the late 1960s, the CSW was relocated to Moravac, the new urban core of an enlarged municipality of over 100,000 inhabitants. In Moravac, the CSW was housed in a hundred-year-old, two-story building that once was a brewery[33] and was supervised

31 See Savelli, "The Peculiar Prosperity of Psychoanalysis in Socialist Yugoslavia," 262, 288; see also Ana Antić, "Getting Rid of 'Little Stalins': The Politics of Children's Mental Health in Cold War Yugoslavia and Europe," paper presented at the "Thinking about Health and Welfare in (Eastern) Europe and Beyond" workshop, London, July 2, 2015; and Karge, in this volume.

32 Interview with social worker Ana, December 9, 2009.

33 The beer cellars in the historical monument (that had been built by an entrepreneurial subject of the Habsburg Empire) were used as a prison in the early "administrative communist" years. Presently, the cellars serve as storage space or to hand out New Year's packages for the users, as there was a shortage of offices in the building.

by the city's social sector. Forty years on, the inhabitants still referred to the municipal welfare administration as "The Old Social" (*Stara socijala*) and the CSW as "The Social" (*Socijala*).

The long-term director (2005–2012), who had obtained her university degree in social work in Belgrade in the 1980s, explained the mandate of "her" CSW in this way:

> First let me tell you what the Center [for Social Work] is dealing with: The center fulfills many tasks connected to social policy, some in the competence of the [central] state respectively the republic, regulated by juridical acts, some in the competence of the city [municipality] itself, for that the lawful basis are the decisions about the rights in the competence of the city [*odluka o pravima iz nadležnosti grada*]. So I do not know what interests you. Is it materially endangered persons or...? We also work with divorces, with delinquents, we do adoptions, custody [*starateljstvo*], placement in institutions. We do everything, [even] foster care [*hraniteljstvo*].[34]

As the quote illustrates, the CSW was a multipurpose institution with many political obligations, legal affiliations, and social responsibilities. According to the CSW's time-honored street work approach, called the "territorial system," each social work professional managed a couple of villages and city streets as their terrain (*teren*), performing all the duties enumerated by the director above. In this way, social worker Ana had been responsible for Gornje Selo.

Yugoslavia always had official unemployment and parts of the population were poor and needy, and it was the mandate of the CSW to care for them.[35] By the 1980s, the CSW gained more responsibilities, as the social security of the population worsened during a decade of economic crisis.[36] At the decade's end, the Yugoslav leadership envisioned the reintroduction of the market economy to rectify the dismal performance of the country's self-managed economy. Therefore, between 1988 and 1991, the Socialist Republic of Serbia reformed its social policy system to meet the anticipated social problems. One innovation was the introduction of a new minimal in-

34 Interview with director of the CSW, July 17, 2009.

35 Woodward, *Socialist Unemployment: The Political Economy of Yugoslavia, 1945–1990*.

36 Sundhaussen, *Jugoslawien und seine Nachfolgestaaten 1943–2011: Eine Ungewöhnliche Geschichte des Gewöhnlichen*, 205–19.

come for families and individuals in 1989. It was to be secured by a generous means-tested benefit called MOP, a newly unified social aid instrument to be managed and disbursed by the CSW.[37] Simultaneously, the CSW administered a new "singular evidence system for users." At this point "the Center for Social Work truly became the central municipal institution of social work, social protection, and social security."[38]

However, in the 1990s the situation deteriorated more dramatically than had been expected in the ambitious law on social protection of 1991.[39] Yugoslavia's secessionist wars disrupted the social and economic fabric of the country and created large streams of refugees.[40] Throughout the 1990s and especially after 2000, the number of unemployed grew, as an emerging semi-peripheral capitalist democracy shifted its economic policies and, following the rather informal privatizations of the 1990s, instituted a tough privatization program.[41] First, the privatizing of industries meant the dismantling of social security provided by the workplace. Second, many privatized industries went bankrupt, while those that survived shed jobs. Third, since 2008 the global financial crisis hit Serbia and diminished the volume of economic activity further. Thus, between 2005 and 2010, "[t]he employment rate fell from 54% to 50.3%, and it is especially low for women (42.2%), and young people aged 15–24 (15%)."[42] Private employers were often in arrears with the payment of insurance premiums, so that workers had difficulties accessing health and pension benefits. Despite rising unemployment, in 2010 the number of people who received unemployment benefits stagnated at a miniscule 1.1 percent, while the number of people living in absolute poverty rose from

37 MOP (Materijalno Obezbeđenje Porodice i Pojedinca) translates as "Material Security for the Family and the Individual." Pioneered in the SR Slovenia in the mid-1980s, it was introduced in Serbia in 1990 and linked to the average wage (40% for one; 60% for two; 75% for three; 90% for four; 100% for five or more family members). In the law on social protection of 1991, MOP was slightly increased (see below).

38 Lakićević, *Socijalna Politika*, 389.

39 Ministry for Work and Social Policy (MWSP), Law on the Social Protection and Safeguarding of the Social Security of the Citizens [Zakon o socijalnoj zaštiti i obezbeđivanju socijalne sigurnosti građana], Sl. glasnik RS 36/91, 79/91, 33/93, 53/93, 67/93, 46/94, 48/94, 52/96, 29/01, 2001, http://www.disabilitymonitor-see.org/documents/legislation/serbia/social_welfare/zak_soc_zast_ser.pdf [last accessed: April 11, 2017].

40 See Sundhaussen, *Jugoslawien und seine Nachfolgestaaten*, 309–442.

41 Organized opposition against the privatizations came from the nationalist-conservative Serbian Radical Party (SRS), a predecessor of the presently austerity-enforcing Serbian Progressive Party (SNS). See Vetta, "'Nationalism Is Back!': 'Radikali' and Privatization in Serbia," in *Headlines of Nation, Subtexts of Class*.

42 Natalija Perišić and Jelena Vidojević, "Path Dependency vs. Transformation: Responses of the Serbian Welfare State to the Crisis," paper presented at a workshop on the "Balkan Precariat," Marija Bistrica, Croatia, November 8–10, 2013, 3.

6.9 to 9.2 percent.[43] Contrary to the unemployment agencies, the CSWs increased their help to the needy, although the coverage of social aid benefits remained small. In the law on social protection of 1991, MOP for a single person had been calculated (even more generously than when it was introduced in 1990) at 50 percent of the average wage. Throughout the 1990s, the value of MOP had deteriorated in parallel with the average wage because of inflation. The net worth of the salaries and of MOP was subsequently not restored to prewar levels, partly because of the low bargaining power of the syndicates. After the opposition overturned Milošević on October 5, 2000, the new government amended the law on social protection in October 2001 and drastically decreased MOP by two-thirds to 16 percent of the average wage.[44]

Starting with the 2001 amendments of the law on social protection, the national social policy began to shift "more and more responsibility toward the families," reducing expenses for the national budget.[45] In 2009, even the World Bank suggested to the Serbian government to significantly increase the spending on MOP (which was at a very low 0.12 percent of GDP).[46] In fact, between 2008 and 2013 the number of households receiving cash welfare benefits and child allowances increased almost 2.5 times from 50,000 to 120,000 households, which amounted to 2 percent of Serbian households or 8.6 percent of the poor.[47]

Internal Political Critique

This adverse constellation provided the background to the trenchant critique of the social workers that Dunja (born in 1955) shared with me. Like many social workers in her generation, Dunja's professional and life experi-

43 Ibid., 3, 6–7. Unemployment benefits were typically paid for the first half year of unemployment only.

44 MWSP, Law on Social Protection 2001, § 10, 11. The 2001 reduction of MOP by two-thirds went through all family sizes. The maximum number of family members to tabulate MOP remained at five, continuing a social policy tradition of disadvantaging large families.

45 Interview with the director, December 8, 2009.

46 In 2009, the World Bank argued for reduced state expenditure combined with a higher efficiency of policy programs and benefits, to counter the effects of the World Financial Crisis on taxes. The World Bank saw MOP as a well-targeted benefit (70 percent of payments went to the poorest quintile), underfinanced in comparison to new EU member states known for low social expenditures (Poland, Latvia, and Estonia). Thus it was recommended to raise the MOP payments per individual and to enlarge the number of recipients. See World Bank, "Srbija: Kako sa manje uraditi više: Suočavanje sa fiskalnom krizom putem povećanja produktivnosti javnog sektora," May 23, 2009, 48–50, http://siteresources.worldbank.org/SERBIAEXTN/Resources/Serbia_PER_srb_web.pdf [last accessed: April 11, 2017].

47 Perišić and Vidojević, "Path Dependency vs. Transformation," 11.

ences made her receptive to the social consequences of the complex changes.[48] She said: "More and more I come to the conclusion that we are 'the usual suspects for everything'" (*dežurni krivci za sve*).[49] I was also told that social issues were "not a priority" for the Serbian state, which was only interested in seeking investment.[50] Indeed, social workers dealt with the most excluded and stigmatized segments of the population and received the brunt of dissatisfaction with economic policies they could not influence.

On one occasion, Dunja observed that the social situation had "only worsened" since she graduated from Belgrade's High School for Social Work in 1980. For six years afterward she had been unemployed, until she found work in the welfare branch of a social enterprise in Moravac.[51] In the mid-1990s, Dunja's enterprise became insolvent and she was part of the workers' delegation that unsuccessfully negotiated the future of their firm. In this way she met the future mayor of Moravac, who was then a union organizer. Dunja became an early member of his party and was employed as his technical secretary. Concomitantly, she also became a municipal supervisory board member (član upravnog odbora) of the CSW.[52] In 2004, Dunja stopped working for the mayor, who had become a minister in the central government and needed less local support. For half a year Dunja worked as an informal elder care giver, then she applied for a position in the CSW. In Dunja's opinion, the then director of the CSW, who feared losing her position because of a scandal at the time, was not aware that Dunja no longer had political connections and employed Dunja, thinking it would make her more secure. However, within a year the director lost her position, and her successor, whom I cited above, instigated a kind of "bullying" of "political opponents."[53] Given their personal differences, Dunja did not shy away from criticizing the present director for "not understanding the essence of social work."[54]

48 Social workers with a high school education formed the majority of the elder generation of CSW professionals. They were ineligible for managing positions, which required a university degree plus five years of practice.

49 Interview with Dunja, September 6, 2013.

50 Interview with Dunja, September 21, 2009.

51 Interview with Dunja, September 16, 2013.

52 Interview with Dunja, September 21, 2009.

53 Ibid.

54 The viewpoint of the director will be elaborated below. Note that Dunja interpreted their professional dissonance not through the generalized corruption discourses. In contrast to other public enterprises, the director of the CSW was hardly well remunerated or in a position for grand embezzlement (*malverzacije*), as Dunja maintained (ibid).

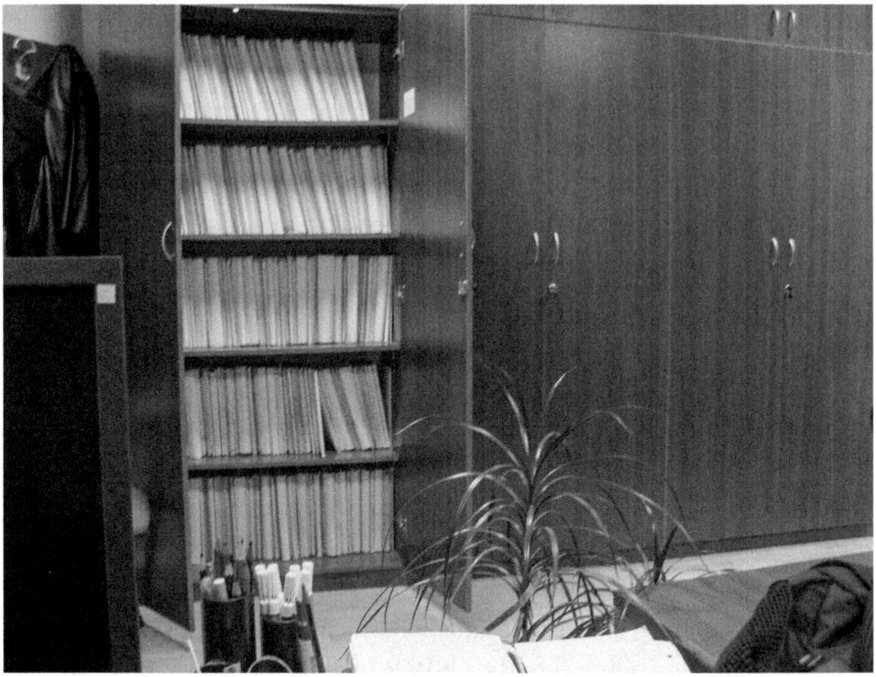

Figure 12.2: *Center for Social Work shelf with active files.* Picture by Andre Thiemann, Serbia December 14, 2009.

What incensed Dunja was the fact that the CSW was now led autocratically, and nobody dared to voice concerns. After the municipal elections in 2009, the director tried to establish an impeccable record of work conducted by the CSW in order to prevent any reason for her to be replaced. According to Dunja, the director controlled her workers with an "iron fist" and exhorted them to spend all their work energy on "formalities." Dunja especially criticized the director's habit of checking every file and returning some (for example, those with sloppy handwriting) to be rewritten. The director's intrusive behavior was linked to the 2008 national regulatory changes in social work procedures,[55] which followed the globalized audit culture of "governing by numbers," i.e., "reducing complex processes to simple numerical indicators and rankings for purposes of management and

55 MWSP, Regulations of the Organization, Normatives, and Standards of Work of the CSW [Pravilnik o organizaciji, normativima i standardima rada centra za socijalni rad], Sl. glasnik RS 59/2008, 39/2011, 1/2012, 2008, http://www.paragraf.rs/propisi/pravilnik_o_organizaciji_normativima_i_standardima_rada.html [last accessed: April 11, 2017].

control."[56] Yet, Dunja alleged that even the supervisors from the Ministry for Work and Social Policy (MWSP) accepted that the rules and regulations were hard to uphold. Yet, when a needy person died of hunger, Dunja quipped, this seemed unimportant to the director because it was not noted by her superiors, but when the time came for the institutional review (*nadzor*), the paperwork had to be flawless.[57]

How, despite these financial and bureaucratic difficulties, did social workers navigate their inclusive politics of distribution? To answer this question, I return to my case study.

Inclusive distribution

Rajko Milović, whom we met in the opening vignette, had lived for a long time in a family situation that his environment found odd. In the 1980s, he had divorced his first wife to remarry and move in with a considerably older widow. The widow's children were given into care via the CSW. This also happened to their two common children later on. After his second wife died, Rajko formed a partnership with her daughter—his stepdaughter—Dejana, who was by then a married housewife and mother in Varošica. In 1999, Rajko and Dejana moved in together in Rajko's half-abandoned paternal house in Gornje Selo, leaving Dejana's children with her husband. That same year their son Ranko was born, who, however, carried the family name of Dejana's then husband (Dejana later divorced to marry Rajko). In 2002, Dejana was pregnant with their third child, and the family approached the CSW for support. After they compiled the required paperwork (a dozen documents from diverse institutions), their application was accepted in 2003.

Social worker Ana intimately knew the Milovići. Ana was one of the most senior employees of the CSW, where she had worked since 1979. Importantly, she had been responsible for Gornje Selo from 1979 until 2007. Born and raised in Moravac in a working-class family, she had studied at the college for social work (*viša škola za socijalni rad*) in Belgrade, where about a hundred students had been enrolled per year.[58] As Ana told me, the Milovići

56 Shore and Wright, "Governing by Numbers: Audit Culture, Rankings and the New World Order," 22.

57 Interview with Dunja, September 21, 2009. To be sure, an external observer thought the director needed to strictly control her rather unruly work force (interview with protocol officer of the mayor, November 2, 2009).

58 Interview with Ana, September 12, 2013.

received a monthly MOP of 10,000 dinar (€100) through the father, Rajko. Child benefits for their four children were collected by the mother, Dejana, from the child benefit section at the municipal "Old Social" and also amounted to circa €100. According to Ana, Dejana lived together with her own "stepfather [*pastor*], old Rajko," and "they would be a case for marriage counseling."[59] Their financial support by the CSW was somewhat unusual, as there were "only three to five users" in Gornje Selo, "because they [village residents] all have property."[60] Ana alluded here to a paragraph in the law on social protection of 1991, according to which possession of half a hectare of property was the eligibility limit for social aid.[61] Before 1991, eligibility had been calculated less restrictively according to the market value of land, as a social worker who was employed in the CSW since 1986 remembered.[62] Thus, in 1991 land had been turned from an asset to a liability concerning eligibility for the MOP, and the majority of villagers became virtually excluded from the major social aid benefit. This exclusionary innovation reflected an ambivalence of urbanites against presumably "un-cultured" villagers that resurfaced during the Wars of 1991–1995.[63] From the perspective of city dwellers, villagers thrived on their plight when they pegged farmers' market food prices to the Deutschmark.[64] Urban policy makers, probably influenced by such resentments, thought that villagers had a resource in land that they could sell if they did not work it (neglecting the volatile market prices of land). Finally, international organizations like the UNHCR, with whom the CSW collaborated after 1991, demanded in their regulations that help was to be given to the landless.[65] This partial overlap of transnational and national urban ideas about rural wealth had potentially dire effects for those small proprietors in mountain villages like Gornje Selo, who

59 Interview with Ana, December 9, 2009. The matrimony of the Milovići was characterized by differences that apparently led to verbal and physical mistreatment. While a private marriage agency in Moravac had closed in the early 2000s, marriage counseling was part of the "professional work" (*stručan rad*) of the CSW.

60 Interview with Ana, December 9, 2009.

61 MWSP, Law on Social Protection 2001, § 12.

62 Interview with Lena, September 30, 2013.

63 Stef Jansen, *Antinacionalizam: Etnografija Otpora u Beogradu i Zagrebu* (Belgrade: Biblioteka XX vek, 2005), chapter 2.

64 Bajić-Hajduković, "Remembering the 'Embargo Cake': The Legacy of Hyperinflation and the UN Sanctions in Serbia," 68. Indeed, one farmer who wanted to remain anonymous told me the early 1990s were "the last time one could live well from agriculture."

65 Interview with Lena, September 30, 2013.

owned poor land of little value and who could not meet their needs from it for lack of (mental or physical) skills and health, machinery, finance, farmhands, or wish to sell their patrimony.

Here we come to the *first bureaucratic error.* Social workers, for the reasons given above, did not check up on village users' landed property, if they were convinced of their neediness and deservingness.[66] Bureaucratically erring in checking their eligibility, social workers were content, for instance, if the cadaster registered no land ownership. In the Milović case, the inheritance of several hectares of woodlands by Rajko and his sister had not been registered.[67] Rajko tried to keep his inheritance a secret, and when his wife, Dejana, told me about the land in an informal interview, he cut her short and ushered me out of the door.[68] However, if the social workers had wanted to, they could have easily known about it. For instance, the clerk of the local council, with whom they collaborated on matters of social aid, had his workplace next door to the Milovići. The point was that no one wanted to formalize this knowledge, as it would involve costly legal proceedings and imperil cash transfers to the needy.

Ever more people had to rely on "the Social," Ana explained, not because of any fault of their own, but "because of the layoffs."[69] The Milovići, who had been marginal workers during late socialism—she a seamstress, he a public greens employee—had been among the first to be fired during the postsocialist privatizations. Therefore, their family was seen as a typical needy case. Furthermore, the Milovići were evaluated as especially deserving because of their (since 2006) four children—echoing the twentieth-century preoccupation with a "proper childhood" and "proper parenting."[70] As represented in the opening vignette, the complex notion of proper parenting included the provision of healthy food, clean and safe housing with enough space for the children, compulsory education, development of the potential

66 Interview with Ana, December 9, 2009.

67 The gap between de jure land ownership and de facto registration was large. The inheritance division procedures were to be initiated by the inheritors and concluded within a year. The legal costs were born by the beneficiaries. One problem was that inheritance upon death occurred as a group right of the children and the spouse. The division of land, house, machinery, etc., often led to quarrels among the inheritors. Legal division therefore strained relations and purses, and it was avoided. Crucially for social workers, land without title could not be legally sold or mortgaged and thus had no official market value.

68 Interview with Dejana and Rajko Milović, October 25, 2010.

69 Interview with Ana, December 9, 2009.

70 Thelen and Haukanes, "Parenting after the Century of the Child: Introduction," 1–2.

of children, and temperance in consumption of drugs like cigarettes, alcohol, etc. Other factors were the physical safety of the children, their nonviolent upbringing, the inculcation of "appropriate" work habits (not stealing), neat clothing, and the possibility of taking a vacation. Proper parenting obviously necessitated money, which the social workers helped needy parents to acquire. However, the financial difficulties of needy and deserving persons like the Milovići were compounded by the fact that the MOP for an "employable person" (*radnosposobno lice*) of €50 per month was perceived as "not enough to live on."[71] Here, Ana referenced the decline of the real value of the MOP during postsocialism. After 2001, aid recipients "had to find work on the side" in order to survive—and that was, of course, not checked on by the CSW, as Ana underlined.[72]

This led to the *second bureaucratic error*. According to the law on social protection, all side income of users needed to be deducted from the MOP payments. The professionals worked the system by summarily deducing the worth of one day of labor (€8.50 in 2009) only. Moreover, mothers in the first year after childbirth had no deductions at all.[73] The minimal enforcement of income deductions was evident in the opening vignette, when Rajko was not scared to tell the psychologist about his occasional income as a mushroom collector and a village undertaker. Such bureaucratic underimplementation was tolerated for years by the director of the CSW.[74] Not double-checking the eligibility of the needy in terms of the ownership of land and not policing their side incomes represented two common methods of inclusive distribution by underimplementing exclusive social policies.[75] Both practices can be understood as the professional discretion of street-level bureaucrats who "mediate aspects of the constitutional relationship of citizens to the state."[76] The underimplementing of the increasingly exclusionary terms of the law on social protection (in the amendments of 2001 and 2005) followed the humanist principles laid out (unchanged) in

71 Interview with Ana, December 9, 2009.

72 Ibid.

73 File on Rajko Milović, MOP decisions (entries for 2003, 2004, 2006, and 2007).

74 As indicated, the director enforced the bureaucratic regulations, which tallied badly with bureaucratic error.

75 A somewhat similar inclusive distribution policy is meanwhile officially developed by central state agencies in five South African states, discussed in Ferguson, *Give a Man a Fish: Reflections on the New Politics of Distribution*, 213–15.

76 Lipsky, *Street-Level Bureaucracy*, 4.

§ 2 of the law. There, a citizen or family in "social need" was defined as one for whom "societal help is essential—with the aim of overcoming social and life difficulties, and the creation of conditions for the fulfillment of basic life needs, inasmuch as these cannot be fulfilled in a different manner, and *on the basis of humanism and human dignity*."[77]

Humanist values formed one resource for social workers to help the needy, reassure themselves of their professionalism, and confront the red tape approach of the director.

Calls for a More Systemic Solution

Proud of her university degree, the director underlined that she had twenty-four years of social work experience and there was nothing she did not already know about it.[78] Previous to her appointment she had been one of the few social workers in the medical sector. She had never been a "field worker" (*terenac*), though, and accordingly did not attach the same central importance to it as did her colleagues. I once overheard a youthful social worker joyfully shout in the CSW car, on her way to visit their users, "The field is the law!" (*Teren je zakon!*). Her exclamation put in a nutshell how social workers valued fieldwork higher than paperwork, because the former allowed a more nuanced feel of the social situation of impoverished people.

The director's position betrayed a peculiar reading of the social fact of large-scale impoverishment when she told me during a joint car ride to a social policy and strategy conference in Belgrade that "people who don't like to work shouldn't receive help."[79] On the other hand, the director had been a student of Dušan Lakićević, and she valued Professor Ana Čekerevac and her approach to social work and social policy highly.[80] Indeed, the director told me during the conference that the local innovations promoted there—which she herself had endorsed previously—created no systemic solutions. In her mind, the idea of reforming the welfare state through local projects,

77 MWSP, Law on Social Protection 2001, § 2, emphasis mine.

78 Interview with director, July 17, 2009.

79 Diary notes, October 16, 2009. How the director understood the social problems of adults influenced her actions when she yielded her position in 2012. She chose to work in the section for adult protection. Later she admitted to colleagues that she had underestimated the amount of work and psychological stress she faced there.

80 Interview with director, November 6, 2009.

municipal social policy strategies, and memoranda of understanding between local state institutions led to quickly outdated solutions. Her experience was that local innovations could not compensate for the absence of systemic agreement among the different working groups of the MWSP.[81] Nonetheless, the director's "productionist" view of need, compounded with her politically insecure position and decreasing faith in local innovation, explained why she advocated systemic solutions and stymied her social workers' local initiatives to expand help to the poor. Bureaucratic error—to help the needy as long as the documentation was impeccable—emerged in this peculiar bureaucratic power constellation as the least common professional denominator "to correct and attenuate certain negative side effects of the market economy."[82]

Conclusion

During the 1990s and early 2000s, an inclusive local social policy emerged in Moravac out of interactive practices within the triple dialectic of the large-scale state and societal transformations, mediated by the local CSW. Each moment of the triad relationally influenced the two others, opening up the possibility for change in the always-emerging local state relation.[83] In this context, the relationship between the Milovići and the CSW was characterized by the tension between professional social work—humanist and fieldwork—and bureaucratic demands of paperwork and recent computer-assisted governing by indices. Social work professionals could choose to work for, along, or against either of these professional and bureaucratic norms. On top of this, the self-will (*Eigensinn*) of the users was sometimes at odds with the bureaucratic-professional struggles, and created additional moments of chaotic creativity. The outcomes were complex shifts in bureaucratic error that resulted in a surprisingly long-term local policy of underimplementing exclusionary national laws and regulations. Thus, out of very muddled struggles emerged the relational modality of inclusive distribution.

This local social policy operated on the idea that the social workers offered material help to impoverished families, giving them the benefit of the

81 Diary notes, October 16, 2009.
82 Lakićević, *Socijalna Politika*, 380.
83 Thiemann, *State Relations*.

doubt regarding the regulations determining eligibility. Thus bureaucratic error operated according to the humanist spirit of the law of 1991, i.e., to ensure the best possible support for poor families in times of politico-economic and social transformation. The main social carrier of this inclusive distribution was the late-socialist generation of high school-educated social workers. Yet, as their policy lacked financial means and political support, social workers needed to select beneficiaries carefully, tending to exclude potential users like refugees or people inhibited to ask for support. Given the fetters imposed on inclusive distribution by national-scale supervision and local micro-management, Dušan Lakićević was proved right that in capitalist class society, humanism can only be partial.[84]

The new law on social protection (2011), unsurprisingly in light of the difficulties to control local bureaucratic erring, was aimed at tightening the definition of social work. Yet, the ensuing curtailment of professional discretion could only create new opportunities for social workers to exercise discretion and commit different forms of "bureaucratic error." However, I will discuss this in another article.

84 In Yugoslav social work practice, however, humanism had remained partial, too, as unpublished archival research suggests (Paul Stubbs, personal communication, May 4, 2016).

COLLECTIVE BIBLIOGRAPHY

Abrams, Bradley. "Hope Died Last: The Czechoslovak Road to Stalinism." In: *Stalinism Revisited: The Establishment of Communist Regimes in East-Central Europe*, ed. Vladimir Tismaneanu (Budapest & New York: Central European University Press, 2009), 345–366.

Adamik, Mária. "Az államszocializmus és a 'nőkérdés': 'A legnagyobb ígéret – a legnagyobb megaláztatás." PhD diss., Budapesti Közgazdasági Egyetem, 2000.

Ajduković, Marina, and Vanja Branica. "Some Reflections on Social Work in Croatia (1945–1989)." In: *Social Care under State Socialism (1945–1989): Ambitions, Ambiguities, and Mismanagement*, ed. Sabine Hering (Opladen: Budrich, 2009), 249–63.

Akrich, Madeleine, and Bernike Pasveer. "Multiplying Obstetrics: Techniques of Surveillance and Forms of Coordination." *Theoretical Medicine* 21 (2000): 63–83.

Anagnost, Ann. "A Surfeit of Bodies: Population and the Rationality of the State in Post-Mao China." In: *Conceiving the New World Order: The Global Politics of Reproduction*, ed. Faye D. Ginsburg and Rayna Rapp (Berkeley: University of California Press, 1995), 22–41.

Antić, Ana. "Heroes and Hysterics: 'Partisan Hysteria' and Communist State-Building in Yugoslavia after 1945." *Social History of Medicine* 27/2 (2014): 349–71.

———. "Psychiatry at War: Psychiatric Culture and Political Ideology in Yugoslavia under the Nazi Occupation." PhD diss., Columbia University, 2012. https://academiccommons.columbia.edu/catalog/ac:174561 [last accessed: April 26, 2017].

Antonakopoulos, George. "The Royal Medical Council of Greece, 1834–1922." *Deltos: Journal of the History of Hellenic Medicine* (2012): 33–36.

Apor, Péter. "Cigányok tere: Kísérlet a kommunista romapolitika közép-kelet-európai összehasonlító elemzésére, 1945–1961." *Aetas* 2 (2009): 69–86.

Apostolopoulos, D. G., and E. N. Fragiskos (eds.), *Νεοελληνικός Διαφωτισμός Βιβλιογραφία 1945–1995*. Athens: National Hellenic Research Foundation [EIE], 1998.

Ash, G. ed. *The Nationalization of Scientific Knowledge in the Habsburg Empire, 1848–1918*. Basingstoke: Palgrave Macmillan, 2012.

Ash, Mitchell. "Wissenschaft und Politik als Ressourcen füreinander." In: *Wissenschaften und Wissenschaftspolitik. Bestandsaufnahmen zu Formationen, Brüche und Kontinuitäten im Deutschland des 20. Jahrhunderts*, ed. Rüdiger vom Bruch and Brigitte Kaderas (Stuttgart: Steiner, 2002), 32–51.

Aust, Martin, Ricarda Vulpius, and Aleksej Miller (eds.). *Imperium inter pares. Rol' transferov v istorii Rossijskoj imperii (1700–1917)*. Moscow: Novoe Literaturnoe Obozrenie, 2010.

Bajić-Hajduković. Ivana. "Remembering the 'Embargo Cake': The Legacy of Hyperinflation and the UN Sanctions in Serbia." *Contemporary Southeastern Europe* 1/2 (2014): 61–79.

Baldwin, Peter. *Contagion and the State in Europe, 1830–1930*. Cambridge: Cambridge University Press, 1999.

Balińska, Marta Aleksandra. "The National Institute of Hygiene and Public Health in Poland 1918–1939." *Social History of Medicine* 9/3 (1996): 427–45.

———. "The Rockefeller Foundation and the National Institute of Hygiene, Poland, 1918–1945." *Studies in History and Philosophy of Biological and Biomedical Sciences* 31/3 (2000): 419–432.

———, and William H. Schneider (eds.). *Ludwik Hirszfeld: The Story of One Life*. Rochester: University of Rochester Press, 2010.

Ballantyne, Tony, and Antoinette Burton. "Introduction: Bodies, Empires and World Histories." In: *Bodies in Contact: Rethinking Colonial Encounters in World History*, ed. Tony Ballantyne and Antoinette Burton (Durham: Duke University Press, 2005), 1–18.

Balsoy, Gülhan. *The Politics of Reproduction in Ottoman Society, 1838–1900*. London: Pickering & Chatto, 2013.

Balz, Viola. *Zwischen Wirkung und Erfahrung. Eine Geschichte der Psychopharmaka. Neuroleptika in der Bundesrepublik Deutschland, 1950–1980*. Bielefeld: Transcript Verlag, 2010.

———. "Terra Incognita: An Historiographic Approach to the First Chlorpromazine Trials Using Patient Records of the Psychiatric University Clinic in Heidelberg." *History of Psychiatry* 22 (2011): 182–200.

———. "'Für einen Aktivisten wie mich muß es in einem sozialistischen Staat doch effektive Medikamente geben'. Psychopharmaka und Konsumenteninteresse in der DDR." *NTM. Zeitschrift für Geschichte der Wissenschaften, Technik und Medizin* 21/3 (2013): 245–71.

Baran, Brigitta, and Gábor Gazdag. "The Fate of the Hungarian Psychiatric Patients during World War II." *International Journal of Mental Health* 35/4 (2006–7): 88–99.

Barany, Zoltan. *The East European Gypsies: Regime Change, Marginality, and Ethnopolitics*. Cambridge: Cambridge University Press, 2002.

Bauer, Bruno. "Semmelweis, Ignaz Philipp" *Neue Deutsche Biographie* (2010): 239–41. http://www.deutsche-biographie.de/pnd118613138.html [last accessed: April 26, 2017].

Beaton, Roderick, and David Ricks (eds.). *The Making of Modern Greece: Nationalism, Romanticism, and the Uses of the Past (1797–1896)*. London: Ashgate, 2009.

Behrends, Jan C. and Martin Kohlrausch (eds.). *Races to Modernity: Metropolitan Aspirations in Eastern Europe, 1890–1940*. Budapest: Central European University Press, 2014.

Beizer, Michael. "'I Don't Know Whom to Thank': The American Jewish Joint Distribution Committees Secret Aid to Soviet Jewry." *Jewish Social Studies* 15/2 (2009): 111–36.

———, and Mikhail Mitsel. *The American Brother: The "Joint" in Russia, the USSR and the CIS*. Jerusalem: The American Jewish Joint Distribution Committee, 2004.

Belzyt, Leszek. *Sprachliche Minderheiten im preußischen Staat 1815–1914*. Marburg: Herder-Institut, 1998.

Bencze, László. *The Occupation of Bosnia and Herzegovina in 1878*. Boulder, CO: Social Science Monographs, 2005.

Benedict, Susan, and Linda Shields (eds.). *Nurses and Midwives in Nazi Germany: The "Euthanasia Programs."* New York: Routledge, 2014.

Benton, Lauren, and Richard J. Ross (eds.). *Legal Pluralism and Empires, 1500–1850*. New York: New York University Press, 2013.

Bergen, Ann, and Alison While. "'Implementation Deficit' and 'Street-Level Bureaucracy': Policy, Practice and Change in the Development of Community Nursing Issues." *Health & Social Care in the Community* 13/1 (2005): 1–10.

Berger, Silvia. *Bakterien in Krieg und Frieden: eine Geschichte der medizinischen Bakteriologie in Deutschland, 1890–1933*. Göttingen: Wallstein, 2009.

Berger, Stefan et al. (eds.). *Nationalizing Empires*. Budapest: Central European University Press, 2015.

Berridge, Virginia. *Temperance: Its History and Impact on Current and Future Alcohol Policy*. York: Joseph Rowntree Foundation, 2005.

———, and Edwards Griffith. *Opium and the People: Opiate Use in Century England*. London & New York: A. Lane/St. Martin's Press, 1981.

Beshkarev, N. A., V. T. Emel'yanov, M. V. Stegantsev, and I. A. Shlyakhov. *V pomoshch' doprizyvniku*. Moscow: Military Publishing House of the Ministry of Defense of the USSR, 1967.

Bespalov, N. G., and I. I. Eliseeva. *Železnye dorogi Rossii v XX veke v zerkae statistiki*. St. Petersburg: Nestor-Istorija, 2008.

Betts, Paul. *Within Walls: Private Life in the German Democratic Republic*. New York: Oxford University Press, 2010.

Blanke, Richard. *Prussian Poland in the German Empire 1871–1900*. Boulder, CO: East European Monographs, 1981.

Bleker, Johanna, and Volker Hess (eds.). *Die Charité. Geschichte eines Krankenhauses*. Berlin: Akademieverlag, 2010.

Blix, Göran. "Charting the 'Transitional Period': The Emergence of Modern Time in the Nineteenth Century." *History and Theory* 45 (2006): 51–71.

Bloch, Sidney, and Peter Reddaway. *Russia's Political Hospitals: The Abuse of Psychiatry in the Soviet Union*. London: Gollancz, 1977.

———. *Soviet Psychiatric Abuse: The Shadow over World Psychiatry*. London: Gollancz, 1984.

Blocker, Jack S., David M. Fahey, and Ian R. Tyrrell (eds.). *Alcohol and Temperance in Modern History: An International Encyclopedia*. Santa Barbara: ABC-CLIO, 2003.

Bock, Gisela. "Equality and Difference in National Socialist Racism." In: *Beyond Equality and Difference: Citizenship, Feminist Politics and Female Subjectivity*, ed. Gisela Bock and Susan James (London: Routledge, 1992), 89–109.

Boeckh, Katrin, and Natali Stegmann. "Veterans and War Victims in Eastern Europe during the 20th Century: A Comparison," *Comparativ. Zeitschrift für Globalgeschichte und Vergleichende Gesellschaftsforschung* 5 (2010): 7–17.

Bohling, Joseph E. "The Sober Revolution: The Political and Moral Economy of Alcohol in Modern France, 1954–1976." PhD diss., Department of History, University of California, Berkeley, 2012, http://digitalassets.lib.berkeley.edu/etd/ucb/text/Bohling_berkeley_0028E_12435.pdf [last accessed: March 28, 2017].

Böhler, Jochen, Wlodzimierz Borodziej, and Joachim von Puttkamer (eds.). *Legacies of Violence: Eastern Europe's First World War*. Munich: Oldenbourg Verlag, 2014.

Boltanski, Luc. *Love and Justice as Competences: Three Essays on the Sociology of Action*. Cambridge: Polity Press, 2012.

———, and Laurent Thévenot. *On Justification: Economies of Worth*. Translated by Catherine Porter. Princeton: Princeton University Press, 2006.

Bourke, Joanna. "Der Heilberuf und das Leiden. Die Erfahrungen der Militärmedizin in den beiden Weltkriegen." In: *Krieg und Medizin*, ed. Melissa Larner (Göttingen: Wallstein S. Verlag, 2009), 119–31.

———. *Dismembering the Male: Men's Bodies, Britain, and the Great War*. London: Reaktion Books, 1996.

Boysen, Jens. "Gezeiten nationaler Identität: Josef von Unruh/Józef Unrug (1884–1973) als Offizier der deutschen und polnischen Marine (1907–1919 bzw. 1919–1947)." In: *After the Fall of Empires: Historical Turning Points and Biographical Experience in Eastern Europe*, ed. Katrin Steffen (Lüneburg: Nordost-Institut, 2015), 103–21.

Bren, Paulina. *The Greengrocer and His TV: The Culture of Communism after the 1968 Prague Spring*. Ithaca: Cornell University Press, 2010.

Brković, Čarna. "Management of Ambiguity: Favours and Flexibility in Bosnia and Herzegovina." *Social Anthropology* 23/3 (2015): 268–82.

Browning, Christopher R., and Lewis H. Siegelbaum. "Frameworks for Social Engineering: Stalinist Schema of Identification and the Nazi Volksgemeinschaft." In: *Beyond Totalitarianism: Stalinism and Nazism Compared*, ed. Michael Geyer and Sheila Fitzpatrick (Cambridge: Cambridge University Press, 2008), 231–65.

Brubaker, Rogers. "Nationalizing States in the 'Old New' Europe—and the New." *Ethnic and Racial Studies* 19/2 (1996): 411–37.

Brunner, Jos. "Will, Desire and Experience: Etiology and Ideology in the German and Austrian Medical Discourse on War Neuroses, 1914–1922." *Transcultural Psychiatry* 37/3 (2000): 295–320.

Brykczynski, Paul. "A Poland for the Poles? Józef Piłsudski and the Ambiguities of Polish Nationalism." In: *Pravo: The North American Journal for Central European Studies* 1 (2007): 1–20.

Buchen, Tim, and Malte Rolf (eds.). *Eliten im Vielvölkerreich: Imperiale Biographien in Russland und Österreich*. Munich: Walter de Gruyter, 2015.

Bucur, Maria. *Eugenics and Modernization in Interwar Romania*. Pittsburgh: University of Pittsburgh Press, 2002.
Buda, Béla et al. "Psychotherapy in Hungary During the Socialist Era and the Socialist Dictatorship." *European Journal of Mental Health* 4.1 (2009): 67–99.
Buklijaš, Tatjana. "Public Anatomies in Fin-de-Siècle Vienna," *Medicine Studies* 2 (2010): 71–92.
———, and Emese Lafferton. "Introduction: Science, Medicine and Nationalism in the Habsburg Empire from the 1840s to 1918." *Studies in History and Philosophy of Biological and Biomedical Sciences* 38 (2007): 679–86.
Bulmer, Martin, Kevin Bales, and Kathryn Kish Sklar. "The Social Survey in Historical Perspective." In: *The Social Survey in Historical Perspective, 1880–1940*, ed. Martin Bulmer, Kevin Bales, and Kathryn Kish Sklar (Cambridge: Cambridge University Press, 1991), 7–9.
Burschel, Peter, and Christoph Marx (eds.). *Reinheit*. Wien: Böhlau, 2011.
Cabanes, Bruno. *The Great War and the Origins of Humanitarianism, 1918–1924*. Cambridge: Cambridge University Press, 2014.
Chahrour, Marcel. "'A Civilizing Mission'? Austrian Medicine and the Reform of Medical Structures in the Ottoman Empire, 1838–1850." *Studies in History and Philosophy of Biological and Biomedical Sciences* 38 (2007): 687–705.
Chodorowski, Jerzy, and Alfred Konieczny (eds.). *Wybór tekstów źródłowych z historii ustroju Polski 1916–1939*. Wrocław: Verlag, 1972.
Christian, Michel. "Le parti et la vie privée de ses membres en RDA." *Politique, culture, société* 7 (2009): 3.
Clarke, John, and Bainton, Dave et al. *Making Policy Move: Towards a Politics of Translation and Assemblage*. Bristol: Policy Press, 2015.
Conrad, Peter. *The Medicalization of Society: On the Transformation of Human Conditions into Medical Disorders*. Baltimore: Johns Hopkins University Press, 2007.
Conrad, Sebastian. *Globalization and the Nation in Imperial Germany*. Cambridge: Cambridge University Press, 2006.
Constantinescu, Doina. "Cotribuţii la studiul de tratament în alcoolismul cronic." PhD diss., Institut de Medicină şi Farmacie Bucureşti, 1990.
Cooter, Roger and Stein, Claudia. *Writing History in the Age of Biomedicine*. New Haven: Yale University Press, 2013.
Courtwright, David T. *Forces of Habit: Drugs and the Making of the Modern World*. Cambridge: Harvard University Press, 2001.
Creese, Mary R. S. and Thomas M. Creese. *Ladies in the Laboratory IV: Imperial Russia's Women in Science, 1800–1900: A Survey of Their Contributions to Research*. Lanham: Rowman & Littlefield, 2015.
Cunningham, Andrew. *The Anatomical Renaissance: The Resurrection of the Anatomical Projects of the Ancients*. Aldershot: Ashgate, 2003.
Cvetkovski, Roland. *Modernisierung durch Beschleunigung: Raum und Mobilität im Zarenreich*. Frankfurt & New York: Campus Verlag Frankfurt, 2006.
Dacome, Lucia. "Women, Wax and Anatomy in the 'Century of Things.'" In: *Spaces, Objects and Identities in Early Modern Italian Medicine*, ed. Sandra Cavallo and David Gentilcore (Oxford: Blackwell Publishing, 2008).
Deák, István. "The Habsburg Empire." In: *After Empire: Multiethnic Societies and Nation-Building: The Soviet Union and the Russian, Ottoman, and Habsburg Empires*, ed. Karen Barkey and Mark von Hagen (Boulder, CO: West View Press, 1997), 129–41.
Degele, Nina, and Sigrid Schmitz. "Somatic Turn?" *Soziologische Revue* 30.1 (2007): 49–58.
Dekel-Chen, Jonathan, David Gaun, Natan M. Meir, and Israel Bartal (eds.). *Anti-Jewish Violence: Rethinking the Pogrom in East European History*. Bloomington: Indiana University Press, 2011.
Demirci, Tuba, and Selçuk Akşin Somel. "Women's Bodies, Demography, and Public Health: Abortion Policy and Perspectives in the Ottoman Empire of the Nineteenth Century." *Journal of the History of Sexuality* 17.3 (2008): 377–420.
Desroisières, Alain. *Die Politik der großen Zahlen*. Berlin: Springer Verlag, 2005.

Dijck, José van. *The Transparent Body: A Cultural Analysis of Medical Imaging.* Seattle: University of Washington Press, 2005.

Diner, Hasia R. *The Jews of the United States, 1654 to 2000.* Berkeley & Los Angeles: University of California Press, 2004.

Dobrivojević, Ivana. *Selo i grad: transformacija agrarnog društva Srbije 1945–1955.* Belgrade: Institut za savremenu istoriju, 2013.

Dodier, Nicolas. "Konventionen als Stützen der Handlung." In: *Soziologie der Konventionen: Grundlagen einer pragmatischen Anthropologie,* ed. Rainer Diaz-Bone (Frankfurt & New York: Campus Verlag, 2001), 69–98.

Douglas, Mary. *Purity and Danger: An Analysis of the Concepts of Pollution and Taboo.* London: Routledge, 2001.

Duraković, Indira. *Serbien und das Modernisierungsproblem: die Entwicklung der Gesundheitspolitik und sozialen Kontrolle bis zum Ersten Weltkrieg.* Frankfurt am Main: Peter Lang Edition, 2014.

Đurčić, Aca, and Samuel Elazar. *Pregled istorije farmacije Bosne i Hercegovine.* Sarajevo: Centralni higijenski zavod, 1958.

Dursun, Selçuk. "Procreation, Family and 'Progress': Administrative and Economic Aspects of Ottoman Population Policies in the 19th Century." *History of the Family* 16 (2011): 160–71.

Ebrahimnejad, Hormoz (ed.). *The Development of Modern Medicine in Non-Western Countries: Historical Perspectives.* Abingdon: Routledge, 2008.

Edele, Mark. *Soviet Veterans of the Second World War: A Popular Movement in an Authoritarian Society, 1941–1991.* Oxford: Oxford University Press, 2009.

Eghigian, Greg. "Was There a Communist Psychiatry? Politics and East German Psychiatric Care, 1945–1989." *Harvard Review of Psychiatry* 10 (2002): 364–68.

Einhorn, Ignacy. *Towarzystwo Ochrony Zdrowia Ludności Żydowskiej w Polsce w latach 1921–1950.* Toruń: Adam Marszałek, 2008.

Eisenbach-Stangl, Irmgard. *Eine Gesellschaftsgeschichte des Alkohols: Produktion, Konsum und soziale Kontrolle alkoholischer Rausch- und Genussmittel in Österreich 1918–1984.* Frankfurt a. M. & New York: Campus Verlag, 1991.

———. "Treatment-Seeking and Treatment-Reluctant Alcoholics: A Two-Class Alcohol-Treatment System in Austria." In: *Cure, Care, or Control: Alcoholism Treatment in Sixteen Countries,* ed. Geoffrey Hunt, Jukka-Pekka Takala, and Harald Klingemann (Albany: State University of New York Press, 1992), 173–90.

Eisenstadt, Shmuel. N. (ed.). "Multiple Modernities," *Daedalus* 129/1 (2000): 1–29.

———, and Bernhard Giesen. "The Construction of Collective Identity." *European Journal of Sociology* 36 (1995): 72–102.

Elekes, Zsuzsanna. "The Development of an Alcohol-Treatment System in Hungary." In: *Cure, Care, or Control: Alcoholism Treatment in Sixteen Countries,* ed. Geoffrey Hunt, Jukka-Pekka Takala, and Harald Klingemann (Albany: State University of New York Press, 1992), 23–38.

Eley, Geoff, and James Retallack (eds.). *Wilhelminism and Its Legacies: German Modernities, Imperialism, and the Meanings of Reform, 1890–1930.* New York & Oxford: Berghahn Books, 2003.

Engel, David. "World War I." In: *The Yivo Encyclopedia of Jews in Eastern Europe.* http://www.yivoencyclopedia.org/article.aspx/World_War_I [last accessed: April 26, 2017].

Engstrom, Eric (ed.). *Figurationen des Experten. Ambivalenzen der wissenschaftlichen Expertise im ausgehenden 18. und frühen 19. Jahrhundert.* Frankfurt/Main: Peter Lang, 2005.

Erčić, Zorka, Dušan Lakićević, and Milorad Milovanović. *Socijalni Rad i Socijalni Radnici: Zbornik Radova Povodom Desetogodišnjice Više škole za Socijalne Radnike u Beogradu (1957–1967).* Belgrade: Visoka škola za socijalne radnike, 1967.

Ernst, Anna-Sabine. *"Die beste Prophylaxe ist der Sozialismus." Ärzte und medizinische Hochschullehrer in der SBZ/DDR 1945–1961.* Münster: Waxmann, 1997.

Etkind, Aleksandr. *Eros of the Impossible: The History of Psychoanalysis in Russia.* Boulder, CO: Westview Press, 1997.

Etzemüller, Thomas (ed.). *Die Ordnung der Moderne. Social Engineering im 20. Jahrhundert.* Bielefeld: Transcript, 2009.

Fayet, Roger (ed.). *Verlangen nach Reinheit oder Lust auf Schmutz? Gestaltungskonzepte zwischen rein und unrein.* Wien: Passagen, 2003.

Ferguson, James. *Give a Man a Fish: Reflections on the New Politics of Distribution.* Durham: Duke University Press, 2015.

Fidelis, Malgorzata. "A Nation's Strength Lies not in Numbers: De-Stalinization, Pronatalism, and the Abortion Law of 1956 in Poland." In: *Geschlechterbeziehungen in Ostmitteleuropa nach dem Zweiten Weltkrieg*, ed. Claudia Kraft (Munich: R. Oldenbourg Verlag, 2008), 203–15.

Fieseler, Beate. "The Bitter Legacy of the 'Great Patriotic War'. Red Army Disabled Soldiers under Late Stalinism." In: *Late Stalinist Russia: Society between Reconstruction and Reinvention*, ed. Juliane Fürst (London/New York: Routledge, 2006), 46–61.

———. [Beate Fizeler]. "'Nishchie pobediteli': invalidy Velikoy Otechestvennoy voyny v Sovetskom Soyuze." *Neprikosnovennyy zapas: debaty o politike i kul'ture* 2/3 (2005): 290–7.

———. "The Wounds of War: Experiences of War-Related Disablement in Soviet Feature Films." In: *Recalling the Past—(Re)constructing the Past: Collective and Individual Memory of World War II in Russia and Germany*, ed. Withold Bonner and Arja Rosenholm (Helsinki: Aleksanteri Institute, 2008), 277–87.

———. "De la 'génération perdue' aux bénéficiaires de la politique sociale? Les invalides de guerre en URSS, 1945–1964." In: *Retour à l'intime au sortir de la guerre*, ed. Bruno Cabanes and Guillaume Piketty (Paris: Tallandier, 2009), 133–48.

———. "Soviet-Style Welfare: The Disabled Soldiers of the 'Great Patriotic War.'" In: *Disability in Eastern Europe and the Former Soviet Union*, ed. Michael Rasell and Elena Iarskaia-Smirnova (London: Routledge, 2014), 18–41.

Fitzpatrick, K. Meghan. "Prostitutes, Penicillin and Prophylaxis: Fighting Venereal Disease in the Commonwealth Division during the Korean War, 1950–1953," *Social History of Medicine* 28.3 (2015): 555–75.

Foucault, Michel. "Governmentality." In: *The Foucault Effect: Studies in Governmentality*, ed. Graham Burchell, Colin Gordon, and Peter Miller (Hemel Hempstead: Harvester Wheatsheaf, 1991), 87–104.

———. *Sicherheit, Territorium, Bevölkerung. Geschichte der Gouvermentalität I.* Frankfurt a. M.: Suhrkamp, 2006.

———. *Society Must Be Defended: Lectures at the Collège de France, 1975–76*, ed. Mauro Bertani and Alessandro Fontana, trans. David Macey. New York: Picador, 2003.

———. *The Birth of Biopolitics: Lectures at the Collège de France, 1978–1979*, ed. Michel Senellart, trans. Graham Burchell. Basingstoke: Palgrave Macmillan, 2008.

———. *The Courage of Truth: Lectures at the Collège de France, 1983–1984*, ed. Frédéric Gros, trans. Graham Burchell. Basingstoke: Palgrave Macmillan, 2011.

———. *The Government of Self and Others: Lectures at the Collège de France, 1982–1983*, ed. Arnold I. Davidson, trans. Graham Burchell. New York: Palgrave Macmillan, 2010.

———. *The Order of Things.* London: Tavistock, 1970.

———. "17 March 1965." In: *Society Must Be Defended: Lectures at the Collège de France, 1975–1976*, ed. Mauro Bertani and Alessandro Fontana, trans. David Macey. New York: Picador, 2003.

Freeland, Jane. "Morals on Trial: State-Making and Domestic Violence in the East German Courtroom." *Perspectives on Europe* 44 (2009): 55–60.

Freis, David. "Curing the Soul of the Nation: Psychiatry, Society, and Psycho-Politics in the German-Speaking Countries, 1918–1939." PhD thesis, European University Institute, 2015.

Friedman, Alexander. "'Der wahre sozialistische Mensch'. Der sowjetische Kampfflieger Aleksej P. Mares'ev (1916–2001) und seine Rezeption in der DDR." In: *Diskriminiert–vernichtet-vergessen. Behinderte in der Sowjetunion, unter nationalsozialistischer Besatzung und im Ostblock 1917–1991*, ed. Alexander Friedman and Rainer Hudemann (Stuttgart: Franz Steiner Verlag, 2016), 511–22.

Frojimovics, Kinga and Géza Komoróczy. *Jewish Budapest: Monuments, Rites, History.* Budapest: Central European University Press, 1999.

Fuchs, Brigitte. "Orientalizing Disease: Austro-Hungarian Policies of 'Race,' Gender and Hygiene in Bosnia and Herzegovina, 1874–1914." In: *Health, Hygiene and Eugenics in Southeastern*

Europe to 1945, ed. Christian Promitzer, Sevasti Trubeta, and Marius Turda (Budapest: Central European University Press, 2011), 57–85.

Gal, Susan, and Gail Kligman. "Reproduction as Politics." In: *The Politics of Gender after Socialism: A Comparative-Historical Essay* (Princeton: Princeton University Press, 2000), 15–36.

Gardikas, Katerina. "Relief Work and Malaria in Greece, 1943–1947." *Journal of Contemporary History* 43 (2008): 493–508.

———. "Health Policy and Private Care: Malaria Sanitisation in Early 20th Century Greece." In: *Health, Hygiene and Eugenics in Southeastern Europe to 1945*, ed. Christian Promitzer, Sevasti Trubeta, and Marius Turda (Budapest: Central European University Press, 2011), 127–142.

———. *Landscapes of Disease: Malaria in Modern Greece*. Budapest: Central European University Press, 2017.

Gawin, Magdalena. *Rasa i nowoczesność*. Warsaw: Neriton. Instytut Historii PAN, 2003.

Gazi, Effi. "'Europe': Writing an Ambivalent Concept in 19th Century Greek Historical Culture." In: *Die Griechen und Europa. Außen- und Innensichten im Wandel der Zeit*, ed. Heppner Heppner and Olga Katsiardi-Hering (Vienna: Böhlau Verlag, 1998), 103–24.

Gelez, Philippe. "Se convertir en Bosnie-Herzégovine." *Süd-Ost Forschungen* 68 (2009): 86–31.

Gestwa, Klaus. "Social und soul engineering unter Stalin und Chruschtschow, 1928–1964." In: *Ordnung der Moderne*, ed. Thomas Etzemüller (Bielefeld: Transcript, 2009), 241–77.

Geyer, Michael. "Ein Vorbote des Wohlfahrtsstaates. Die Kriegsopferversorgung in Frankreich, Deutschland und Großbritannien nach dem Ersten Weltkrieg." *Geschichte und Gesellschaft* 9.2 (1983): 230–77.

Geyer, Dietrich. *Klio in Moskau und die sowjetische Geschichte*. Heidelberg: University of Heidelberg, 1985.

Giddens, Anthony. *The Consequences of Modernity*. Oxford: John Wiley & Sons, 2013.

Giomi, Fabio. "Daughters of Two Empires: Muslim Women and Public Writing in Habsburg Bosnia and Herzegovina (1878–1918)." *Aspasia: The International Yearbook of Central, Eastern and Southeastern European Women's and Gender History* 9 (2015): 1–18.

———."Forging Habsburg Muslim Girls: Gender, Education and Empire in Bosnia and Herzegovina (1878–1918)." *History of Education* 44/3 (2015): 274–92.

Göckenjan, Gerd. *Kurieren und Staat machen. Gesundheit und Medizin in der bürgerlichen Welt*. Frankfurt a. M.: Suhrkamp, 1985.

Goltermann, Svenja. *Die Gesellschaft der Überlebenden. Deutsche Kriegsheimkehrer und ihre Gewalterfahrungen im Zweiten Weltkrieg*. Munich: Pantheon, 2011.

Gordon, Linda. *Heroes of Their Own Lives: The Politics and History of Family Violence: Boston, 1880–1960*. New York: Viking, 1988.

Granick, Jaclyn. "Waging Relief: The Politics and Logistics of American Jewish War Relief in Europe and the Near East, 1914–1918." *First World War Studies* 5/1 (2014): 55–68.

Gromulska, Marta. "Ludwik Hirszfeld in the National Institute of Hygiene 1920–1941." *Przegląd Epidemiologiczny* 68 (2014): 695–702.

Gross Solomon, Susan. "The Expert and the State in Russian Public Health: Continuities and Changes across the Revolutionary Divide." In: *The History of Public Health and the Modern State*, ed. Dorothy Porter (Atlanta: Editions Rodopi, 1994), 183–223.

Guillemain, Hervé, and Stéphane Tison. *Du front à l'asile, 1914–1918*. Paris: Alma, 2013.

Hacking, Ian. "How Should We Do the History of Statistics?" In: *The Foucault Effect: Studies in Governmentality*, ed. Graham Burchell, Colin Gordon, and Peter Miller (Chicago: University of Chicago Press, 1991), 181–96.

———. "Making up People." *London Review of Books* 20/16 (2006): 23–6.

———. *Rewriting the Soul: Multiple Personality and the Sciences of Memory*. Princeton: Princeton University Press, 1995.

———. *The Taming of Chance*. Cambridge: Cambridge University Press, 1990.

———. *The Social Construction of What?* Cambridge, MA: Harvard University Press, 1999.

———. *Was heißt soziale Konstruktion? Zur Konjunktur einer Kampfvokabel in den Wissenschaften*. Frankfurt a.M.: Fischer Taschenbuch, 1999.

Hagen, William W. *Germans, Poles and Jews. The Nationality Conflict in the Prussian East 1772–1914*. Chicago: University of Chicago Press, 1980.

Hahn, Robert A., and Marcia Claire Inhorn. "Introduction." In: *Anthropology and Public Health: Bridging Differences in Culture and Society*, ed. Robert A. Hahn and Marcia Claire Inhorn (Oxford: Oxford University Press, 2009), 1–34.

Hähner-Rombach, Sylvelyn. *Sozialgeschichte der Tuberkulose: Vom Kaiserreich bis zum Ende des 2. Weltkrieges unter besonderer Berücksichtigung Württembergs*. Stuttgart: Steiner, 2000.

Halliwell, Martin. *Therapeutic Revolutions: Medicine, Psychiatry, and American Culture, 1945–1970*. New Brunswick: Rutgers University Press, 2013.

Hancock, Philip et al. *The Body, Culture and Society: An Introduction*. Buckingham: Open University Press, 2000.

Hanebrink, Paul A. *In Defense of Christian Hungary: Religion, Nationalism and Antisemitism*. Ithaca & London: Cornell University Press, 2006.

Haney, Lynne. *Inventing the Needy: Gender and the Politics of Welfare in Hungary*. Berkeley: University of California Press, 2002.

———. "'But We Are Still Mothers': Gender, the State, and the Construction of Need in Postsocialist Hungary." In: *Uncertain Transition: Ethnographies of Change in the Postsocialist World*, ed. Michael Burawoy and Katherine Verdery (Lanham: Rowman & Littlefield, 1999), 151–84.

Harrison, Mark. "Disease, Diplomacy and International Commerce: The Origins of International Sanitary Regulation in the Nineteenth Century." *Journal of Global History* 1 (2006): 197–217.

Harsch, Dona. *Revenge of the Domestic: Women, the Family and Communism in the German Democratic Republic*. Princeton: Princeton University Press, 2007.

Hartmann, Betsy. *Reproductive Rights and Wrongs: The Global Politics of Population Control*. Boston: South End Press, 1995.

Heimann, Siegfried. *Der Preussische Landtag 1899–1947: Eine politische Geschichte*. Berlin: Ch. Links, 2011.

Heinemann, Isabel. "Social Experts and Modern Women's Reproduction: From 'Working Women's Neurosis' to the Abortion Debate, 1950–1980." In: *Inventing the "Modern American Family": Family Values and Social Change in 20th Century United States*, ed. Isabel Heinemann (Frankfurt a. M.: Campus, 2012), 124–51.

Heller, Mária, Dénes Némedi, and Ágnes Rényi. "Népesedési viták Magyarországon 1960–1986." In: *Népesedési viták Magyarországon 1960–1986*, ed. István Monigl (Budapest: KSH, 1991), 13–125.

Hentschel, Christhardt. "Einführung. Der Militärdienst für Juden und die Verheißung der Emanzipation." *Simon Dubnow Yearbook* 12 (2013): 95–10.

———. *Jeder Bürger Soldat. Militär, Juden und die Zweite Polnische Republik zwischen Geschichte und Gegenwart*. Göttingen: Vandenhoeck & Ruprecht (forthcoming).

Henze, Charlotte. *Disease, Health Care and Government in Late Imperial Russia: Life and Death on the Volga, 1823–1914*. London: Routledge, 2011.

Herczl, Moshe Y. *Christianity and the Holocaust of Hungarian Jewry*. New York: New York University Press, 1993.

Hering, Sabine and Waaldijk, Berteke (eds.). *Guardians of the Poor, Custodians of the Public: Welfare History in Eastern Europe, 1900–1960*. Opladen: Barbara Budrich Publishers, 2006.

Herrn, Rainer, and Laura Hottenrott (eds.). *Die Charité zwischen Ost und West 1945–1992. Zeitzeugen erinnern sich*. Berlin: Bebra Verlag, 2010.

Hervé, Guillemain, and Stéphane Tison. *Du front à l'asile. 1914–1918*. Paris: Alma, 2013.

Herzfeld, Michael. "The Absent Presence: Discourses of Crypto-Colonialism." *South Atlantic Quarterly* 101/4 (2002): 341–371.

Hess, Volker (ed.). *Normierung der Gesundheit. Messende Verfahren der Medizin als kulturelle Praktik um 1900*. Husum: Matthiesen Verlag, 1997.

Heywood, Anthony. *Engineer of Revolutionary Russia: Iurii V. Lomonosov (1876–1952) and the Railways*. Surrey & Burlington: Ashgate, 2011.

Hirschfeld, Gerhard. "Der Erste Weltkrieg in der deutschen und internationalen Geschichtsschreibung," *Aus Politik und Zeitgeschichte* 29–30 (2004): 3–12.

Hoffmann, David L., and Timm, Annette F. "Utopian Biopolitics: Reproductive Policies, Gender Roles, and Sexuality in Nazi Germany and the Soviet Union." In: *Beyond Totalitarianism: Stalinism and Nazism Compared,* ed. Michael Geyer and Sheila Fitzpatrick (Cambridge: Cambridge University Press, 2008), 87–130.

Hösler, Joachim. *Die sowjetische Geschichtswissenschaft 1953 bis 1991. Studien zur Methodologie- und Organisationsgeschichte.* Munich: Verlag Otto Sagner, 1995.

Huber, Valeska. "The Unification of the Globe by Disease? The International Sanitary Conferences on Cholera, 1851–1894." *The Historical Journal* 49 (2006): 453–76.

Huerkamp, Claudia. *Der Aufstieg der Ärzte im 19. Jahrhundert. Vom gelehrten Stand zum professionellen Experten: Das Beispiel Preußens.* Göttingen: Vandenhoeck & Ruprecht, 1985.

Hull, Isabel V. *Sexuality, State and Civil Society in Germany, 1700–1815.* Ithaca: Cornell University Press, 1996.

Hull, Matthew S. *Government of Paper: The Materiality of Bureaucracy in Urban Pakistan.* Berkeley: University of California Press, 2012.

Hunt, Geoffrey, Jukka-Pekka Takala, and Harald Klingemann (eds.). *Cure, Care, or Control: Alcoholism Treatment in Sixteen Countries.* Albany: State University of New York Press, 1992.

Hüntelmann, Axel C. *Hygiene im Namen des Staates. Das Reichsgesundheitsamt 1876–1933.* Göttingen: Wallstein, 2008.

Iarskaia-Smirnova, Elena, and Pavel Romanov. "Heroes and Spongers: The Iconography of Disability in Soviet Posters and Film." In: *Disability in Eastern Europe and the Former Soviet Union,* ed. Michael Rasell and Elena Iarskaia-Smirnova (London & New York: Routledge, 2014), 67–96.

Inglot, Tomasz, Dorottya Szikra, and Cristina Rat. "Continuity and Change in Family Policies of the New European Democracies: A Comparison of Poland, Hungary and Romania." Working Papers of the National Council for Eurasian and East European Research (NCEEER), 2011.

Institute of Medicine (US). *Broadening the Base of Treatment for Alcohol Problems: Report of a Study by a Committee of the Institute of Medicine, Division of Mental Health and Behavioral Medicine.* Washington, DC: National Academy Press, 1990.

Ioanid, Radu. *The Holocaust in Romania: The Destruction of Jews and Gypsies under the Antonescu Regime.* Chicago: Ivan R. Dee, 2000.

Jansen, Stef. *Antinacionalizam: etnografija otpora u Beogradu i Zagrebu.* Belgrade: Biblioteka XX. vek, 2005. vol. 152.

Jarausch, Konrad Hugo (ed.). *Care and Coercion: The GDR as Welfare Dictatorship.* New York: Berghahn Books, 1999.

———. "Realer Sozialismus als Fürsorgediktatur. Zur begrifflichen Einordnung der DDR." *Aus Politik und Zeitgeschichte* 20 (1998): 33–46.

Jessen, Ralph. *Akademische Elite und kommunistische Diktatur. Die ostdeutsche Hochschullehrschaft in der Ulbrich-Ära.* Göttingen: Vandenhoeck und Ruprecht, 1999.

Johler, Reinhard, Christian Marchetti, and Monique Scheer (eds.). *Doing Anthropology in Wartime and Warzones: World War One and the Cultural Sciences in Europe.* Bielefeld: Transcript, 2010.

Johnson, Sam. "Breaking or Making the Silence?: British Jews and East European Jewish Relief, 1914–1917." *Modern Judaism* 30/1 (2010): 95–119.

Judson, Pieter M. *The Habsburg Empire: A New History.* Cambridge, MA: Harvard University Press, 2016.

Kalinová, Lenka. *Konec nadějím a nová očekávání: K dějinám české společnosti v letech 1969–1993.* Prague: Academia, 2012.

Kamarás, Ferenc. "Születési mozgalom és termékenység az elmúlt 125 évben," *Statisztikai szemle* 74 (1996): 662–79.

———. "Terhességmegszakítások Magyarországon." *Data archive of TÁRKI Social Research Institute.* http://www.tarki.hu/adatbank-h/nok/szerepvalt/Kamaras-99.html [last accessed: April 26, 2017].

Karge, Heike. "Making Sense of War Neurosis in Yugoslavia." In: *Psychological Trauma and the Legacies of the Great War,* ed. Peter Leese and Jason Crouthamel (London: Palgrave Macmillan, 2016): 217–35.

———. *Steinerne Erinnerung—versteinerte Erinnerung? Kriegsgedenken im sozialistischen Jugoslawien.* Wiesbaden: Harrassowitz, 2010.

Karlinksy, Nahum. "Jewish Philanthropy and Jewish Credit Cooperatives in Eastern Europe and Palestine up to 1939: A Transnational Phenomenon?" *Journal of Israeli History* 27/2 (2008): 149–70.

Kassow, Sam. "On the Jewish Street 1918–1939." In: *Polin: 1000 Year History of Polish Jews*, ed. Barbara Kirshenblatt-Gimblett and Antony Polonsky (Warsaw: Museum of the History of the Polish Jews, 2014), 227–85.

Kasumović, Amila. "Prilog povijesti marginalnih skupina u Bosni i Hercegovini u doba austrougarske uprave: prostitutke." *Historijski zbornik* 60 (2007): 161–78.

Katzburg, Nathaniel. *Hungary and the Jews: Policy and Legislation, 1920–1943*. Ramat-Gan: Bar-Ilan University Press, 1981.

———. "Louis Marshall and the White Terror in Hungary. 1919–1920." *American Jewish Archives* 45/1 (1993): 1–12.

Kęsik, Jan. *Naród pod bronią. Społeczeństwo w programie polskiej polityki wojskowej 1918–1939*. Wrocław: Wydawnictwo Uniwersytetu Wrocławskiego, 1998.

———. *Wojsko polskie wobec tężyzny fizycznej społeczeństwa 1918–1939*. Wydawn: Akademii Wychowania Fizycznego we Wrocławiu, 1996.

Kienitz, Sabine. *Beschädigte Helden: Kriegsinvalidität und Körperbilder 1914–1923*. Paderborn: Ferdinand Schöningh, 2008.

Kind-Kovács, Friederike. "Compassion for the Distant Other: Children's Hunger and Humanitarian Relief in Budapest in the Aftermath of WWI." In: *Rescuing the Vulnerable: Poverty, Welfare and Social Ties in Nineteenth- and Twentieth-Century Europe*, ed. Beate Althammer, Lutz Raphael, and Tamara Stazic-Wendt (New York: Berghahn Books, 2016), 129–59.

Kingston-Mann, Esther. "Statistics, Social Science, and Social Justice: The Zemstvo Statisticians of Pre-Revolutionary Russia." In: *Russia in the European Context, 1789–1914: A Member of the Family*, ed. Susan P. McCaffray and Michael Melancon (New York: Palgrave Macmillan, 2005), 113–39.

Kitromilides, Paschalis M. "Tradition, Enlightenment and Revolution: Ideological Change in Eighteenth and Nineteenth Century Greece." PhD diss., Harvard University, 1978.

———. "'Imagined Communities' and the Origins of the National Question in the Balkans." In: *Modern Greece: Nationalism and Nationality*, ed. Martin Blinkhorn and Thanos Veremis (Athens: Sage-Eliamep, 1990), 23–66 (first published in this volume in a special issue of *European History Quarterly* 19 (1989): 131–34).

———. *Enlightenment, Nationalism, Orthodoxy: Studies in the Culture and Political Thought of Southeastern Europe*. Aldershot: Variorum, 1994.

Klajn, Hugo. *Ratna Neuroza Jugoslovena*. Beograd: Tersit, 1995.

Kleemann, Christoph (ed.). *Niemiecki Wschód*. Poznań: Poznańska Biblioteka Niemiecka, 2014.

Kligman, Gail. "Political Demography: The Banning of Abortion in Ceausescu's Romania." In: *Conceiving the New World Order: The Global Politics of Reproduction*, ed. Faye D. Ginsburg and Rayna Rapp (Berkeley: University of California Press, 1995), 234–55.

Knabe, Ferdinand. *Sprachliche Minderheiten und nationale Schulpolitik in Preußen zwischen 1871 und 1933*. Münster: Waxmann, 2000.

Kochan, Thomas. *Blauer Würger: So trank die DDR*. Berlin: Aufbau-Verlag, 2011.

Kohlrausch, Martin, Katrin Steffen, and Stefan Wiederkehr (eds.). *Expert Cultures in Central Eastern Europe: The Internationalization of Knowledge and the Transformation of Nation States since World War I*. Osnabrück: Fibre, 2010.

Kontogiorgi, Elisabeth. *Population Exchange in Greek Macedonia: The Rural Settlement of Refugees 1922–1930*. Oxford: Oxford University Press, 2006.

Kowalski, Tadeusz. *Mniejszości narodowe w siłach zbrojnych Drugiej Rzeczypospolitej Polskiej (1"918–1939)*. Toruń: Wydawnictwo Adam Marszałek, 1998.

Kreševljaković, Hamdija. *Sarajevo za vrijeme austrougarske uprave (1878–1918)*. Sarajevo: Archiv Grada Sarajeva, 1969.

Kreuder-Sonnen, Katharina. "Wie die Mikroben nach Warschau kamen." *NTM* 20.3 (2012): 157–80.

Krotofil, Maciej. "Ukraińcy w Wojsku Polskim w okresie międzywojennym." In: *Mniejszości narodowe i wyznanione w siłach zbrojnych Drugiej Rzeczypospolitej*, ed. Zbignies Karpus and Waldemar Rezmer (Toruń: Wydawnictwo Uniwersytetu Mikołaja Kopernika, 2001), 153–75.

Labbé, Morgane. "'Reproduction' as a New Demographic Issue in Interwar Poland." In: *A World of Populations: Transnational Perspectives on Demography in the Twentieth Century*, ed. Heinrich Hartmann and Corinna R. Unger (New York & Oxford: Berghahn Books, 2014), 36–57.

Labisch, Alfons. *Homo Hygienicus Gesundheit und Medizin in der Neuzeit*. Frankfurt a. M. & New York: Campus Verlag, 1992.

Labouvie, Eva. *Beistand in Kindsnöten: Hebammen und weibliche Kultur auf dem Land (1550–1910)*. Frankfurt a. M.: Campus Verlag, 1999.

Lakićević, Dušan. *Socijalna politika*. Belgrade: Savremena administracija, 1991.

Lang, Branko, and Jasna Srdar. "Therapeutic Communities and Aftercare Clubs in Yugoslavia." In: *Cure, Care, or Control: Alcoholism Treatment in Sixteen Countries*, ed. Geoffrey Hunt, Jukka-Pekka Takala, and Harald Klingemann (Albany: State University of New York Press, 1992), 53–64.

Langewiesche, Dieter. "Das Jahrhundert Europas. Eine Annäherung in globalhistorischer Perspektive." *Historische Zeitschrift* 296/1 (2013): 29–48.

Latour, Bruno. *We Have Never Been Modern*, trans. Catherine Porter. Cambridge, MA: Harvard University Press, 2012.

Laverychev, V. Y. "Trends towards State Monopoly in Pre-Revolutionary Russia's Railways." *Journal of Transport History* 6/2 (1985): 37–47.

Lazaroms, Ilse Josepha. "Marked by Violence: Hungarian Jewish Histories in the Wake of the White Terror, 1919–1922." *Zutot: Perspectives on Jewish Culture* 11 (2014): 39–48.

Le Bonhomme, Fanny. "Au croisement des logiques politiques et médicales: les 'patients-camarades' des services psychiatriques de la Charité (Berlin-Est, République démocratique allemande, 1959–1964)." *Cultures et Conflits* 90 (2013): 21–38.

———. "Viols en temps de guerre, psychiatrie et temporalités enchevêtrées. Expériences de femmes violées par les soldats de l'Armée Rouge entre la fin de la Seconde Guerre mondiale et le début de la période de paix (République démocratique allemande, 1958–1968)." *Guerres mondiales et conflits contemporains* 257 (2015): 53–74.

Leese, Peter. *Shell Shock: Traumatic Neurosis and the British Soldiers of the First World War*. Basingstoke & New York: Palgrave Macmillan, 2002.

"Leiden's Anatomical Theater: Pure Science or Vulgar Spectacle?" Leiden University website, July 15, 2014, http://www.news.leiden.edu/news-2014/anatomical-theatre.html [last accessed: April 26, 2017].

Lemke, Thomas. *Biopolitics: An Advanced Introduction*. New York: New York University Press, 2011.

Lemm, Vanessa and Vatter, Miguel. *The Government of Life: Foucault, Biopolitics, and Neoliberalism*. New York: Fordham University Press 2014.

Lengwiler, Martin, and Jeannette Madarász (eds.). *Das präventive Selbst. Eine Kulturgeschichte moderner Gesundheitspolitik*. Bielefeld: Transcript, 2010.

Lerner, Paul. "Psychiatry and Casualties of War in Germany, 1914–18." *Journal of Contemporary History* 35/1 (2000): 13–28.

Leskošek, Vesna. "Social Policy in Yugoslavia between Socialism and Capitalism." In: *Social Care under State Socialism (1945–1989): Ambitions, Ambiguities, and Mismanagement*, ed. Sabine Hering (Opladen: Budrich, 2009), 239–48.

Leuenberger, Christine. "Socialist Psychotherapy and Its Dissidents." *Journal of the History of the Behavioral Sciences* 37/3 (2001): 261–73.

Levine, Harry G. "The Discovery of Addiction: Changing Conceptions of Habitual Drunkenness in America." *Journal of Studies on Alcohol* 39 (1978): 143–74.

Lipsky, Michael. *Street-Level Bureaucracy: Dilemmas of the Individual in Public Services*. New York: Russell Sage Foundation, 1980.

Lloyd, G. E. R. *Disciplines in the Making: Cross-Cultural Perspectives on Elites, Learning, and Innovation*. Oxford: Oxford University Press, 2009.

Loudon, Irvine. *Death in Childbirth: An International Study of Maternal Care and Maternal Mortality, 1800–1950.* Oxford: Clarendon Press, 1992.

Löwy, Ilana. "The Social History of Medicine: Beyond the Local." *Social History of Medicine* 20/3 (2007): 465–81.

Maier, Charles. "Transformations of Territoriality." In: *Transnationale Geschichte: Themen, Tendenzen und Theorien*, ed. Gunilla Budde, Sebastian Conrad, and Oliver Janz (Göttingen: Vandenhoeck & Ruprecht, 2006), 32–56.

Majerus, Benoît. *Parmi les fous. Une histoire sociale de la psychiatrie au XXe siècle.* Rennes: PUR, 2014.

Majtényi, Balázs, and György Majtényi. *A Contemporary History of Exclusion: The Roma Issue in Hungary from 1945 to 2015.* Budapest: Central European University Press, 2016.

Malach, Henry. "Die Individualtherapie Karl Leonhards—Rekonstruktion und Vergleich mit verhaltenstherapeutischen Methoden der 50er und 60er Jahre." PhD diss., University of Berlin/Charité, 2009.

Marks, Sarah. "From Experimental Psychosis to Resolving Traumatic Pasts: Psychedelic Research in Communist Czechoslovakia, 1954–1974." *Cahiers du Monde russe* 1 (2015): 53–76.

———, and Mat Savelli (eds.). *Psychiatry in Communist Europe.* Basingstoke: Palgrave Macmillan, 2015.

———, and Mat Savelli (eds.). "Communist Europe and Transnational Psychiatry." In: *Psychiatry in Communist Europe*, ed. Mat Savelli and Sarah Marks (Basingstoke: Palgrave Macmillan, 2015), 1–26.

Marks, Steven G. *Road to Power: The Trans-Siberian Railroad and the Colonization of Asian Russia, 1850–1917.* Ithaca: Cornell University Press, 1991.

Marung, Steffi, and Katja Naumann (eds.). *Vergessene Vielfalt. Territorialität und Internationalisierung in Ostmitteleuropa seit der Mitte des 19. Jahrhunderts.* Göttingen: Vandenhoeck & Ruprecht, 2014.

Mašić, Izet. *Korjeni medicine i zdravstva u Bosni i Hercegovini.* Sarajevo: AVICENA, 2004.

Matanović, Damir. *Grad na granici: slobodni vojni komunitet Brod na Savi od sredine 18. do sredine 19. stoljeća.* Slavonski Brod: Hrvatski institut za povijest, 2008.

Matusik, Przemysław. "Idea pracy organicznej w Poznańskiem w dobie Karola Marcinkowskiego." *Karol Marcinkowski i jego czasy. Kronika Miasta Poznania* 3 (1996): 66–84.

Mazumdar, Pauline M. "Blood and Soil: The Serology of the Aryan Racial State." *Bulletin of the History of Medicine* 64/2 (1990): 187–219.

McCagg, William O. "On Habsburg Jewry and Its Disappearance." In: *Studies in Contemporary Jewry: The Jews and the European Crisis*, ed. Jonathan Frankel, Peter Y. Medding, and Ezra Mendelsohn (New York: Oxford University Press, 1988), 84–95.

———. *A History of Habsburg Jews, 1670–1918.* Bloomington: Indiana University Press, 1989.

McCrea, Heather. *Diseased Relations: Epidemics, Public Health, and State-Building in Yucatán, Mexico, 1847–1924.* Albuquerque: University of New Mexico Press, 2010.

McIntosh, Tania. *A Social History of Maternity and Childbirth: Key Themes in Maternity Care.* London & New York: Routledge, 2012.

Meir, Natan. "From Communal Charity to National Welfare: Jewish Orphanages in Eastern Europe before and after World War I." *East European Jewish Affairs* 39/1 (2009): 19–34.

Melegh, Attila. "Living to Ourselves: Localising Global Hierarchies in State-Socialist Hungary in the 1970s and 1980s." *Journal of Modern European History* 9/2 (2011): 263–83.

———. *On the East/West Slope: Globalization, Nationalism, Racism and Discourses on Eastern Europe.* Budapest: Central European University Press, 2006.

Mendelsohn, Ezra. *The Jews of East Central Europe between the World Wars.* Bloomington: Indiana University Press, 1983.

Merridale, Catherine. "The Collective Mind: Trauma and Shell-Shock in Twentieth-Century Russia." *Journal of Contemporary History* 35.1 (2000): 39–55.

Mespoulet, Martine. "Pratique de l'enquéte et construction du savoir statistique en Russie à la fin du XIXe siécle." *Genèses* 53/3 (2003): 96–118.

———. "Professional'naja etika zemskich statistikov i formy ich otnošenija k vlasti (1880–1922)." In: *Vlast' i nauka, učenye i vlast': 1880-e–načalo 1920-x godov: Materialy meždunarordnogo naučnogo kollokviuma*, ed. N. N. Smirnov et al. (St. Petersburg: Bulanin, 2003), 112–23.

———. *Statistique et révolution en Russie. Un compromis impossible (1880–1930)*. Rennes: Presses Universitaires de Rennes, 2001.

Meurs, Wim Van and Müller, Dietmar (eds.). *Institutionen und Kultur in Südosteuropa*. Munich: Verlag Otto Sagner, 2014.

Meyer, Eva. "Zum Phantasma der Selbstgeburt." In: *Vordenker. Webforum für Innovatives in Wissenschaft, Wirtschaft und Kultur/Webforum for Innovative Approaches in Sciences, Economy and Culture*, ed. J. Paul (Winter 2008/2009): 16–17. http://www.vordenker.de/ggphilosophy/eva-meyer_zum-phantasma-selbstgeburt.pdf [last accessed: April 26, 2017].

Mezey, Barna (ed.). *A magyarországi cigánykérdés dokumentumokban, 1422–1985*. Budapest: Kossuth, 1986.

Micale, Mark S., and Paul Frederick Lerner (eds.). *Traumatic Pasts: History, Psychiatry, and Trauma in the Modern Age, 1870–1930*. Cambridge & New York: Cambridge University Press, 2001.

Michaels, Paul A. *Curative Powers: Medicine and Empire in Stalin's Central Asia*. Pittsburgh: University of Pittsburgh Press, 2003.

Michl, Susanne. *Im Dienste des "Volkskörpers." Deutsche und französische Ärzte im Ersten Weltkrieg*. Göttingen: Vandenhoeck & Ruprecht, 2007.

Maier, Charles. "Transformations of Territoriality 1600–2000." In: *Transnationale Geschichte. Themen, Tendenzen und Theorien*, ed. G. Budde, S. Conrad, and O. Janz (Göttingen: Vandenhoeck & Ruprecht, 2006), 32–55.

Mikanowski, Jacob. "Dr. Hirszfeld's War: Tropical Medicine and the Invention of Sero-Anthropology on the Macedonian Front." *Social History of Medicine* 25/1 (2011): 103–21.

Mikkonen, Simo, and Pia Koivunen (eds.). *Beyond the Divide: Entangled Histories of Cold War Europe*. New York: Berghahn Books, 2015.

Miller, Alexei, and Alfred J. Riebe (eds.). *Imperial Rule*. Budapest: Central European University Press, 2004.

Miller, Martin A. *Freud and the Bolsheviks: Psychoanalysis in Imperial Russia and the Soviet Union*. New Haven: Yale University Press, 1998.

Miłosz, Czesław. *Wyprawa w Dwudziestolecie*. Cracow: Wydawnictwo Literackie, 1999.

Mol, Annemarie. *The Body Multiple: Ontology in Medical Practice*. Durham: Duke University Press, 2002.

———. *The Logic of Care: Health and the Problem of Patient Choice*. London: Routledge, 2008.

Molik, Witold. "The Elites of the Polish National Movement in Prussian Poland in the Late 19th and Early 20th Centuries." *Polish Western Affairs* 34/2 (1993): 61–80.

———. *Inteligencja polska w Poznańskiem w XIX i początkach XX wieku*. Poznań: Wydawnictwo Poznańskie, 2009.

Mossé, Philippe. "The Rise of Alcohology in France: A Monopolistic Competition." In: *Cure, Care, or Control: Alcoholism Treatment in Sixteen Countries*, ed. Geoffrey Hunt, Jukka-Pekka Takala, and Harald Klingemann (Albany: State University of New York Press, 1992), 205–22.

Mossensohn Shefer, Miri. *Ottoman Medicine: Healing and Medical Institutions, 1500–1700*. Albany: State University of New York Press, 2009.

Moulin, Anne Marie, and Yeşim Işıl Ülman. *Perilous Modernity: History of Medicine in the Ottoman Empire and the Middle East from the 19th Century Onwards*. Istanbul: The Isis Press, 2010.

Müller, Klaus-Dieter. "Die Ärzteschaft im staatlichen Gesundheitswesen der SBZ und der DDR 1945–1989." In: *Geschichte der deutschen Ärzteschaft*, ed. Robert Jütte (Cologne: Deutscher Ärzte-Verlag, 1997), 243–73.

Müller-Jahncke, Wolf-Dieter. "Hoffmannstropfen." In: *Enzyklopädie Medizingeschichte*, ed. Werner E. Gerabek et al. (Berlin: De Gruyter, 2005), 610.

Mycielska, Dorota. "Drogi życiowe profesorów przed objęciem katedr akademickich w niepodległej Polsce." In: *Inteligencja Polska XIX i XX wieku*, ed. Ryszard Czepulis-Rastenis (Warsaw: Polska Akademia Nauk. Instytut Historii, 1981), vol. 2, 244–90.

Mydlarski, Jan. "Seroantropologia." In: *Ludwik Hirszfeld*, ed. Hanna Hirszfeldowa, Andrzej Kelus, and Feliks Milgrom (Wrocław: Wrocławskiego Towarzystwo Naukowe, 1956, 65–68.

Newlands, Emma. *Civilians into Soldiers: War, the Body and British Army Recruits, 1939–45*. Manchester: Manchester University Press, 2014.

Newman, John Paul. *Yugoslavia in the Shadow of War: Veterans and the Limits of State Building, 1903–1945*. Cambridge: Cambridge University Press, 2015.

Nicholls, James. *The Politics of Alcohol: A History of the Drink Question in England*. Manchester: Manchester University Press, 2009.

Nikolow, Sybille. "Die Nation als statistisches Kollektiv. Bevölkerungskonstruktionen im Kaiserreich und in der Weimarer Republik." In: *Wissenschaft und Nation in der europäischen Geschichte*, ed. Ralph Jessen and Jakob Vogel (Frankfurt a. M.: Campus Verlag, 2002), 235–59.

Oberfield, Zachary. *Becoming Bureaucrats: Socialization at the Front Lines of Government Service*. Philadelphia: University of Pennsylvania Press, 2014.

Oişteanu, Andrei. *Inventing the Jew: Antisemitic Stereotypes in Romanian and Other Central-East European Cultures*. Lincoln: University of Nebraska Press, 2009.

Okey, Robin. *Taming Balkan Nationalism: The Habsburg "Civilizing Mission" in Bosnia, 1878–1914*. Oxford: Oxford University Press, 2007.

Osterhammel, Jürgen. *The Transformation of the World: A Global History of the 19th Century*, trans. Patrick Camiller. Princeton: Princeton University Press, 2014.

Otáhal, Milan. *Normalizace, 1969–1989: Příspěvek ke stavu bádání*. Prague: Ústav pro Soudobé Dějiny AV ČR, 2002.

Panzac, Daniel. *Population et santé dans l'Empire ottoman (XVIIIe–XXe siècles)*. Istanbul: Isis, 1996.

Parin, Paul. *Es ist Krieg und wir gehen hin. Bei den jugoslawischen Partisanen*. Hamburg: Europ. Verl.-Anst., 1997.

Patek, Philipp. "Die Entwicklung der Anatomie in Düsseldorf. Von der Akademie für praktische Medizin zur Universität Düsseldorf." PhD diss., University of Dusseldorf, 2010.

Patriarca, Silvana. *Numbers and Nationhood: Writing Statistics in Nineteenth-Century Italy*. Cambridge: Cambridge University Press, 1996.

Pawlowsky, Verena. *Mutter ledig—Vater Staat: das Gebär- und Findelhaus in Wien 1784–1910*. Innsbruck: Studien Verlag, 2001.

Pence, Katherine, and Paul Betts. "Introduction." In: *Socialist Modern: East German Everyday Culture and Politics*, ed. Katherine Pence and Paul Betts. Ann Arbor: University of Michigan Press, 2008.

Pető, Andrea, and E. Kossuth. "Women's Rights in Stalinist Hungary: The Abortion Trials of 1952–53." *Hungarian Studies Review* 29/1–2 (2002): 49–76.

Petrovsky-Stern, Yohanan. *Jews in the Russian Army 1827–1917: Drafted into Modernity*. Cambridge & New York: Cambridge University Press, 2009.

Phillips, Laura L. "Gendered Dis/ability: Perspectives from the Treatment of Psychiatric Casualties in Russia's Early Twentieth Century Wars." *Social History of Medicine* 20 (2007): 333–50.

Pinnow, Kenneth M. *Lost to the Collective: Suicide and the Promise of Soviet Socialism, 1921–1929*. Ithaca: Cornell University Press, 2010.

Plamper, Jan. "Fear: Soldiers and Emotion in Early Twentieth-Century Russian Military Psychology," *Slavic Review* 68.2 (2009), 259–83.

———. *The History of Emotions: An Introduction*. Oxford: Oxford University Press, 2015.

Poldrugo, Flavio, and Roberto Urizzi. "The Italian Paradox: Treatment Initiatives and Falling Alcohol Consumption." In: *Cure, Care, or Control: Alcoholism Treatment in Sixteen Countries*, ed. Geoffrey Hunt, Jukka-Pekka Takala, and Harald Klingemann (Albany: State University of New York Press, 1992), 191–204.

Polonsky, Antony. *The Jews in Poland and Russia, Vol. III: 1914–2008*. Oxford: Littman, 2012.

Pomogyi, László. *Cigánykérdés és cigányügyi igazgatás a polgári Magyarországon*. Budapest: Osiris, Századvég, 1995.

Poovey, Mary. *A History of Modern Fact: Problems of Knowledge in the Sciences of Wealth and Society*. Chicago & London: University of Chicago Press, 1998.

———. *Making a Social Body: British Cultural Formation, 1830–1864*. Chicago: University of Chicago Press, 1995.

Porter, Dorothy. *Health, Civilization and the State: A History of Public Health from Ancient to Modern Times*. London: Routledge, 1999.

———. *The History of Public Health and the Modern State*, ed. Dorothy Porter. Atlanta: Editions Rodopi, 1999.

Porter, Theodore M. "Statistical and Social Facts from Quetelet to Durkheim." *Sociological Perspectives* 38/1 (1995): 15–26.

Posłuszna, Małgorzata. "Stan sanitarno-higieniczny wsi polskiej w okresie II Rzeczypospolitej." In: *Z dziejów zdrowia publicznego*, ed. Jan Nosko (Łódź: Instytut Medycyny Pracy, 2006), 273–87.

Promitzer, Christian, Sevasti Trubeta, and Marius Turda (eds.). *Health, Hygiene and Eugenics in Southeastern Europe to 1945*. Budapest: Central European University Press, 2011.

Pravilova, Ekaterina. *A Public Empire: Property and the Quest for the Common Good in Imperial Russia*. Princeton: Princeton University Press, 2014.

Prince, Ruth J., and Marsland, Rebecca (eds.). *Making and Unmaking Public Health in Africa: Ethnographic and Historical Perspectives*. Athens: Ohio University Press, 2014.

Proctor, Robert N. *The Nazi War on Cancer*. Princeton: Princeton University Press, 1999.

Prusin, Victor Alexander. *Nationalizing a Borderland: War, Ethnicity, and Anti-Jewish Violence in East Galicia, 1914–1920*. Tuscaloosa: University of Alabama Press, 2005.

Raphael, Lutz. "Die Verwissenschaftlichung des Sozialen als methodische und konzeptionelle Herausforderung für eine Sozialgeschichte des 20. Jahrhunderts," *Geschichte und Gesellschaft* 22.2 (1996): 165–93.

Rechter, David. "Galicia in Vienna: Jewish Refugees in the First World War." *Austrian History Yearbook* 28 (1997): 113–30.

Reichman, Henry. *Railwaymen and Revolution: Russia, 1905*. Berkeley: University of California Press, 1987.

———. "The 1905 Revolution on the Siberian Railroad." *Russian Review* 47 (1988): 25–48.

Revel, Jacques. "Présentation." In: *Jeux d'échelles. La micro-analyse à l'expérience*, ed. Jacques Revel (Paris: Seuil, 1996), 7–14.

Rezmer, Waldemar. "Służba wojskowa Żydów w siłach zbrojnych Drugiej Rzeczypospolitej." In: *Mniejszości narodowe i wyznaniowe w siłach zbrojnych Drugiej Rzeczypospolitej 1918–1919*, ed. Zbigniew Karpus and Waldemar Rezmer (Toruń: Wydawnictwo Uniwersytetu Mikołaja Kopernika, 2001), 97–121.

Roberts, Dorothy. *Killing the Black Body: Race, Reproduction and the Meaning of Liberty*. New York: Pantheon Press, 1997.

Rohdewald, Stefan. "Mimicry in a Multiple Postcolonial Setting: Networks of Technocracy and Scientific Management in Piłsudksi's Poland." In: *Expert Cultures in Central Eastern Europe. The Internationalization of Knowledge and the Transformation of Nation States since World War I*, ed. Martin Kohlrausch, Katrin Steffen, and Stefan Wiederkehr. (Osnabrück: fibre Verlag, 2010), 63–84.

Rodogno, Davide, Francesca Piana, and Shaloma Gauthier. "Shaping Poland: Relief and Rehabilitation Programmes Undertaken by Foreign Organizations, 1918–1922." In: *Shaping the Transnational Sphere: Experts, Networks and Issues from the 1840s to the 1930s*, ed. Davide Rodogno, Bernhard Struck, and Jakob Vogel (New York & Oxford: Berghahn Books, 2015), 259–78.

Röger, Maren. *Kriegsbeziehungen: Intimität, Gewalt und Prostitution im besetzten Polen 1939 bis 1945*. Frankfurt a. Main: S. Fischer, 2015.

Rose, Nikolas. *Powers of Freedom: Reframing Political Thought*. Cambridge: Cambridge University Press, 1999.

Rolf, Malte. *Imperiale Herrschaft im Weichselland. Das Königreich Polen im Russischen Imperium (1864–1915)*. Berlin: De Gruyter Oldenbourg, 2015.

Rosenqvist, Pia, and Noriko Kurube. "Dissolving the Swedish Alcohol-Treatment System." In: *Cure, Care, or Control: Alcoholism Treatment in Sixteen Countries*, ed. Geoffrey Hunt, Jukka-Pekka Takala, and Harald Klingemann (Albany: State University of New York Press, 1992), 65–86.

Rotskoff, Lori. *Love on the Rocks: Men, Women, and Alcohol in Post-World War II America, Gender and American Culture*. Chapel Hill: University of North Carolina Press, 2002.

Rowney, Don K., and Eugene Huskey (eds.), *Russian Bureaucracy and the State: Officialdom from Alexander II to Vladimir Putin*. Basingstoke: Palgrave Macmillan, 2009.

Rüb, Dorothea et al. *Aller Anfang*. Wien: Österreichisches Museum für Volkskunde, 2002.

Rutar, Sabine (ed.). *Beyond the Balkans: Towards an Inclusive History of Southeastern Europe*. Berlin: Lit Verlag, 2013).

Ruthner, Clemens et al. (eds.). *WechselWirkungen: Austria-Hungary, Bosnia-Herzegovina and the Western Balkans, 1878–1918*. New York: Peter Lang, 2015.

Sachße, Christoph, and Florian Tennstedt. *Soziale Sicherheit und soziale Disziplinierung: Beiträge zu einer historischen Theorie der Sozialpolitik*. Frankfurt a. M.: Suhrkamp, 1986.

Sarasin, Philipp. *Reizbare Maschinen: Eine Geschichte des Körpers 1765–1914*. Frankfurt a. M.: Suhrkamp, 2003.

———. et al. *Bakteriologie und Moderne: Studien zur Biopolitik des Unsichtbaren, 1870–1920*. Frankfurt a. M.: Suhrkamp, 2007.

Savelli, Mat. "The Peculiar Prosperity of Psychoanalysis in Socialist Yugoslavia." *Slavonic and East European Review* 91/2 (2013): 262–88.

Scheer, Tamara. "Austro-Hungarian Occupation Regimes in the Balkans (1915–1918): The Organisation of the 'Health Front'." In: *Medicine Within and Between the Habsburg and Ottoman Empires 18th–19th Centuries*, ed. Teodora Daniela Sechel (Bochum: Winkler, 2011), 213–232.

Schenk, Frithjof Benjamin. "Imperiale Raumerschliessung: Die Beherrschung der russischen Weite." *Osteuropa* 55/3 (2005): 33–45.

———. *Russlands Fahrt in die Moderne: Mobilität und sozialer Raum im Eisenbahnzeitalter*. Stuttgart: Franz Steiner Verlag, 2014.

Scheutz, Martin. "Demand and Charitable Supply: Poverty and Poor Relief in Austria in the 18th and 19th Centuries." In: *Health Care and Poor Relief in 18th and 19th Century Southern Europe*, ed. Ole Peter Grell, Andrew Cunningham, and Bernd Roeck (Burlington: Ashgate, 2005), 52–95.

Schlich, Thomas. "Negotiating Technologies in Surgery: The Controversy about Surgical Gloves in 1890s." *Bulletin for the History of Medicine* 87 (2013): 170–97.

Schutte, Christoph. "Deutsche und Polen in der Provinz Posen. Überlegungen zur Relevanz gegenseitiger Lernprozesse." In: *Vom Gegner lernen. Feindschaften und Kulturtransfer im Europa des 19. und 20. Jahrhunderts*, ed. Martin Aust and Daniel Schönpflug (Frankfurt a. M.: Campus Verlag, 2007), 114–36.

———. *Die Königliche Akademie in Posen (1903–1919) und andere kulturelle Einrichtungen im Rahmen der Politik zur "Hebung des Deutschtums."* Marburg: Herder-Institut, 2008.

Schwartz, Michael. *Sozialistische Eugenik. Eugenische Sozialtechnologien in Debatten und Politik der deutschen Sozialdemokratie 1890–1933*. Bonn: Dietz, 1995.

Sdvižkov, Denis. *Das Zeitalter der Intelligenz. Zur vergleichenden Geschichte der Gebildeten in Europa bis zum Ersten Weltkrieg*. Göttingen: Vandenhoeck & Ruprecht, 2006.

Sechel, Daniela Teodora. *Medicine within and between the Habsburg and Ottoman Empires: 18th–19th Centuries*. Bochum: Winkler, 2011.

———. "Contagion Theories in the Habsburg Monarchy (1770–1830)." In: *Medicine within and between the Habsburg and Ottoman Empires: 18th–19th Centuries*, ed. ibid. (Bochum: Dieter Winkler, 2011), 55–77.

Serrier, Thomas. *Provinz Posen, Ostmark, Wielkopolska. Eine Grenzregion zwischen Deutschland und Polen 1848–1914*. Marburg: Herder-Institut, 2005.

Shapira, Michael. "The Psychological Study of Anxiety in the Era of the Second World War." *Twentieth Century British History* 24/1 (2013): 31–57.

Shephard, Ben. *A War of Nerves: Soldiers and Psychiatrists, 1914–1994*. London: Pimlico, 2002.

Shore, Cris, and Susan Wright. "Governing by Numbers: Audit Culture, Rankings and the New World Order," *Social Anthropology* 23/1 (2015): 22–28.

Silvermann, Lisa. *Becoming Austrian: Jewish Culture between the World Wars*. Oxford: Oxford University Press, 2012.

Skála, Jaroslav. *Lékařův maraton: Ber a dávej*. Prague: Český spisovatel, 1998.
Smajić, Ramiza. *Bosanska krajina: Historija, legende i mitovi*. Sarajevo: Dobra knjiga, 2009.
Smith, Theresa C., and Thomas A. Oleszczuk. *No Asylum: State Psychiatric Repression in the Former USSR*. New York: New York University Press, 1996.
Sokolova, Vera. "Planned Parenthood behind the Iron Curtain: Sterilization of Romani Women." In: *Cultural Politics of Ethnicity: Discourses on Roma in Communist Czechoslovakia*, ed. Andreas Umland (Stuttgart: Ibidem-Verlag, 2008), 207–46.
Solovyova, A. M. "The Railway System in the Mining Area of Southern Russia in the Late Nineteenth and Early Twentieth Century." *Journal of Transport History* 5/1 (1984): 66–81.
Soyer, Daniel. "Transnationalism and Americanization in East European Jewish Immigrant Public Life." In: *Imagining the American Jewish Community*, ed. Jack Wertheimer (Brandeis: Brandeis University Press, 2007), 47–66.
Sparks, Tricia. *The Body Soviet: Propaganda, Hygiene and the Revolutionary State*. Madison: University of Wisconsin Press, 2008.
Spencer, Ian Henry. "An Investigation of the Relationship of Soviet Psychiatry to the State." PhD diss., University of Glasgow, 1997.
Spode, Hasso. "Germany." In: *Alcohol and Temperance in Modern History: An International Encyclopedia*, ed. Jack S. Blocker, David M. Fahey, and Ian R. Tyrrell (Santa Barbara: ABC-CLIO, 2003), 257–63.
Stambolieva, Marija. "Conclusion: The Post-Yugoslav Welfare States—From Legacies to Actor Shaped Transformations." In: *Welfare States in Transition—20 Years after the Yugoslav Welfare Model*, ed. Marija Stambolieva and Stefan Dehnert (Sofia: Friedrich-Ebert-Stiftung, 2011), 345–64.
Stawecki, Piotr. "Kilka uwag o roli wojska w procesach integracyjnych i dezintegracyjnych II Rzeczypospolitej." In: *Drogi integracji społeczeństwa w Polsce XIX–XXw*, ed. Henryk Zieliński (Warsaw: Polska Akademia Nauk, 1976), 193–215.
Steffen, Katrin. "Experts and the Modernization of the Nation—The Arena of Public Health in Poland in the First Half of the 20th Century." *Jahrbücher für Geschichte Osteuropas* 61/4 (2013): 574–90.
———. "Migration, Transfer und Nation: Die Wissensräume polnischer Naturwissenschaftler im 20. Jahrhundert." In: *Europäische Wissenschaftskulturen und politische Ordnungen in der Moderne (1890–1970)*, ed. Gangolf Hübinger (Munich: De Gruyter Oldenbourg, 2014), 185–205.
———. "Ludwik Hirszfeld, the Great War, and Seroanthropology: Expectations and Unfulfilled Promises." *Ab Imperio* 2 (2016): 125–52.
———, and Martin Kohlrausch. "The Limits and Merits of Internationalism. Experts, the State and the International Community in Poland in the First Half of the Twentieth Century." *European Review of History* 16 (2009): 715–37.
Stegmann, Natali. *Kriegsdeutungen—Staatsgründungen—Sozialpolitik. Der Helden- und Opferdiskurs in der Tschechoslowakei, 1918–1948*. Munich: Oldenbourg, 2010.
Steinmetz, George. "Empires, Imperial States, and Colonial Societies." In: *Concise Encyclopedia of Comparative Sociology*, ed. Masamichi Sasaki et al. (Leiden: Brill, 2014), 58–74.
Stessel, Zahava Szász. *Wine and Thorns in Tokay Valley: Jewish Life in Hungary: The History of Abaújszantó*. Madison: Fairleigh Dickinson University Press, 1995.
Stewart, Michael. "Communist Roma Policy, 1945–1989 as Seen through the Hungarian Case." In: *Between Past and Future: The Roma of Central and Eastern Europe*, ed. Will Guy (Hertfordshire: University of Hertfordshire, 2001), 71–92.
Strobel, Angelika. "Die Gesundung Russlands: Hygienepropaganda in der Provinz um 1910." *Jahrbücher für Geschichte Osteuropas* 61 (2013): 531–551.
Stubbs, Paul. "Performing Reform in South East Europe: Consultancy, Translation and Flexible Agency." In: *Making Policy Move: Towards a Politics of Translation and Assemblage*, ed. John Clarke et al. (Bristol: Polity, 2015), 65–93.
Sundhaussen, Holm. *Jugoslawien und seine Nachfolgestaaten 1943–2011: Eine ungewöhnliche Geschichte des Gewöhnlichen*. Wien: Böhlau, 2012.
Süß, Sonja. *Politisch missbraucht? Psychiatrie und Staatssicherheit in der DDR*. Berlin: Links, 1998.

Szajkowski, Zosa. "Private and Organized American Jewish Overseas Relief, 1914–1938." *American Jewish Historical Quarterly* 57 (1967): 52–106.

———. "'Reconstruction' vs. 'Palliative Relief' in American Jewish Overseas Work (1919–1939)." *Jewish Social Studies* 32/1 (1970): 14–42.

Szikra, Dorottya. "A szociálpolitika másik arca: Fajvédelem és produktív szociálpolitika az 1940-es évek Magyarországán." *Századvég* 48/2 (2008): 35–77.

Tampakis, Kostas. "Onwards Facing Backwards: The Rhetoric of Science in Nineteenth-Century Greece." *The British Journal for the History of Science* 47 (2014): 217–37.

Tessaris, Chiara. "The war relief work of the American Jewish Joint Distribution Committee in Poland and Lithuania, 1915–1918." *East European Jewish Affairs* 40/2 (2010): 127–44.

Thelen, Tatjana, and Haldis Haukanes. "Parenting after the Century of the Child: Introduction." In: *Parenting after the Century of the Child: Travelling Ideals, Institutional Negotiations and Individual Responses*, ed. ibid. (Farnham: Ashgate, 2010), 1–11.

———, and Rosie Read. "Introduction: Social Security and Care after Socialism: Reconfigurations of Public and Private." *Focaal* 50 (2007): 3–18.

———, Larissa Vetters, and Keebet von Benda-Beckmann. "Introduction to Stategraphy: Toward a Relational Anthropology of the State." *Social Analysis* 58/3 (2014): 1–19.

———, Andre Thiemann, and Duška Roth. "State Kinning and Kinning the State in Serbian Elder Care Programs." *Social Analysis* 58/3 (2014): 107–23.

Ther, Philipp. "Vom Gegenstand zum Forschungsansatz. Zentraleuropa als kultureller Raum." In: *Schauplatz Kultur—Zentraleuropa. Transdisziplinäre Annäherungen*, ed. Johannes Feichtinger, Elisabeth Großegger, and Gertraud Marinelli-König (Innsbruck: Studien Verlag, 2006), 55–63.

Thévenot, Laurent. "Die Pluralität kognitiver Formate und Engagements im Bereich zwischen dem Vertrauten und dem Öffentlichen." In: *Soziologie der Konventionen: Grundlagen einer pragmatischen Anthropologie*, ed. Rainer Diaz-Bone (Frankfurt a. M.: Campus-Verlag, 2011), 255–74.

Thiemann, Andre. "'It Was the Least Painful to Go into Greenhouse Production': The Moral Appreciation of Social Security in Post-Socialist Serbia." *Contemporary Southeastern Europe* 1/2 (2014): 24–41.

———. "State Relations: Local State and Social Security in Central Serbia." PhD diss., Martin-Luther University Halle/Saale, 2016.

Thom, Betsy. *Dealing with Drink: Alcohol and Social Policy: From Treatment to Management*. London & New York: Free Association Books, 1999.

———, and Virginia Berridge. "'Special Units for Common Problems': The Birth of Alcohol Treatment Units in England." *Social History of Medicine* 8/1 (1995): 75–93.

Thorne, M. Benjamin. "Assimilation, Invisibility, and the Eugenic Turn in the 'Gypsy Question' in Romanian Society, 1938–1942." *Romani Studies* 21/2 (2011): 177–206.

Thum, Gregor. "Imperialists in Panic: The Evocation of Empire at Germany's Eastern Frontiers around 1900." In: *Helpless Imperialists: Imperial Failure, Fear and Radicalization*, ed. Maurus Reinkowski and Gregor Thum (Göttingen: Vandenhoeck & Ruprecht, 2013), 137–62.

Tilse, Mark. *Transnationalism in the Prussian East: From National Conflicts to Synthesis, 1871–1914*. Basingstoke: Palgrave Macmillan, 2011.

Todorova, Maria. *Imagining the Balkans*. New York: Oxford University Press, 2009.

Trencsényi, Balázs, Dragos Petrescu, Cristina Petrescu, Constantin Iordachi, and Zoltán Kántor (eds.). *Nation-Building and Contested Identities: Romanian and Hungarian Case Studies*. Budapest: Regio Books, 2001.

Trischler, Helmuth, and Martin Kohlrausch. *Building Europe on Expertise: Innovators, Organizers, Networkers*. New York: Palgrave Macmillan, 2014.

Turczynski, Emanuel. *Sozial- und Kulturgeschichte Griechenlands im 19. Jahrhundert*. Mannheim and Möhnesee: Bibliopolis, 2003.

Turda, Marius. *Eugenics and Nation in Early 20th Century Hungary*. London: Palgrave Macmillan, 2014.

———. "'To End the Degeneration of a Nation': Debates on Eugenic Sterilization in Inter-war Romania." *Medical History* 53 (2009): 77–104.

———. "The Nation as Object: Race, Blood, and Biopolitics in Interwar Romania." *Slavic Review* 66/3 (2007): 413–41.

———. "Focus on Social History of Medicine in Central and Eastern Europe." *Social History of medicine* 21/2 (2008): 395–401.

———. "Private and Public Traditions of Health Care in Central and South-Eastern Europe, from the Nineteenth to the (Mid-)Twentieth Centuries." In: *Healthcare in Private and Public from the Early Modern Period to 2000*, ed. Paul Weindling (New York: Routledge, 2015).

———. *The History of East-Central European Eugenics, 1900–1945: Sources and Commentaries.* London: Bloomsbury Academic, 2015.

———. "In Pursuit of Greater Hungary: Eugenic Ideas of Social and Biological Improvement, 1940–1941," *Journal of Modern History* 85/3 (2013): 558–591.

———, and Paul J. Weindling (eds.). *Blood and Homeland: Eugenics and Racial Nationalism in Central and Southeast Europe, 1900–1940.* Budapest & New York: Central European University Press, 2007.

Turkowska, Justyna A. "Im Namen der 'großen Kolonisationsaufgaben': Das Hygiene Institut in Posen (1899–1920) und die preußische Hegemonialpolitik in der Ostmark." *Jahrbücher für Geschichte Osteuropas* 61/4 (2013), 552–73.

Turner, Bryan. *Medical Power and Social Knowledge.* London: Sage, 1987.

Unger, Dieter. *Alkoholismus in der DDR: Die Geschichte des Umganges mit alkoholkranken Menschen in der ehemaligen DDR im Zeitraum 1949 bis 1989.* Halle: Projekte-Verlag Cornelius, 2011.

Vandendriessche, Joris, Evert Peeters, and Kaat Wils (eds.). *Scientists' Expertise as Performance: Between State and Society, 1860–1960.* London: Pickering & Chatto, 2015.

Vernon, James. "The Ethics of Hunger and the Assembly of Society: The Techno-Politics of the School Meal in Modern Britain." *American Historical Review* 110/3 (2005): 693–725.

Vetta, Théodora. "'Nationalism Is Back!': 'Radikali' and Privatization in Serbia." In: *Headlines of Nation, Subtexts of Class*, ed. Don Kalb and Gábor Halmai (New York: Berghahn, 2011), 37–56.

Vowinckel, Annette, Marcus M. Payk, and Thomas Lindenberger (eds.). *Cold War Cultures: Perspectives on Eastern and Western European Societies.* Oxford: Berghahn Books, 2012.

Vulpius, Ricarda. "The Emergence of an Imperial Identity in the Russian Empire." In: *Cultural Transfers: Encounters and Connections in the Global 18th Century*, ed. Matthias Middell (Leipzig: Leipziger Universitätsverlag, 2014), 185–210.

Walkenhorst, Peter. *Nation-Volk-Rasse. Radikaler Nationalismus im Deutschen Kaiserreich 1890–1914.* Göttingen: Vandenhoeck & Ruprecht, 2007.

Wehler, Hans-Ulrich. "Polenpolitik im Deutschen Kaiserreich." In: *Krisenherde des Kaiserreiches 1871–1918* (Göttingen: Vandenhoeck & Ruprecht, 1979), 174–202.

Weindling, Paul. "Public Health and Political Stabilization: The Rockefeller Foundation in Central and Eastern Europe between the Two World Wars." *Minerva* 31/3 (1993): 253–67.

———. "From Disease Prevention to Population Control: The Realignment of Rockefeller Foundation Policies in the 1920s to 1950s." In: *American Foundations and the Coproduction of World Order in the Twentieth Century*, ed. John Krige and Helke Rausch (Göttingen: Vandenhoeck & Ruprecht, 2012), 127–8.

——— (ed.). *Healthcare in Private and Public from the Early Modern Period to 2000.* New York: Routledge, 2015.

Wendland, Anna Veronika. "Randgeschichten? Osteuropäische Perspektive auf Kulturtransfer und Verflechtungsgeschichte." *Osteuropa* 58/3 (2008): 95–116.

Wessely, S. "Twentieth-Century Theories on Combat Motivation and Breakdown." *Journal of Contemporary History* 41/2 (2006): 268–86.

White, William L. *Slaying the History of Addiction Treatment and Recovery in America.* Bloomington: Chestnut Health Systems/Lighthouse Institute, 1998.

Wienemann, Elisabeth. "Hundert Jahre betriebliche Suchtprävention: Visionen und Wirken der Mäßigkeitsbewegung in der Arbeitswelt." In: *Der Geist der Deutschen Mäßigkeitsbewegung: Debatten um Alkohol und Trinken in Vergangenheit und Gegenwart*, ed. Karl Wassenberg and

Sabine Schaller (Halle: Mitteldeutscher Verlag, 2010), 114–43.
Wierzbicki, Marek. "Białorusini w Wojsku Polskim (1921–1939)." In: *Mniejszości narodowe i wyznaniowe w siłach zbrojnych Drugiej Rzeczypospolitej 1918–1919*, ed. Zbigniew Karpus and Waldemar Rezmer (Toruń: Wydawnictwo Uniwersytetu Mikołaja Kopernika, 2001), 153–75.
Wigen, Einar. "Ottoman Concepts of Empire," *Contributions to the History of Concepts* 8.1 (2013): 43–66.
Wildgrube, Christiane et al. "Psychological Trauma in German, Serbian and British Psychiatry since 1945: A Comparison of Textbooks." In: *Transnational Psychiatries: Social and Cultural Histories of Psychiatry in Comparative Perspective, c. 1800–2000*, ed. Waltraud Ernst and Thomas Mueller (Newcastle: Cambridge Scholars, 2010), 244–71.
Wilson, Ross J. *New York and the First World War: Shaping an American City*. Burlington: Ashgate, 2014.
Winter, Jay. "Shell-shock and the Cultural History of the Great War." *Journal of Contemporary History* 35/1 (2000): 7–11.
Winterbottom, Anna E. "Of the China Root: A Case Study of the Early Modern Circulation of Materia Medica." *Social History of Medicine* 28/1 (2015): 22–44.
Withuis, Jolande, and Annet Mooij (eds.). *The Politics of War Trauma: The Aftermath of World War Two in Eleven European Countries*. Amsterdam: Aksant, 2010.
Wittrock, Björn. "Modernity: One, None, or Many? European Origins and Modernity as a Global Condition." *Daedalus* 129/1 (2000): 31–60.
Wolff, Larry. *Inventing Eastern Europe: The Map of Civilization on the Mind of the Enlightenment*. Stanford: Stanford University Press, 1994.
Woodward, Susan. *Socialist Unemployment: The Political Economy of Yugoslavia, 1945–1990*. Princeton: Princeton University Press, 1995.
Young, Allan. *The Harmony of Illusions: Inventing Post-Traumatic Stress Disorder*. Princeton: Princeton University Press, 1995.
Yuval-Davis, Nira. *Gender and Nation*. Los Angeles: Sage, 1997.
Zakythinos, Dionysios A. *The Making of Modern Greece: From Byzantium to Independence*, trans. K. R. Johnstone. Oxford: B. Blackwell, 1976.
Zalshik, Rakefet, and Nadav Davidovitch. "Taking and Giving: The Case of the JDC and OZE in Lithuania 1919–1926." *East European Jewish Affairs* 39/1 (2009): 57–68.
Zarifi, Maria. "Modernizing through Medicine: Knowledge Transfer and Scientific Networks between Greece and Germany in the Long 19th Century." *Zeitschrift für Balkanologie* 50/1 (2014): 99–118.
Zaviršek, Darja. "Engendering Social Work Education under State Socialism in Yugoslavia." *British Journal of Social Work* 38/4 (2008): 734–50.
Zelepos, Ioannis. *Die Ethnisierung griechischer Identität 1870–1912*. Munich: R. Oldenburg Verlag, 2002.
Zimmermann, Susan. "Gender Regime and Gender Struggle in Hungarian State Socialism." *Aspasia: International Yearbook for Women's and Gender History of Central, Eastern and South Eastern Europe* 4 (2010): 1–24.
"Zirkulationen." *Nach Feierabend, Zürcher Jahrbuch für Wissensgeschichte* 7 (2011).
Zola, Gary Philip, and Marc Dollinger. *American Jewish History: A Primary Source Reader*. Waltham: Brandeis University Press, 2014.
Zylberman, Patrick. "Fewer Parallels Than Antitheses: René Sand and Andrija Stampar on Social Medicine, 1919–1955." *Social History of Medicine* 17.1 (2004): 77–92.

LIST OF CONTRIBUTORS

Sara Bernasconi defended her PhD in history in July 2017 at the University of Zurich with a dissertation about Habsburg's Midwives in Bosnia and Herzegovina. Her PhD project was funded by the Research Fund of the University of Zurich, including a yearlong research stay in Bosnia and Herzegovina. She studied History and Slavic Linguistics at the Universities in Zurich, Basel, and Zagreb. She is interested in the history of the Balkans, gender and women's history, history of migrations, historical anthropology and digital humanities.

Alexander Friedman is a lecturer at the University of Saarland and the Sciences Po Paris in Nancy (French-German European campus). He is also a WP coordinator of the research project WW2CRIMESONTRIAL1943-91(CERCEC Paris, EHESS-CNRS) and a researcher for the documentary projects "Jews in the Third Reich" by Yad Vashem (Jerusalem) and "Resistance in the Rhineland, 1933–1945" (LVR-Institute of Regional Studies, Bonn). His research and teaching are focused on Russian and Soviet History, National Socialism, the history of Jews in Eastern Europe, as well International Relations in the twentieth century. He is the author of *Deutschlandbilder in der weißrussischen sowjetischen Gesellschaft 1919–1941: Propaganda und Erfahrungen* (Stuttgart: Franz Steiner Verlag, 2011), and co-editor of *Diskriminiert – vernichtet – vergessen: Behinderte und Kranke in der Sowjetunion, in den besetzten sowjetischen Gebieten und im Ostblock* (Stuttgart: Franz Steiner Verlag, 2016).

Heike Karge is Assistant Professor at the Chair for Southeast and East European History, University of Regensburg. She earned her PhD in 2006 at the EUI in Florence with a thesis on Second World War memory cultures in socialist Yugoslavia, published as *Steinerne Erinnerung - versteinerte Erinnerung? Kriegsgedenken im sozialistischen Jugoslawien* (Wiesbaden: Harrassowitz, 2010); revised and translated into Serbocroatian as *Sećanje u kamenu – okamjeno sećanje?* (Beograd: Biblioteka XX Vek, 2014). Her research interests lie in the field of cultural and social history of the twentieth century in Eastern and Southeastern Europe, mainly on remembrance cultures, the social history of medicine, and the history of war trauma. She is currently exploring the history of soldiers' mental breakdown in war in the Yugoslav societies from the First World War onwards.

Friederike Kind-Kovács is Assistant Professor at the Chair for Southeast and East European History, University of Regensburg and a postdoctoral fellow of the Graduate School for East and Southeast European Studies (Regensburg/Munich). She published in 2014 *Written Here, Published There: How Underground Literature Crossed the Iron Curtain*, which won the 2015 University of Southern California Book Prize in Cultural and Literary Studies. She co-edited in 2013 *Samizdat, Tamizdat and Beyond: Transnational media during and after socialism*. She is currently writing her second monograph, entitled *Budapest's Starving Children: Famine and Humanitarian Relief after the Great War*. In the academic year 2017/18 she will be a research fellow at the Imre Kertész Kolleg Jena.

Fanny Le Bonhomme is an associate researcher at the Centre Marc Bloch in Berlin. She graduated in history from the University Rennes 2 in France. She defended her doctoral thesis, entitled *Psychiatry and society in the German Democratic Republic: Stories of Patients from the Charité Psychiatry and Neurology Clinic (East-Berlin, 1960–1968)*, at the University Rennes 2 and the University of Potsdam in 2016. Between 2013 and 2016, she was an associate PhD candidate at the Center for Contemporary History in Potsdam. Her latest publications include "'Le Mur lui est monté à la tête.' Construction du mur de Berlin et basculement dans la maladie," *Le Mouvement social* 253 (2015), 31–47, and "Viols en temps de guerre, psychiatrie et temporalités enchevêtrées. Expériences de femmes violées par les soldats de l'Armée Rouge entre la fin de la Seconde Guerre mondiale et le début de la période de paix," *Guerres mondiales et conflits contemporains* 257 (2015), 53–74.

Katrin Steffen is a Faculty Member at the Nordost-Institute Lüneburg at University of Hamburg. Previously, she worked at the German Historical

Institute in Warsaw and the University of Halle. She received her Ph.D. from the Free University of Berlin, published in 2004 as *Jewish Polishness: Ethnicity and the Nation mirrored in the Polish-Jewish Press 1918–1939* (in German). She is the author of "Experts and the Modernization of the Nation: The Arena of Public Health in Poland in the First Half of the 20th Century," *Jahrbücher für Geschichte Osteuropas* 61/4 (2013), 574–90, and co-author of *Expert Cultures in Central Eastern Europe: The Internationalization of Knowledge and the Transformation of Nation States since World War I* (Osnabrück: Fibre, 2010). She is currently working on a double biography of Ludwik Hirszfeld und Jan Czochralski.

Angelika Strobel is a PhD student in Eastern European history at the university of Zurich with a forthcoming thesis, *Russia's Recovery: Technologies, Medialities, and Agents in the Railway and Zemstvo Medicine, 1905–1914*. Her publications include "Die Gesundung Russlands: Hygienepropaganda in der Provinz um 1910" in *Jahrbücher für Geschichte Osteuropas* 2013/4, 531–51. Her areas of interest are the political and social history of the Russian empire, historical epistemology, and historical anthropology of the state and its public services.

Andre Thiemann is a junior core fellow at the Institute for Advanced Studies, Central European University, Budapest. Between 2009 and 2013, he was part of the Volkswagen project "Local State and Social Security in Hungary, Romania and Serbia" at the Max Planck Institute for Social Anthropology in Halle, Germany, and conducted 18 months of fieldwork in Serbia. In 2016, he received his PhD in Social Anthropology at the Martin-Luther University Halle-Wittenberg. He investigates the mutual constitution of state and society through social security, infrastructural, and work relations. His research interests comprise the anthropology of the state, and relational and spatial theory.

Justyna A. Turkowska is a Lecturer at the Department of East European History at the University of Gießen. Previously, she was a research assistant at the Institute of History of Medicine at the University of Bonn and a research fellow at the Herder Institute for Historical Research on East Central Europe in Marburg. She studied history, political science, and sociology in Warsaw, Berlin and Hannover. She earned her PhD in 2016 from the University of Gießen with a project on the medical mastery and dissemination patterns of sociohygienic issues in the Prussian Polish-German province of Posen from the 1880s until 1920. Her areas of interests are history of science and social and cultural history of Eastern Europe in its global context.

Eszter Varsa is fellow at the Leibniz Institute for East and Southeast European Studies (IOS) at Regensburg. She gained her PhD in 2011 in Comparative Gender Studies from Central European University in Budapest with a thesis entitled *Gender, 'Race'/Ethnicity, Class and the Institution of Child Protection in Hungary, 1949–1956*. Her research deals with gender and the history of (child) welfare, health education, and Roma in Cold War Central Eastern Europe. She taught at the Gender Studies and History Departments at Central European University. Her latest publication is "'The (final) solution of the Gypsy-question': Continuities in Discourses about Roma in Hungary, 1940s–1950s," *Nationalities Papers* 45, 1 (2017): 114–130.

Esther Wahlen holds a PhD from the European University Institute in Florence and an MA in East European studies from Regensburg University (Germany). In spring 2015, she was a visiting scholar at the Department of History at the University of California, Berkeley. In her dissertation project, Esther investigated the politics of alcohol in Romania and Czechoslovakia in the 1970s and 1980s. She is currently working on turning her PhD thesis into a book. Esther works as an information specialist at the Goethe Institut in Munich.

Maria Zarifi is a senior lecturer of History and Philosophy of Science at the Hellenic Open University in Greece. She has lectured at the University of Athens, the University of Thessaly in Greece, and the University of Regensburg in Germany. She was fellow at FRIAS in Freiburg, the Institute for East and Southeast European Studies (IOS) in Regensburg, and the Heidelberg Centre for Transcultural Studies. Her research interests focus on science and imperialism, science and nationalism, medicine, public health, and modernity. She has published in peer reviewed collective volumes and several journals and is the author of *Science, Culture and Politics: Germany's Cultural Policy and Scientific Relations with Greece 1933–1945* (Saarbrücken: AV Akademikerverlag GmbH & Co. KG, 2010).

INDEX

For Product Safety Concerns and Information please contact our EU representative GPSR@taylorandfrancis.com Taylor & Francis Verlag GmbH, Kaufingerstraße 24, 80331 München, Germany

Batch number: 10725853

Printed by Printforce, the Netherlands